Cultural Evolution and its Discontents

People worry that computers, robots, interstellar aliens, or Satan himself – brilliant, stealthy, ruthless creatures – may seize control of our world and destroy what's uniquely valuable about the human race. *Cultural Evolution and its Discontents* shows that our cultural systems – especially those whose last names are "ism" – are already doing that, and doing it so adeptly that we seldom even notice. Like other parasites, they've blindly evolved to exploit us for their own survival. Creative arts and humanistic scholarship are our best tools for diagnosis and cure.

The assemblages of ideas that have survived, like the assemblages of biological cells that have survived, are the ones good at protecting and reproducing themselves. They aren't necessarily the ones that guide us toward our most admirable selves or our healthiest future. Relying so heavily on culture to protect our uniquely open minds from cognitive overload makes us vulnerable to hijacking by the systems that co-evolve with us.

Recognizing the selfish Darwinian functions of these systems makes sense of many aspects of history, politics, economics, and popular culture. What drove the Protestant Reformation? Why have the Beatles, *The Hunger Games*, and paranoid science fiction thrived, and how was hip-hop co-opted? What alliances helped neoliberalism out-compete Communism, and what alliances might enable environmentalism to overcome consumerism? Why are multiculturalism and university-trained elites provoking working-class nationalist backlash? In a digital age, how can we use numbers without having them use us instead?

Anyone who has wondered how our species can be so brilliant and so stupid at the same time may find an answer here: human mentalities are so complex that we crave the simplifications provided by our cultures, but the cultures that thrive are the ones that blind us to any interests that don't correspond to their own.

Robert N. Watson received his B.A. *summa cum laude* from Yale and his Ph.D. with Highest Honors from Stanford, and was Associate Professor of English at Harvard before moving to UCLA, where he has been Chair of the Faculty of Letters and Science and Vice-Provost for Educational Innovation, and is now Distinguished Professor of English. He is the author of prize-winning scholarly books, and poems in the *New Yorker* and many other journals. He has been awarded Guggenheim and NEH fellowships, as well as visiting fellowships at Trinity College, Cambridge, and Christ Church College, Oxford, and prizes for excellence in teaching and public service.

Literary Criticism and Cultural Theory

For a full list of titles published in the series, please visit www.routledge.com

Cultural Evolution and its Discontents

Cognitive Overload, Parasitic Cultures, and the Humanistic Cure

Robert N. Watson

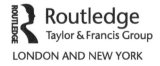

Routledge
Taylor & Francis Group

LONDON AND NEW YORK

First published 2019 by Routledge

2 Park Square, Milton Park, Abingdon, Oxfordshire OX14 4RN
52 Vanderbilt Avenue, New York, NY 10017

Routledge is an imprint of the Taylor & Francis Group, an informa business

First issued in paperback 2019

Library of Congress Cataloging-in-Publication Data
A catalog record for this title has been requested

ISBN: 978-0-367-03024-7 (hbk)
ISBN: 978-0-367-47656-4 (pbk)

Typeset in Sabon
by codeMantra

Contents

List of Figures

Acknowledgments

I owe special thanks on this project to Russ Abbott, Sydney Alairys, H. Clark Barrett, Philip Boche, Tommy Bourgeois, Sara Burdorff, Andrea Collins, Julien Crockett, Patricia Cuarenta, Emily Davidson, Rob Dorit, Sabrina Feldman, Anna George, Bill Germano, Katherine Kahn, Tae-Yeoun Keum, Eloise Lemay, John R. Levine, Dan Magida, Claire McEachern, Jack Ramsey, Mary Roach, Rip Roach, Michelle Salyga, Michael Salzman, Debora Shuger, Chris Stephan, Dana Cairns Watson, David Watson, and Jonathan Watson – and to UCLA for demonstrating so compellingly the value of a public university.

1 Culture vs. Anarchy

Meaningful resistance to dominator culture demands of all of us a willingness to accurately identify the various systems that work together to promote injustice, exploitation, and oppression. To name interlocking systems of domination is one way to disrupt our wrong-minded reliance on dualistic thinking. Highlighted, these interlocking systems tend to indict us all in some way, making it impossible for any of us to claim that we are absolutely and always victims, calling attention to the reality of our accountability, however relative. ... asserting agency, even in small ways, is always the first step in self-determination. It is the place of hope.
—bell hooks, *Writing Beyond Race*[1]

The main business of humanity is to do a good job of being human beings, not to serve as appendages to machines, institutions, and systems.
—Kurt Vonnegut, *Player Piano*[2]

People worry that computers and robots, or interstellar aliens, or Satan himself – brilliant, crafty, stealthy, ruthless creatures – may seize control of our world and destroy what is uniquely valuable about the human race. This book shows that our cultural systems – especially those whose last names are "ism" – are already doing that, and doing it so adeptly that we seldom even notice. Like other parasites, they have blindly evolved to exploit us for their own survival, and we need to be alert, creative, and determined in our resistance. If you have ever wondered how our species can be so smart and so foolish at the same time, this book offers an explanation: human mentalities are so complex that we crave the simplifications provided by cultural constructs, but the cultural constructs that thrive are the ones that divert us from any interests that don't correspond to their own.

Cultures – roughly, the beliefs, values, entertainments, and manners of our communities – are presumed innocent. Wonderfully diverse though they are, they generally reflect what their members have assumed or decided is good and true. What people have failed to notice is that the assemblages of ideas that have survived, like the assemblages of biological cells that have survived, are the ones skilled at protecting and replicating themselves – not necessarily the ones that guide us toward our most admirable selves or our healthiest future. That has been a costly blind spot. Fortunately, it is also a curable blind spot.

So, this is a book about cultural evolution and its discontents. It offers what I hope is an interesting and plausible explanation of why human beings suffer from cognitive overload, why that overload necessitates culture, how culture evolves to control us, why that control turns societies against creative minds, and what all that means for politics, education, scholarship, and the arts in the 21st century. Beyond the better-known advantages human beings derive from humanistic learning and artistic creativity, these endeavors allow us to evaluate, regulate, and sometimes replace the evolving systems that we empower, at some cost and risk, to protect us from the unique openness of human consciousness. Intellectuals can be both valuable and vulnerable because they tend to resist the resulting conformist pressures of tribalism that collude with forces such as capitalism, fascism, neoliberalism, communism, and institutional religions that have evolved ingenious mechanisms to protect themselves from competing ideas while protecting their true believers from discomforting complexity and ambiguity. Whether democracy itself can survive in this sociopolitical ecosystem, and coexist with ideals of kindness and justice – ideals so fundamentally human that they are already visible in infants – has become an open and urgent question worldwide, as new reactionary alliances rise to power and could take any of several radically different directions. This book will offer readers a fresh perspective on their own tribal certainties – a perspective that may allow them to recognize common enemies instead of demonizing rival tribes.

The bubble that each wing of American politics believes the other is trapped in – campus snowflakes and their radical professors on one side, Fox News dittoheads on the other – can be more productively understood as idea clusters that are dangerously good at gathering and retaining their carriers. Democrats may – without surrendering their understandable loathing of Donald Trump – begin to sympathize with the aspects of Trumpism that protest the way a rampant neoliberal economic system benefits only the elites, as career politicians of both mainstream parties (despite their moral posturing) serve the self-replicating desires of the money system that feeds them rather than serving the best interests of their human constituencies. Leftists may also notice where their investment in some causes becomes partly a doctrinaire self-congratulatory reflex, and where some well-intentioned big-government programs perpetuate themselves rather than producing a net gain for a society. Christian fundamentalist Republicans may recognize the progressive campaigns against poverty and consumerism as reflecting some of their religion's first and deepest values, such as succoring the poor and warning more privileged souls against the seductions of materialism. Conservatives may see that entrenched economic interests have superficially mimicked and thereby co-opted their value system to enlist them in shortsightedly protecting profits instead of stabilizing our wondrous and indispensable biosphere. They may also notice that racism and sexism can function through them even though they feel no racial animosity or gender prejudice, while, on the opposite wing, identity politics activists may, by the same insights, realize that labeling as "hate" every view that doesn't conform to their latest program is neither intellectually valid nor tactically wise. And all citizens can realize that they aren't obliged to make the moral compromises that a system – a nation, a religion, an economic structure – supposedly embodying their ideals has made for its own survival.

Some major social problems will remain unsolvable, and some serious self-betrayals inevitable, unless we recognize them as the natural product of systems with a talent for making us serve them rather than serving what is best about ourselves and best for each other. With obviously dysfunctional social structures flourishing all around the world, such that suffering communities cannot seem to escape them, we need to understand why. It suits some people to blame the victims as simply lacking sufficient moral character, intelligence, and determination to escape. Personal responsibility is certainly important, but this book is emphasizing a different answer: when a system, or one strain of a system, comes along, that happens to have a talent for perpetuating itself through generations of human carriers even when it creates a disease in those carriers, that is the system likely to persist, by a fundamental Darwinian logic. Such systems can be ingenious seducers and puppeteers without having any conscious intent, just as many tiny biological parasites are.

The systems may also be deployed with malicious intent. Governments and other sociopolitical actors (notably the Kremlin) have started to realize they can inject dangerous parasites into the cultural systems of their enemies. So the danger of memetic forces is no longer only through side effects of their own Darwinian self-protectiveness. They can be engineered into a kind of virus warfare sprayed into enemy territory to sicken its citizenry, turning them into a population of civil-warring bots, or turning them into consumers rather than citizens.

Recent evolutionary anthropology and archeology have shown convincingly that a massive increase in the brainpower of our ancestors made cultural learning feasible. What this book seeks to add is that cultural learning then had to make massive brainpower manageable, or at least tolerable. Those same fields have shown compellingly how indispensable cultural transmission is to the success of our species.[3] What this book seeks to add is that our dependency on culture sometimes causes our costliest failures. It is risky to hire institutions with a stake in their own persistence to manage the balance between control and freedom – a task that is central to the thriving of our species and our individual selves.

* * * * * * * * * * * *

Before those main features, let me provide a movie trailer that offers a fabulous insight into the terrors of knowledge when it is unbounded by the limits human culture provides. It is literally fabulous: a fable, a story from which a deep warning eventually emerges:

Indiana Jones and the Kingdom of the Crystal Skull – the latest install-ment of Steven Spielberg's hit movie franchise, with a screenplay by David Koepp – shows the heroic archeologist Dr. Jones on the trail of a trans-parent cranium that may have the power to grant world dominion, and hence is fiercely pursued by the brilliant but ruthless Dr. Irina Spalko on behalf of the Soviet empire. A longtime colleague of Indy's named Oxley has already been driven insane by exposure to the skull, but – using enig-matic quotations from T. S. Eliot and John Milton, which Dr. Spalko (as a no-nonsense Russian scientist) cannot understand – Oxley does manage to tell Indy to return the skull to the underground temple from which it had been stolen. That temple's antechamber is crammed with cobwebbed artifacts from many ancient civilizations, which the crystal-skulled beings – now themselves ancient artifacts pursued by archeologists – had collected to study the range of human cultures. We are thus confronted with multiculturalism squared, a panorama of diversity in factorial: "There are artifacts from every era of early history," observes an amazed Indiana Jones; "Macedonian. Sumerian … Etruscan. Babylonian … Early Egyptian …. Collectors. They were archeologists."

With the skull finally mounted back on its skeleton among a dozen others – maybe a weird version of Christ and his Apostles at a Last Supper, maybe just an evocation of the superstitious fear of the number 13 – the eggheads resume a timeless conversation and promise to reveal a "big gift." "Tell me everything you know," is Dr. Spalko's rash demand: the intellectual analogue to the Soviet will to world empire, tying the movie's theme nicely to its plot. Indy rolls out his signature gut-instinct warning: "I've got a bad feeling about this." The temple spins itself into a vortex that Oxley identifies as "A pathway to another dimension," and again Jones senses the danger: "I don't think we want to go that way," he says, leading his group out a side passage.

But the entranced Spalko, epitomizing human curiosity, stands in the center and persists: "I want to know. I want to know. Tell me. I'm ready. I want to know." The movie then cuts to Mac, a treacherous archeolo-gist, greedily snatching up a variety of the artifacts in the antechamber, fatally encumbering his escape. It is a different mistake from the one Spalko is making, but finally not so different: they are both gathering too many different forms and frames of knowledge for a human being to bear.

We return to Spalko, as strange wisps from all 13 skulls invade her eyes. "I can see," she exults; "I can see!" But, as the saying goes, she ain't seen nothing yet. The crystal creatures rotate and combine into what now looks like a conscious single being who concentrates its knowing gaze on her, like a genie granting a foolish wish in a fairy tale. "No more," she begs; "Cover it. Cover it!" But the discovery is relentless, and omniscience is a major headache. Flames shoot out of her eye sockets, and with a scream of anguish she explodes into tiny particles that the vortex consumes.

The collective wisdom of the temple, at once a summation of the human past and a terrifying futuristic alien vehicle, is then smashed to bits and dissolved in a flood that leaves a tranquil lake, covering over the alien traces, the dangerous knowledge, and the alternative dimensionality – "like a broom to their footprints," says Oxley. The scene becomes a retraction of the whole archeological enterprise, a renunciation of Jones's professorial determination to unearth secret knowledge no matter what the risks. "Knowledge was their treasure," Indy concludes, but there can evidently be too much of a good thing, and the heroes are all relieved to see that treasure reburied. This seems remarkably similar to the conclusion of the blockbuster first Indiana Jones movie, *Raiders of the Lost Ark*, where the power-hungry villains are Nazis rather than Soviets, but their rash peek into forbidden superhuman knowledge also sent flames through their eye sockets, evaporating all the evildoers before sealing itself back up.

So – as this, conceived as the last Indiana Jones movie, slips back from an unsettling adventure to a formulaic comic ending – nothing is left for Indy but assimilation back into the most normative modes of domesticity. He heads back to 1950s small-town America, marries his long-lost sweetheart under the guidance of a Protestant minister and the beatific gaze of their all-Caucasian friends, embraces the role of fatherhood he had neglected in his daring and arcane research, and returns to his college as an associate dean. His nickname, which hinted at heroic independence, yields to the formal form that absorbs him in a conservative Midwestern state. The world is safe from the transparent skull.

※ ※ ※ ※ ※ ※ ※ ※ ※ ※ ※

What was so dangerous about it anyway? I want to suggest it might be the same thing that makes intellectuals and great artworks and universities so beautifully dangerous, so resented for their assaults on common values and common sense, but also so persistent through modern human history. In human evolution, as in the movie, the amazing oversized cranium is both a treasure and a threat – and one that can either resist or abet tyranny.

The climax of the film offers an allegory of the problem of the human mind – and most other artworks respond to that same problem. We are designed (as Steven Pinker's research has shown[4]) to see through two eyeholes, not omnidirectionally through a crystal skull. Just as our physical view is limited in order to permit adequate attention to what is in front of us and coming near enough to matter, so our mental system is limited also, lest we become inundated with experience. There is a thrill, but also a lurking threat, in the question William Blake asks in "The Marriage of Heaven and Hell": "How do you know but ev'ry Bird that cuts the airy way, / Is an immense world of delight, clos'd by your senses five?" Vision that expands to the visionary can be glorious but also overwhelming in its scope. We take in certain frequencies through those sensory channels, and our intellectual range is similarly constrained – usually to our benefit, as evolutionary models would predict, but (this book will argue) also to our peril because enemies can lurk in our blind spots.

Cognitive overload is a human-nature problem now widely mistaken for an Information Age problem. Prophets of the digital era warn that "We are producing data at a rate that already outstrips our ability to store them and outpaces our ability to catalog, analyze, and archive these data in meaningful ways."[5] But all that is really new is that we are recording more of that information electronically and disseminating it more quickly and widely: none of us have ever been able to catalog, analyze, and archive all the waves of information that flood in through our senses and slosh around our minds. The noumenal world – the world in itself, beyond our perceptual filters – is infinitely complex, and already was so before we packed our view of it with subatomic particles and their indeterminacies. Toward the end of her masterpiece, *Middlemarch*, George Eliot observed that

> If we had a keen vision and feeling of all ordinary human life, it would be like hearing the grass grow and the squirrel's heart beat, and we should die of that roar which lies on the other side of silence. As it is, the quickest of us walk about well wadded with stupidity.[6]

So there is a cognitive trade-off. According to some (admittedly controversial) theories, genetically based illnesses such as sickle-cell anemia and Tay-Sachs disease became entrenched in a lineage by protecting against malaria and tuberculosis, respectively.[7] A genetic variant that encourages osteoarthritis may have survived by helping some people survive in colder climates.[8] Our dangerously expandable consciousness may be similarly a side effect of an evolutionary advantage sufficient to make it worth enduring under some circumstances, because it has protected our adaptability to rapidly changing social and physical worlds. But the expandability of human consciousness can provoke a backlash against openness of mind, whether the expansion arrives in the form of heightened sensory receptivity, multiculturalism, or academic freedom.

The original equipment firmware of *Homo sapiens* is advantageously adaptable but also dangerously so. It allows too many complicated, fuzzy-logical, and potentially conflicting programs to run simultaneously in our brains, and it is vulnerable to hijacking by alien programs for their own benefit. A chief task of culture, broadly conceived – along with the transfer of knowledge useful for survival – is to set firewalls around a world-view or belief-system, and to give shape to the deluge of data offered by the internal and external worlds.[9]

Cultures – "systems of concepts or ideas which guide thought and conduct"[10] – soothe the thorny tangle of cognition and smooth the rough edges of our social imbrications. The creative arts – a part of culture sometimes dismissed as functionless – help us evolve mentally within those constraints to fit the changing circumstances of our species while also brokering the tension between a cacophonous world and our limited ability to make sense of it. Scholarship in the humanities – another part of culture sometimes deemed essentially useless – highlights the changes and contradictions in human consciousness, enabling us to make informed choices about which mutations to nurture and which to cease feeding. Primarily, however, culture is a force that stabilizes a community by encouraging a consensus on how the field of possible ideas and behavior should be limited.

While the immense capacity of the human brain and the malleable structure of its thinking have given our species unique opportunities, there is a catch in the bargain – a bug in the system. As Hamlet puts it, "there's the rub ... what dreams may come?" Our talent for imagination and for prudential and abstract thought risks overwhelming not only our mental capacities but also our morale with some equivalent of a computer stuck calculating infinities or dividing by zero – especially, as for Hamlet, in the bony or ghostly face of mortality. When he first finds the Crystal Skull, Indiana Jones spends almost two minutes staring into that face, often in poses highly reminiscent of the most famous pose in theater history: Hamlet contemplating the skull of Yorick, the court jester from his childhood. Both heroes are gravely imperiled by the unbearably limitless truths a skull might tell them, especially if they start seeing through its eyes. The wise Horatio warns Hamlet not to "consider too curiously" the implications of Yorick's remains (5.1.205).[11] What a ghost might tell Hamlet, his father's spirit warns, can destroy through the ears as well as the eyes:

> I could a tale unfold whose lightest word / Would harrow up thy soul, freeze thy young blood, / Make thy two eyes like stars start from their spheres / ... / But this eternal blazon must not be / To ears of flesh and blood.
>
> (1.5.15–22)

The dangerous burden conveyed by that message stands in for the hidden dangers of excessive information of any kind, making Hamlet stand in for any of us, as readers have almost always and almost everywhere felt that he does. Even within the conduct of mundane daily life, even with the help of evolved psychological modules, there is just too much to think about: too much to know and too many ways of knowing. Replacing so many creaturely instincts and simple appetites with conscious choices, as evolution has done, risks turning us into endless overthinkers (another Hamlet problem), putting our functionality as well as our sanity at risk. Hamlet's action stops, and at times his sanity totters, in his soliloquies – but those soliloquies are so famous because they epitomize a fundamental human struggle that modern individualism and the accompanying emphasis on psychology have intensified. In recent centuries, humankind has invested millions of songs and poems, and countless intimate and therapeutic conversations, in attempts to understand and communicate its own dissonant emotions.

Escaping from emotionality to the supposed harbor of rationality hardly protects us from the incalculable turbulence underlying our experience. Building a rational contemplative function atop the more reflex-like functions of the human mind only aggravates the problem. We are constantly obliged to decide, usually preconsciously, how to "chunk" incoming data and what kind of mental filters and normalizing algorithms to use in order to avoid being inundated (in perception and in memory) by the specificities of each instance at each moment. This process constitutes a never-ending negotiation between the (sensual) workers and the (cognitive) management, but with the help of culture we can usually keep the factory running productively. The problems people with schizophrenia have functioning in society appear to correlate strongly with deficits in their filtering of external stimuli. Obsessive-compulsive disorders as well as paranoia often appear to be runaway versions of the imposition of patterns. In other words, the voluntary calibrating of the scale between seeing order or seeing chaos, between seeing correspondences and generalizations or instead seeing instances in all their particularities, is another risk-laden opportunity for the human mind.

It is also a revealingly chronic problem in the construction of artificial intelligence.[12] Sheldon Klein, a professor of computer science and linguistics at the University of Wisconsin, comments that

> Contemporary artificial-intelligence researchers find the problem of computing human behavior by rules intractable ... the time it takes to make such computations can increase exponentially or even combinatorially with the size and heterogeneity of the knowledge system .... The problem of making such computations ... can be solved if appropriate constraints apply to the structure of the rules. There seems to be evidence that systems of such constraints were invented in the Upper Paleolithic .... The evidence can be found in the material and symbolic artefacts of a variety of cultures, and the

major sources are classification schemes, divination systems, iconographie [sic] systems, language structures, and shamanistic, mythic, or religious systems.[13]

The modern human mind evidently could not function without culture – and it is therefore (this book asserts) to some extent a hostage in the drive of cultural forms toward self-perpetuation.

The distinguished (if controversial) cognitive scientist Philip Lieberman has recently argued that genetic changes in the hominoid group affected "the caudate nucleus – the basal ganglia structure that is the neural engine that confers creativity." Furthermore, "'highly accelerated regions' (HARs) of the human genome that differ from the Neanderthal genome … appear to be associated with cognition. Their 'cost' is that they seem to be associated with schizophrenia, autism, and other mental illnesses."[14] If so, then the unique aspects of the human brain produce creativity, indecision, and insanity – and cultural filters, which seek to control all three. We may not be the only species that has produced radically magnified intelligence; we may just be the only species in which it has, thus far, survived.[15] "So wise so young, they say, do never live long," observes Shakespeare's Richard III (3.1.79) – and we are still a very young species.

Human consciousness is therefore more malleable than that of other animals. Like them, we certainly have some built-in protocols for simplifying data and allocating attention. For example, cross-cultural studies indicate that the way we sort the spectrum of visual wavelengths into color bands may be partly hard-wired.[16] As in other areas, however, we seem to have a much greater capacity for disabling or overriding those cognitive constraints than other species generally do; and cultures vary widely in their vocabulary of colors, which seems to affect even how they see. Ancient Greek and Roman cultures often sorted colors more by saturation levels than by hues, and Isaac Newton divided the humanly visible spectrum into seven colors to align it with other systems his culture had divided into seven, such as musical notes, metals, planets, and days of the week. Joseph Henrich reports that (for speakers of English) "acquiring eleven basic color terms improves our ability to distinguish between colors with different verbal labels, although it also degrades our ability to distinguish shades with the same label"[17]; that degradation, I believe, is for the overburdened mind a defense against the infinitude of wavelengths even within our visible spectrum.

Evolutionary psychology sometimes tends to exaggerate the ratio of hard wiring to cultural shaping in the human mind. A landmark 2010 study showed that "visual perception, fairness, cooperation, spatial reasoning, categorization and inferential induction, moral reasoning, reasoning styles, self-concepts and related motivations, and the heritability of IQ" all vary much more widely across cultures than many social scientists had assumed. Those scientists underestimated the impact of culture because they mostly compared subjects from "Western, Educated, Industrialized, Rich, and Democratic" societies; the acronym WEIRD wittily reinforces the warning against presuming such subjects represent some ideal human norm.[18] (Admittedly, this book has similar limitations, reflecting the world I was raised in and the canon I was taught.) Even the epigenetic profiles of identical twins diverge sharply if they encounter different environments; even when such twins are raised together, those profiles differ by age 5.[19] I agree heartily with the evolutionary psychologists when, in their battle against constructivist social scientists, they say the human mind must have *a priori* structures in place to begin sorting and prioritizing information and possible responses. But I seriously doubt that such structures are sufficient to the task. The astonishing diversity of human cultures indicates it is more important that there be a shared culture than that the culture have any particular attributes, contents, or configuration.

My emphasis on the burdens of human perception has been challenged on the grounds that our nearest common ancestors seem untroubled by their encounters with perceptible reality despite lacking our cultural filters. That does not strike me as a refutation, however, since it could on the contrary suggest that species lacking *Homo sapiens*' uniquely open and complex mentality have no need for guidance as elaborate as human cultures provide.

The human mind's daily to-do list is daunting. One theory associates the growth of hominoid brains with the burdensome obligation of this highly communal species to imagine people not physically present.[20] The social as well as physical habitats experienced by *Homo sapiens* are far more varied than those of most non-human species.[21] Furthermore, those other species lack the powers of language that allow us to explore each others' inner selves, receive many generations of lived experience, and (especially) to fantasize hypothetical worlds in addition to the real one: mental enterprises that at times overwhelm even our relatively vast cognitive capacity.

Hence the risks played out in the fictions of Jorge Luis Borges such as "Funes the Memorious," where iterative remembering – hyperthymesia – fatally congests the mind and thereby the heart. A pair of 2017 studies in the distinguished journal *Science* confirm earlier findings that a major purpose of sleep is forgetting: shrinking synapses and pruning away connections built up during the waking hours, the noise of which might otherwise drown out more important signals or patterns.[22]

As for Dr. Spalko in that underground temple of temples, part of the problem is the sheer accumulation of information over time. A prominent recent study on mice suggests that deficits in long-term memory may reflect not a loss of the ability to record information but rather a loss of the ability to clear or choose space in the crowded brain for new information by forgetting the old; any new data thus becomes as hard to read as new writing on an already-scribbled page.[23] The chief function of one gene that is "present only in hominoids" is apparently "to mop up the neurotransmitter glutamate after neurons have fired, so preparing the way for the neuron to be able to fire again," leading some scientists to believe that "it may play an important role in facilitating the greater cognitive abilities of hominoids compared to those of simians."[24] Like much speculation linking uniquely human genes to uniquely human behaviors, this claim is questionable, but it does suggest that the art of forgetting, of clearing mental pathways, may be crucial in preventing mental overload.

Furthermore, a new study of visual process suggests that the brains of elderly people are actually no worse at many learning skills than the brains of the young, except that they lose the ability to exclude distracting peripheral information; only the younger subjects ceased attending to moving dots around the main information once those dots fell into predictable patterns. This useful youthful narrowing of focus resembles the work of culture in sorting large portions of reality (by myths, for example) into familiar containers to prevent cognitive overload.[25] Another new study suggests that autism may be produced by a failure to prune away neural spines, leaving the brain "overloaded with stimuli"; "an oversupply of synapses in at least some parts of the brain … may help explain some symptoms like oversensitivity to noise or social experiences."[26] Medical science is thus beginning to recognize the problems of overburdened minds, from childhood to senility. Borges's Funes has a further problem, however: his mind is so swarmed with every instance of every perception of every object that he cannot generalize and achieve ideas.[27] Or consider Borges's "The Library of Babel," with its terror of a plentitude of information, which is ultimately no information at all. If human experience is not arranged, it is deranged.

From this perspective, increasing data-flow is not always as beneficial as triumphalist theories of technological mastery would predict. What has happened in the Information Age – and, I would say, in the accompanying hectic eras of entertainment and globalization – is a collective version of the overload that would be the daily experience of any ordinary person without the guidance of culture. Certain forms of data are certainly pressed on us much more frequently in the 21st century, and more frequently marked as data, but the world received without a mediating screen has always been overwhelming for the human mind.[28] According to studies performed in several countries over the past century, we register more than 10,000,000 bits of information per second through our senses, but our conscious minds can manage only about 100 per second.[29] It makes for a daunting, tottering inbox.

A distinguished psychologist has recently observed that "the upper limits of attention are in the order of about 120 bits per second," and that

> Out of the millions of bits of potential information present in the environment, attention selects an infinitesimal subset and assimilates it into consciousness, thus creating a distinct experience, such as fear, awe, love, understanding, doubt, or jealousy. It is not surprising that William James wrote that our lives consist of those things that we have attended to. What *is* surprising is that this fundamental insight was so little appreciated by psychologists over the past hundred years. On what basis do we decide what to pay attention to? And how do we order experiences out of what has been attended to?[30]

My answer is that we depend heavily on our cultures to guide that allocation of attention, and our cultures can therefore insulate us within their assumptions.

We settle for "lossy compression": the kind of compromise audiophiles lament in MP3s, but adequate to convey the melody – and the melody helps us remember more than we could otherwise. The ability of the human brain to store information is astonishing, but its ability to register it all and index it all for conscious recall is much more limited – and mercifully so. Mechanisms of selective attention and recollection are indispensable.

I believe that the main threat of cognitive overload comes not from the flood of trivial, transient distractions offered by the Internet but from an expansion of the available ways of thinking, judging, and believing. That problem has been aggravated by modern trends (most visible in advanced Western nations) toward open and tolerant societies that (1) support free speech and a free press, (2) believe everyone should have all opportunities, (3) separate government from religion, (4) are reluctant to prosecute seemingly victimless offenses, (5) have large immigrant communities, and (6) indulge in arts that aspire to originality. A culture – or, in its condensed form, a cult – narrows down the limitless perceptual and behavioral possibilities to a manageable few, telling you that there are correct ways to evaluate and feel and act in each situation. Lowered expectations are certainly a problem in some advanced societies in the 21st century, but so is a lowered ability to know what to expect. As Alexis de Tocqueville commented, people can "get used to anything except living in a society that does not share their manners."[31] Most primates could join a faraway tribe and know exactly how to behave, but the churchmen banish Mark Twain's Connecticut Yankee, despite all his good intentions, from King Arthur's court.

Culture is a flow regulator on the broad-gauge conduit of human consciousness. Without it, there are just too many things to perceive and imagine, too much information and too many angles from which to see it, and too many taxonomies into which it could be sorted. On the last point, the relevant Borges piece is "The Analytical Language of John Wilkins," which imagines a Chinese encyclopedia organized by categories that would strike most readers as randomly crisscrossing mismatched associative categories (in a way that again resembles some common malfunctions in schizophrenia). Some optimists predict that the reduced obligations of memory in the era of Google searches and smartphone calendars will free up our capacity for greater cognitive and hence cultural flexibility[32]; but that probably overestimates the proportion of mental work such factual memorization really occupies.

When a group agrees to shut down most of its censoring faculties for the sake of generating new ideas, that process is aptly called brainstorming. Shakespeare's King Lear relinquishes many familiar and comforting illusions out in the thunderstorm, and his new clarity of perception quickly becomes indistinguishable from madness. The great cultural anthropologist Clifford Geertz has argued that "nearly all those characteristics of man's existence which are most graphically human: his thoroughly encephelated nervous system, his incest-taboo-based social structure, and his capacity to create and use symbols ... emerged together" during the Ice Age, indicating that "man's nervous system does not merely enable him to acquire culture, it positively demands that he do so if it is going to function at all."

Culture is therefore not a mere supplement; not just a diversion but a way of diverting surplus information. Geertz's overstatement should not blind us to the insight underlying his claim that "A cultureless human being would probably turn out to be ... a wholly mindless and consequently unworkable monstrosity."[33] When infants or toddlers become "overstimulated," caretakers expect a tantrum or a nap. Lacking any other frame by which to limit the inflow of experience, the little person whose cultural filters are barely developed usually either gets mad or shuts down. Oddly, few people seem to notice that many big persons display the same pair of responses when culture fails to prevent input from becoming overload: madness, or a flight into willful blinkering (or both, in some cases of fundamentalist violence), or sedative drugs.

We may assume that ancient Athenians led very simple lives by our modern standards. But they were an experimental democracy emerging from a world of tyrannical hierarchies, a culture that valued intellectual exploration, and an ambitious sea-faring economy that brought them into contact with many other types of societies that had formerly developed in isolation.[34]

So it is no mere coincidence that Athens was also the source of so much great drama, since one key function of both comedies and tragedies is to explore the dysfunctions and lurking contradictions in cultural rules by showing persons trapped in those conflicting dictates. Plato's *Laws* shows how strong the drive therefore became for cultural unity, arguing that a "State and polity come first, and those laws are best, where there is observed as carefully as possible throughout the whole State the old saying that 'friends have all things really in common'." Furthermore, in Plato's ideal state,

> so far as possible it is contrived that even things naturally 'private' have become in a way 'communized,' – eyes, for instance, and ears and hands seem to see, hear, and act in common, – and that all men are, so far as possible, unanimous in the praise and blame they bestow, rejoicing and grieving at the same things, and that they honour with all their heart those laws which render the State as unified as possible.

Only then can citizens "dwell pleasantly."[35]

No wonder "A wealth of anthropological data suggests that human groups possess considerable cultural inertia" so that – even centuries later – some groups continue to resemble the culture from which their ancestors emigrated more than they resemble the culture of their current neighbors.[36] The sense of civic duty among Americans of European descent, for example, correlates quite strongly with those of the countries of their settler ancestors.[37] This is true even when the cultural legacy appears maladaptive: for example, the violent culture of masculine honor in the southeast United States, a legacy from social conditions of centuries ago may not comport well with modern weaponry, any more than the unpredictable movements that squirrels evolved to evade predators serve them well in a world of motor vehicles that have no hunger for squirrel meat.[38]

No wonder, also, that the undifferentiated swirl of sound proves intolerable to some of the profoundly deaf who receive artificial hearing (usually through cochlear implants) after adolescent brain development is complete. A similar fate may await recipients of a new type of visual implant that adds frequencies to the spectrum normally seen by human beings. Even basic sensory experience can be unbearably complicated without some training in ways of sorting it into segments and meanings, and choosing what to perceive and what to ignore. If the system for managing sounds cognitively is not awoken and attuned when it emerges developmentally, what for most people is ordinary reality can become excruciating. These sensory problems offer an analogy to the problems that would torment a human mind unguarded by the conservative work of culture.

No wonder, either, that (regardless of race) people in the grip of poverty, which has recently been shown to impose a massive cognitive burden,[39] have trouble escaping the grip of destructive cultural formations that make it all the more difficult to escape poverty. The capacity for resistance may be nearly exhausted before the battle even begins against entrenched malfunctions such as gambling (in the United States, mostly as state lotteries, formerly as "playing the numbers"; in Ghana, by Chinese machines), unhealthy diets, violence in young men and teen pregnancy in young women, disincentives for education, and abuse of both legal and illegal drugs. The Nation of Islam, for all its off-putting attributes, can be understood as an attempt to provide Detroit and then other inner cities with an alternative culture claiming ancient roots and offering strict rules that resisted those malfunctions. Other systems evolve to exploit that vulnerability: payday loans, for instance, which depend on a practical alliance with larger predatory banking systems and with an illusory ideology of free choice. Less-than-worthless private universities use algorithms to target impoverished single mothers who are desperate for some hope of escaping their predicaments.[40] This may be one reason why offering prisoners higher education – which I will be arguing expands the mind's ability to bear awkward cognitive loads – has proven so much more effective than other programs at reducing recidivism and increasing quality of life.[41]

And no wonder, finally, that many sensitive people – reportedly an ever-increasing proportion in modernized societies – retreat into the private cultures of compulsive ritual behavior as a mode of soothing and control. Consider also the surging popularity of videos that induce autonomous sensory meridian response (ASMR), which provides the hypnotic delights of a kind of painless masochism, as a kind, gentle, wise, confident, lovely, and completely unthreatening soft voice takes over guiding the listener's experience. The problem of "cognitive load" has been extensively studied as an obstacle to be minimized in the workplace and the classroom, but I believe these situations of directed learning are only the most obvious and instrumental instances of a task nearly ubiquitous in waking human life. This book explores the way that task of taming cognitive overload – never more than provisionally completed – shapes our institutions and ideologies.

Our noses cease to notice persistent scents so that we can attend to new ones, and, for a similar purpose of reducing cognitive load, cultures similarly become a nearly undetectable background. A new place's odors or a new country's customs therefore seem vivid as well as strange. Our sensory array has evidently developed a system like the "elimination prints" detectives collect from regular members of a household, to make it easier to recognize the crucial fingerprints of the intruder rather than becoming overwhelmed by all the innocent fingerprints around the crime scene.

Admittedly, the modern world has become busier than it was for ancient hunter-gatherers, as agriculture both demanded and produced local stability, while modern industrial capitalism accelerated exchange and (abetted by Protestantism, as Max Weber famously argued,[42] though Japan has endured similar transformations) demanded tireless exertion toward practical productivity. What persists, however, through the massive shifts from systems run by ritual and (at some point) scripture to a system run largely by science is the need for systematic, normalizing channels of thought. The invention of writing neither initiated nor erased humanity's appetite for some ordering authority outside the individual mind. It does not take a Henry James novel to understand that even a seemingly ordinary moment of social interaction among human beings can be fraught with many subtle but consequential complexities.[43] It may be argued that high Victorian society was a high-water mark of constructed social delicacy, but perhaps James was recording a fact about human interaction that had become more visible under those mores, rather than a fact that was wholly new.

Discussions of the evolutionary aspect of human culture generally emphasize its ability to accelerate and distribute innovation, but it also has to slow down innovation and block out novel signals from different cultures. A conservative tendency is therefore not surprising and can be healthy if pursued with alertness to changing conditions and a heart that stays open even if the mind begins to contract. The need for shared channeling and control explains why 21st-century societies that are otherwise dismissive of the past nonetheless regress to archaic cultural traditions (as my first Interchapter will assert). Some of this regression takes the stark form of backlash: recent increases in toleration for diversity in sexuality, and accompanying retreats from longstanding regimens of gender, have predictably provoked intense resistance to same-sex marriage, birth control, and gender transitions – and perhaps, as proxies for masculinity, resistance to gun control, and energy efficiency as well.

Clearly, recognizing and remedying the problem of gender dysphoria is very important and long overdue. Yet, having been raised by Dr. Barbara Bellow Watson, the founder of one of the first university women's studies programs as second-wave feminism arose 50 years ago, I still struggle with the insistence of many transgender advocacy groups that human brains are compellingly binary in gender. Longstanding patriarchal traditions insisted that there was a thing called a woman (corresponding to XX chromosomes, though the genetics are not quite that simple) which necessarily brought along with it a whole set of identifying markers that were inherent in it, not merely socially imposed. The current progressive view, at least as articulated by many activists, insists that some people (despite their XY chromosomes) cannot be who they really are unless they become a woman with many of those same markers. I am not equating these two positions ethically; I believe the activist position is often compelled by the violence by which the patriarchal one is imposed. The horrific level of assaults on transgender persons, and suicides among them, makes some concessions to gender essentialism perfectly justifiable. But even the progressive argument that insists on allowing people to situate themselves on a continuum between male and female implies that there is an anchoring point at each end of that continuum. It brings a simplifying rubric to bear on the complexities of gender and sexuality.[44]

It seems noteworthy that the repressive fundamentalist regime in Iran actively promotes gender transitions as a way to eradicate homosexuality. On the Indian subcontinent, a third gender called *hijra* protects the categories, and Albanian women willing to become "sworn virgins" are allowed to take on the social identity of men. In some Native America plains tribes, boys who opted out of the violent role of warrior "were called *berdache*, 'women-men.' They wore woman's clothing, did woman's work, married men, stuffed their clothes to look pregnant, and even cut themselves to imitate menstruation."[45] These are all ways for heteronormative regimes to avoid any acknowledgment of same-sex desire and gender fluidity.

* * * * * * * * * * *

Like so many others who were teenagers then, I grew up awestruck by the "counterculture" of the late 1960s. I see now, however, that despite the radical liberationist rhetoric it deployed against conservative tendencies, that movement actively strove to import cultures – preferably ones with ancient roots and elaborate disciplines – to replace the one it was rejecting. Indian forms (including yoga, meditation, sitar music, and even particular forms of vegetarianism and pacifism) were popular, as were bits of Taoism, and splinters from Celtic and Native American belief and ritual. This need of people outside the dominant culture for alternative foundations – often ancient and mystical – may also explain the persistent interest in astrology, tarot cards, and pagan rituals in gay communities.[46]

Extreme social movements apparently need to offer this kind of reassuring substitution: for example, "French Revolutionaries trying to free themselves of existing coordinations might try to efface recent history by appealing to a 'mythic present' or trump it by appealing to the even older ideals of ancient Greece."[47] A letter written in 2010 makes an unremarkable, even fussily old-fashioned literary-scholarly request: "if there are any brothers with you who know about poetic metres, please inform me, and if you have any books on the science of classical prosody, please send them to me." What makes the letter remarkable is that the preceding sentence requests a recommendation for a suitable candidate to lead "a big operation inside America" and that the letter was written by Osama bin Laden, the architect of the 9/11 attacks.[48] This represents an unwelcome challenge to the view that poetry inculcates gentleness, but a confirmation of my belief that political revolutionaries feel a need to compensate with traditional cultural formalities.

Syria's most famous living poet, Adonis (Ali Ahmad Said Esber), took a secularist stand against any revolution based in mosques rather than in laity, thinking that a fundamentalist takeover would only create a worse authoritarianism than that of Bashar al-Assad. This seems to correlate meaningfully with Adonis's controversial practice and advocacy of poems in experimental forms when "almost all poetry in Arabic, from the pre-Islamic period onward, had been composed in fixed metres." Criticized by those who wanted "to safeguard the 'unity' of Arabic culture," Adonis therefore dug back into the poetic history "to discover a 'modernist' counter-heritage buried within the classical heritage itself."[49] Again, the radical position had to defend itself by claiming a deep link to traditional culture. My point is that freeing themselves of existing conditions would not have required these importations unless, for the 1789 or 2010 radicals as for the 1968 ones, being entirely free of normative traditions was actually intolerable.

The Puritan revolution in 17th-century England was determined to root out rituals, which they felt blocked a true and direct encounter with God, but the resulting lack of shared and set forms of thinking and practice, however liberating at first, proved intolerable. They believed that the absolute authority of the Bible would be a more than adequate substitute for the traditions of the populace, but it did not prove so, partly because of the inherent subjectivity of reading. The difference between the characteristic cognitive styles of the revolutionaries and the more orderly, conservative styles of the royalists is reflected in the main schools of poetry from the period.[50] That history offers lessons about the way different responses to cognitive overload shape political divisions in 21st-century societies, as the left preaches tolerance, diversity, relativism, and liberation, whereas the right (apart from its libertarian branch) offers fundamentalist religion, incarceration, sexual regulation, reverence for financial bottom lines, and nostalgia for the old orders of gender and social hierarchy.

James C. Scott's masterful *Weapons of the Weak* shows that successful revolutionary moments are seldom fueled – at least among the popular masses, who are essential to that success – by some messianic, millennial, or even just high-ideological vision of the future. Instead, the foundation of most successful revolutions is a widespread resentment among the populace that old norms are being violated by the privileged. Antonio Gramsci, Michel Foucault, and many less famous radical theorists argue that the masses are in the grip of an ideological order created by the powerful to keep them subjugated, which is then naturalized and mystified beyond their power to penetrate until a radical thinker comes along to awaken them to a glorious alternative. Scott demonstrates the opposite: underclasses tend to be very well aware of the way the system is falling short of the society's ideals of fairness. In fact, it is the privileged who are trapped in "false consciousness" because they must pay lip service to longstanding traditions of justice while violating them as needed under a new order (such as capitalism and/or imperialism).[51] Again, revolutionary movements need a foundation in traditional order and values, and depend on it for their footing and force.

Within what proclaimed itself a movement of antinomian resistance in the late 1960s ran a compensating appetite for normalizing signals: clothing and hair, rituals of music (with its exalted deities) and drugs, shared slang, and presumptions of political solidarity all served to provide a soothing conformism within the nonconformist ethic. The "free your head" movement may have installed different filters of thought, but it didn't actually manage to do without them. No one could tell these cultural radicals what to do – except perhaps the I Ching hexagrams. The paradox is nicely captured in the title of Jack Kerouac's 1958 Beatnik novel *The Dharma Bums*: an oxymoron which sets the ancient Indian term against contemporary American slang, and the concept of order and law against messy indiscipline. Even now, the bar scene for cool young adults in Los Angeles (led by the aptly named 1933 Group) is laden with nostalgic Americana. Brooklyn is full of hipsters sporting beards and flannel shirts from a mountain-man era of American logging; many queer women choose a similar aesthetic. Experienced guides for psychedelic trips on LSD or psilocybin tend to surround the psychic traveler with a collection of cultural artifacts as mixed and crowded as the chamber where Indiana Jones finds the Crystal Skull, apparently so that the dangerously unlocked mind can find some reassuring landmarks in its field of vision.[52]

Bob Dylan's sneering, defiant, drug-fueled efforts (taking up the legacy of Allen Ginsberg and the Beats) to carry the decrepit body of post-World War II American culture to its grave and vivify a new one produced an astonishing cluster of transformative art in 1965–66, as he left behind the folk ballad and its received traditions of form, content, and instrumentation. His Nobel Prize in literature, half a century later, confirms how important that work was. But Dylan apparently found the pressure unbearable, and after disappearing into small-town domesticity for a few years, began instead – to the puzzled dismay of his radical followers – leaning ever more heavily on highly traditional forms of that culture: country and western music, the Christian Bible, conservative Judaism, and what Greil Marcus's book about Dylan's "Basement Tapes" has aptly called "the old, weird America" of accumulated folklore. This retreat resembles the retreat of Indiana Jones. We might say of culture what Dylan himself sang of love, as he withdrew from hip Greenwich Village to upstate life and from psychedelic electric guitarists to old-boy Nashville studio musicians: "No matter what you think about it / You just won't be able to do without it / Take a tip from one who tried."[53]

I am not dismissing these resistance movements by pointing out that they resorted to reviving or importing other cultural norms. The question,

I will argue, is not whether to have such norms, but instead which ones to deploy to steer a dominant culture in healthier directions.

Some Introductory Definitions and Conclusions

Out of the thousands of different kinds of garments in the world, how did you choose to put on the ones you are now wearing? Out of the millions of foods, how did you end up eating the ones you did for breakfast? When someone said "Good morning" to you, how did your sleepy head decide which of the billions of available utterances would be your reply?

These weren't self-evident or worldwide choices. They weren't even exactly your choices, and they probably weren't optimal choices either. But you didn't have to spend your morning figuring them out. Human beings have given cultural systems wide authority over our thinking and behavior because neither individual cognition nor social cooperation would be manageable without such guidance. A tension between the unique complexity and openness of the human mind on the one hand and the problem of sustaining group cohesion and personal sanity on the other makes us take many things for granted. Prominent among the survival skills of cultures (as of many living creatures) is their ability to camouflage themselves as permanent facts of nature.

The creative arts, the humanities, and other peculiar forms of resistant intellectualism help a society recognize and resist that blind enslavement in two ways. These practices inculcate a tolerance for complexity rather than simplification, thereby reducing the cognitive pressure that causes people to subjugate themselves to cultural norms. The same practices provide reminders of lasting human attributes and values, and of alternative ways of organizing consciousness and society, as touchstones for testing whether current cultural forces should be respected or, instead, challenged.

Anthropology makes clear that cultures serve to pass along information about how to perform various tasks essential for survival and thriving. My addendum is that – as epistemology and cognitive science make clear – this transmission must include information about how to filter information: about how to choose what to perceive, and how to frame and judge and prioritize what is perceived. We need to not notice everything, and for the most part we need to not notice the same things our neighbors are not noticing. To have an identity and a community, and neither of them at war with themselves – in short, to avert inward or outward chaos – human beings need culture to sort the world, and to shape a shared reality. Developing a human mind may be less like filling an empty cabinet (as the influential philosopher John Locke described it in the 17th century) than like climbing up a viewing tower with fixed binoculars at the top, as at many officially designated vista points, aimed at what a society has deemed the essential sights. That illusion of unity is precious even inside the individual mind, as modules of perception and intellection situated around the brain are coordinated nearly seamlessly in order to sustain each person's sense of being a self in relation to a world.

But those cultural systems become rigid and even coercive as people's fear of losing control (psychologically or socially) empowers a complex assemblage of rules and rituals, which evolves over generations into a form that protects itself as well as the community. Sometimes, it screens off alternatives we need later; its simplifying and coercive functions have side effects that can override better possibilities and can ally themselves with human tyrants. As Wallace Stevens wrote in "The Man with the Blue Guitar,"

> behold
> The approach of him whom none believes,
> Whom all believe that all believe,
> A pagan in a varnished car.
> Roll a drum upon the blue guitar ....
>
> (Stanza X)[54]

These lines imply that the need to maintain a culture's mythologies by mutual affirmation breeds a cult of dictatorship and a rise of militarism, even though each citizen may silently suspect those grand mythologies are bright, shining lies. Such mythologies are like many dangerous leaders (in a painfully complex and intractable world) who say, follow me and empower me, march to my drum, and in return I will keep you safe and confirm your prejudices as truth.

Some of humanity's most serious problems in the 21st century arise from our failure to recognize that cultures – not just biological creatures – undergo Darwinian evolution, meaning that the cultural forms that survive are the ones that are most successful in steering our energies toward their own replication rather than our thriving. The vast majority of scholarship on cultural evolution examines how it works in human populations; I am interested instead in how cultural evolution works on cultures. For example, where Daniel Smail rightly observes that "The mutual interests between believers and cultures appear to be distinctly symbiotic,"[55] I want to add that that appearance of symbiosis may be delusory: there is a probably symbiotic relationship between clergy and the religion itself, but the believers may not actually benefit. Where Stephen Shennan rightly argues that "selection on people can operate through selection on their cultural traditions," my questions are, how does selection on cultural traditions shape those traditions and how does that competition deform humanity?

In the Preface to *Culture and Anarchy* (1869), the renowned English poet and cultural critic Matthew Arnold recommended culture – "the best that has been thought and said" – as the greatest

> help out of our present difficulties ... turning a stream of fresh and free thought upon our stock notions and habits, which we now follow staunchly but mechanically, vainly imagining that there is a virtue in following them staunchly which makes up for the mischief of following them mechanically.

This book has some similar goals, but also recognizes that, in opposing anarchy, culture is necessarily wary of "fresh and free thought," and that this tension is formative of individuals as well as of societies. I am trying to offer, in a speculative rather than a scientific mode, a new way of thinking about the relations among some essential functions of human experience, from the very basic to the very arcane.

My title borrows from Sigmund Freud's *Civilization and Its Discontents*, which explores the tension between the instinctive drives (toward both love and violence) of individuals and the constraints of social life. Freud here points out that people refuse to recognize "the social source of suffering":

> We do not admit it at all; we cannot see why the regulations made by ourselves should not, on the contrary, be a protection and a benefit for every one of us. And yet, when we consider how unsuccessful we have been in precisely this field of prevention of suffering, a suspicion dawns on us that here, too, a piece of unconquerable nature may lie behind – this time a piece of our own psychical constitution. When we start considering this possibility we come upon a contention which is so astonishing that we must dwell upon it. This contention holds that what we call our civilization is largely responsible for our misery, and that we should be much happier if we gave it up and returned to primitive conditions.[56]

Freud's book sought to attribute human unhappiness to civilization's necessary repression of those evolved biological drives. My book calls attention instead to the way certain evolved drives of civilization itself – certain self-reproducing institutions and practices – create unnecessary human suffering by repressing our healthiest ethical instincts and aesthetic appetites. Freud sees civilization as a device we have invented to reduce our suffering that now causes most of our suffering. I see a similar paradox in what I am calling culture: we have invented it partly to reduce the difficulty of our experience, but it often makes our lives more difficult, or at least less rewarding. As Freud believes that "a person becomes neurotic because he cannot tolerate the amount of frustration which society imposes on him in the service of its cultural ideals,"[57] I believe that the moral character of a society of persons becomes distorted, and its intellectual character delimited, by cultural norms imposed in the service of simplified and coordinated life – norms we fail to recognize as rivals of higher aspirations.

This book will explain the dynamics of this problem through a trio of color-coded elements, referring back to them periodically as a kind of shorthand. The Crystal Skull symbolizes the dangers of cognitive overload produced by the plasticity that is unique to human consciousness. The Blue Guitar symbolizes the function of artistic creativity in giving us a grasp on that unruly mental multiplicity without strangling the life out of it; as the Stevens poem puts it, "The blue guitar / Becomes the place of things as they are, / A composing of senses of the guitar" (Stanza VI). Such creativity can sort human experience into forms that are not only tolerable but beautiful: forms that shape consciousness in ways that revive human ideals rather than empowering cultural parasites. This is the happier alternative to the Red Scare, which epitomizes the defense mechanisms against complexity that manifest themselves as conformism, jingoism, and anti-intellectualism. Those overreactions conspire to repress potentially liberatory consciousness and enslave us to self-perpetuating cultural models. Matthew Arnold himself envisioned a severely ordered society as a precondition for refined human achievements, and therefore saw culture as "the most resolute enemy of anarchy."[58] My point is nearly the converse: that, by preventing an anarchy of consciousness, a healthy culture can make a less authoritarian state tolerable because (to take a more positive view of a phenomenon observed by Foucault) much of the necessary work of ordering has already been accomplished without forcible policing. A persistent theme of this book will be that, in many aspects of human life, including mental health, democratic government, artistic creativity, and education, sustaining the delicate balance between freedom and control, and between novelty and tradition, is crucial. The trick is choosing what to relinquish and what to retain so as to produce a healthy kind of coherence.

* * * * * * * * * * * *

Several key terms in my argument have obscure or multiple meanings, so let me briefly define what they mean in this book. A **meme** is a transmittable piece of cultural information, often analogized with a gene in studies of cultural evolution; Richard Dawkins proposed "memetics" as a science partially parallel with genetics. A **memeplex** is a systematic aggregation of memes that has the power to replicate itself through human carriers. Although in some cases (such as linguistics) it seems possible to trace the evolution of individual memes, this book is more concerned with these larger assemblages:

concepts that have become symbiotic with institutional embodiments. The small-unit memes that travel within these memeplexes benefit reproductively from the thriving of the aggregate and can also spread, virus-like, into other memeplexes that have compatible receptors. Many social phenomena function as memeplexes, and they may reside within a culture or across several. They may take many forms – religions, fashions, sports, universities, corporations, political movements, economic systems, etc. – and as such their dynamics have been studied in a variety of academic disciplines. I am not saying that all pieces of information or all aspects of culture should be understood as Darwinian entities (or Lamarckian entities, to the extent that transmission includes acquired characteristics and guided variation). What I am saying is that it would be helpful to understand the Darwinian functions of entities – on the boundary between organisms and organizations – that must survive and reproduce by enlisting human carriers or else go extinct.

By a **culture**, I mean a mutually reinforcing system of ideas, rules, values, and practices adopted by a community – and there can be many overlapping cultures and communities. My main interest is in the tension between two competing functions of culture. One is conservationist and usually appears as ritual or some more diffuse version of conformism, winning adherents and advocates by protecting people from uncertainty and complexity. The opposing force is innovative and transformative, attempting to offer new ideas and values; it strives to reshape the dominant memeplexes, and wins adherents and advocates by allowing a fuller exercise of our capacities and by making available models better adapted to the changing circumstances of persons and societies. I will be emphasizing the role of humanistic scholarship and creative arts in providing this oppositional force, which is sometimes concentrated in **high culture** – the more sophisticated arts disproportionately practiced and patronized by an educated elite – but is by no means limited to that category or universal within that category (my own sensibilities rarely rise above upper-middlebrow, as this book will make only too clear). Culture helps a community share systems of perceiving, believing, and behaving, and helps exclude the infinite alternatives as simply wrong – all of which promotes unity, which promotes group survival, which renews the cycle by promoting the culture. These systems supplement the role of the evolved psychological routines of the human mind in taming our experience into tolerably simplified forms. By setting norms, this basic cultural function offloads enough cognitive load that high symbolic creativity becomes possible. High symbolic creativity, in turn, permits enough selective innovation in the cognitive and social norms for them to adapt to changing circumstances. I am especially concerned, however, with the way some cultural entities evolve into groupings (and memes into memeplexes) that, to put it in biological terms, are mutualist with each other – that is, each benefitting the other's survival – while becoming parasitic to their human carriers.[59]

Capitalism, for example, is a competitive system under which the means of production are owned by private corporations or individuals, rather than by a public collective or by the wage laborers who produce value. That value is measured by price, maximized as profit, and skimmed off as capital (accumulated possessions) by the owners. **Consumer capitalism** is capitalism's alliance with a culture that identifies the prime goals of human life as the acquisition and consumption of the commodities produced by capitalism, especially industrial capitalism, and especially under the influence of advertising.

By **neoliberalism,** I mean a kind of mutual defense treaty between capitalism and a plutocratic version of government that extends these allied memeplexes imperially and imperiously into many areas of human experience. Rising to power in the English-speaking world under the political leadership of Margaret Thatcher and Ronald Reagan, and the economic theories of Friedrich Hayek and Milton Friedman, it asserts that property rights are the most essential rights, that economic competition must be the main organizing fact of life, and (the starkest difference from classical liberalism) that public spheres should therefore be privatized to allow the genius of the profit motive to improve the functionality of societies. Under the guise of rational neutrality and reduced government regulation, it thus allies itself with the established privileges of race, class, and gender, viewing them not as residual structures of injustice but as a continuously earned superiority that cannot be erased without damaging the salubrious efficiencies of a laissez-faire marketplace. From a right-wing perspective, that system has proven itself to be the greatest engine of innovation, prosperity, and peaceful interaction between nations in recorded history. From a left-wing perspective, however, neoliberalism's endorsement of competition without government meddling is conveniently hedged. It assumes that a decent government must prevent the physically strong from brutalizing the physically feeble – an obvious moral imperative – but should never hinder the economically strong from brutalizing the economically feeble.[60] Gangs of impoverished teenagers cannot be allowed to mug corporate Chief Executive Officers for their bulging wallets, but the CEOs can give those teenagers no plausible means of survival other than alienated labor, the profits from which go disproportionately to the CEO.

A **society** is a group of persons, usually sharing a geographic area and a political system (hence, a state) and a set of cultures (which overlap and interact in various ways, affecting the kinds of guidance individuals in that society receive). The first half of this book calls attention to a function – and, most importantly, a malfunction – of cultures as they co-evolve with human minds and turn us into tribes and nations. The second half then calls attention to the ways societies may choose – with informed consent, as conditions change – the cultural forms we believe are healthiest for our community, and resist or revise the others.

By **evolution**, I mean what Darwin calls "descent with modification" – that is, inheritance susceptible to changes over generations – steered by differential reproduction, meaning the fact that some versions or portions of the entity will reproduce themselves more successfully than others. Not all traits are passed along, or passed along unchanged, from parents to offspring, and some of those offspring will be better adapted than others to survive and reproduce in a given environment, so their traits will become more prevalent in the population by what Darwin called "natural selection." The genetic functions of biological evolution emphasized by neo-Darwinism may be absent from cultural evolution, but the process of heredity with variation allows both kinds of entities to evolve by unconscious selection.

By **the humanities**, I mean academic fields that principally study the products of human culture – such as philosophy, languages (including complex forms of reading and writing), and the historical and aesthetic aspects of art forms – often in critical, subjective, speculative, and imaginative modes, as opposed to the empirical scientific study of social or natural phenomena. By widely varied means, scholars in these fields seek and transmit knowledge that often lacks immediate practical applications but allows us to recognize and reconsider our values. Ideally, they offer usefully indirect ways of understanding ourselves as well as past and present others, and give us a nuanced account of our traditions and our languages. The humanities provide instruments of collective memory and validations of personal experience while refining non-technical aspects of consciousness whose goal is not certainty. They explore human nature without claiming to encompass the unique emergent properties of each human being and human interaction. They therefore tend to inculcate flexibility of intellectual, emotional, and spiritual response, while also teaching the ability to appreciate and analyze expressions or experiences of irreducible complexity.

* * * * * * * * * * * *

Human beings need culture (I have been suggesting) to narrow the wide field of possible perception, thought, and behavior that is our most significant evolutionary peculiarity. This helps to explain reactionary tribalism. I now want to argue that culture therefore co-evolves with us, and the cultures that have survived and spread tend to have good strategies for self-replication with just enough plasticity and variability to adapt to new conditions over time. They also – like predatory animals – have good strategies for assimilating the energies of rivals: for swallowing others to enlarge themselves and prolong the existence of their structuring identities. Human beings and cultures depend on each other to survive, and they each engage in niche construction to make the other into an environment that will sustain them. Peter J. Richerson and Robert Boyd, eminent collaborators in the study of cultural evolution, describe culture as "a sophisticated cognitive *and* social system evolved to finesse the problem that information costs preclude a general purpose, problem-solving system inside every individual's head."[61] But cultures sometimes find it advantageous to exploit that problem rather than merely finessing it.

Imaginative arts and flexible languages are relatively safe ways human consciousness has found to create and endure mutations in order to remain adaptable to new conditions. Liberal arts education and humanistic scholarship (if imaginatively but rigorously practiced) perform a version of the artificial selection often practiced in the strategic breeding of plants and domestic livestock: selecting the most adaptive memeplexes to be reproduced, or at least by selecting what parts of their latent cultural epigenome should be activated in a particular environment to preserve what we value about our humanity.

What produces the canon of high culture must therefore be a skill conjoined with an attitude, rather than a dogma. Such a canon serves students, ideally, not as an assembly of divine scriptures that demand blind reverence but as a deeply diverse group of examples that suggest how to develop a canon for their own generation, with awareness of their local memes but not limited or enslaved to any memeplex. That canon may provide a haven for humane recognitions and sympathies that such complexes seek to suppress. The winnowing should therefore not be narrowly programmatic, but instead an open search for markers of qualities including intricacy, courage, beauty, empathy, insight, humor, imagination, and the articulation of a deep and/or unique sensibility. Neoplatonism, in both its pagan and Christian traditions, urged people to recognize the divine qualities underlying their earthly love objects; I am similarly arguing that we can identify criteria that are neither obscure nor inflexible by identifying the qualities we love in the people we love most happily. Those criteria can serve as touchstones to check the value of our cultural formations; or, by a different metaphor, compasses to guide us through forests of memetic trees.

Ingenious neuroscientific experiments have shown that the brain's "reward center" is actually dual: one bestows pleasure when we get something we wanted, the other when we get something we recognize as fundamentally good.[62] So my distinction between addictive drives that cultures can inculcate and more lasting valuations may not be wholly arbitrary and unfounded. The humanities seek a fulfillment of human potential – what Aristotle would have called our "finality" (*finem*), the ideal purpose toward which we instinctively strive – not merely the passive playing out of mechanisms that grow in and around us into malignancies, and enmesh our virtues in their self-replicating devices. Like cancers, memeplexes corrupt individuals (persons rather than cells) into reproducing them, to the overall harm of the body (in this case, the social aggregate, metaphorically termed "the body politic" by political theorists since medieval times), evading the defenses of the immune system (an alert social conscience).

Let me be clear from the start that my Darwinian model of social systems disavows the politically regressive tradition associated with Francis Galton (and less justly with Herbert Spencer). Alfred Kroeber has shown, following on the work of Franz Boas, that recognizing the co-evolutionary functions of culture is the best refutation of so-called Social Darwinists who deduce racial inferiority from what are largely cultural differences and postcolonial after-effects (which, my argument suggests, are all the more devastating because of their forcible disruption of cultural coherence). I am not seeking to endorse modern conservatism, but instead to explain its meaningful (though far from absolute) correlation with the conservation of existing cultural norms.

Nor am I supporting the simplistic and deterministic versions of evolutionary psychology that discourage progress toward (for example) human equality; I am interested in the power of culture and our ability to influence it, not in the supposedly immutable and insuperable power of some posited atavistic human nature that precludes conscious and conscientious choice. In fact, recognizing that evolutionary success is not a marker of inherent moral or practical superiority may help us recognize that the increasing dominion of certain configurations of industrial capitalism – for example, the self-serving, self-preserving powers of the large-scale banking system and its human and digital symbionts – should not be presumed good or necessary. Let me also emphasize that I am certainly not saying my argument explains everything about culture, arts, memes, or humanities. All four terms are understood in unmanageably multiple ways.[63] But I believe that what follows may illuminate a largely overlooked dynamic with major implications for evolutionary psychology, for cultural studies generally, for universities, and for human freedom in the multicultural and politically divisive world of our new century.

This is a book for people who want to understand why human society is often such a mess and are not satisfied with blaming it all on Eve nibbling fruit from the Tree of the Knowledge of Good and Evil, or any other explanatory backstory that resigns us to the weird dysfunctions of our world, and that deems disobedience to the overarching powers of the world presumptively a sin and/or a folly. A major obstacle to understanding the weirdness and curing the dysfunctions is precisely our tendency to sort the world into good and evil, rather than seeking a more complicated analysis of social functions. I am interested instead in the causes, diagnosis, and treatment of cultural forms that have become parasites on our species. This epidemiology becomes all the more essential in an era of rapid communication through social media and mass media, which speed up the spread of cultural forms while also subjecting those forms to constant challenge from other perspectives (unless Facebook filters them out). We are living in an agar-primed Petri dish for accelerating evolutionary competition among memes.

Interchapter: Modern Medievalism

Accompanying the garish political manifestations of anxiety about modern cultural complications (such as religion-based bans, border walls, and hate crimes based on race and gender) is a pattern of softer atavism. The need for established cultural guidance can make us behave oddly and regressively – a fact that is worth demonstrating at some length here because if that need can make us play pointless, self-distorting roles, and deny history, it can certainly do so in ways dangerous to our humanity. Evolutionary psychologists attribute various social dysfunctions to a mismatch between the modern First World and ancient mental modules adapted to Pleistocene societies.[1] Wisdom teeth that no longer fit modern jaws are a physical equivalent. My point is that what unhelpfully endures from previous eras despite having become maladaptive is often a cultural formation rather than a psychological or physiological one: a social code, rather than a behavior or body coded in DNA.

Andy Warhol's oft-quoted remark that, in the future, everyone will be famous for 15 minutes, could be revised to observe that many people now work largely for the privilege of posing as aristocrats of a bygone era for an occasional hour. Whether or not we agree with Bruno Latour's slightly less famous dictum that "we have never been modern," it is remarkable how often we choose still to be medieval. That is, the need for scripts is so overwhelming, and the culture therefore so slow to change, that the First World sometimes looks like a massive Renaissance Faire, still nostalgically replicating feudalism half a millennium after its functional demise.

People spend their working weeks as servants within the commercial world, where the boss or the customer must always be deemed right, as if money were just social class in a volatile form. They tolerate this subjugation and self-denigration for the survival of their families, but they are willing to invest some of their pay in making someone else play servant to them when they go shopping, where they receive "customer service," or (especially) out to a nice restaurant on special occasions, where they will be called Sir or Ma'am, as they sit in old-fashioned costumes practical only for signaling status (as King Lear says at 2.5.69–70, "Nature needs not what thou gorgeous wear'st, / Which scarcely keeps thee warm"), give their "orders" (in French, commander) to the person "serving" them, and sometimes eat from heavy silverware under simulated candlelight in lavishly paneled halls. When the wild rebel British rock stars of the 1960s became rich, they promptly bought themselves old aristocratic mansions. Most Christians still choose to address their God as "Lord" – a term otherwise out of favor in the United States for centuries ("lording it" is not admired, nor generally are landlords beloved). As Tocqueville observed nearly two centuries

ago, "The surface of American society is covered with a layer of democratic paint, but from time to time one can see the old aristocratic colors
breaking through."[2]

This craving, not for any durable high status but for a stable repertoire
of status-determinative behaviors, is a much more fundamental human
need than has been recognized. We often meet that need in otherwise
useless or even destructive ways precisely because we are unwilling or
unable to recognize that it is controlling us more than we are controlling
it. Upwardly mobile American citizens materialize their social progress
by building McMansions instead of houses practical for modern life.
Like Blanche DuBois clinging to the aura of Belle Reve in Tennessee
Williams's A Streetcar Named Desire, they move into gated communities with incongruous landed-lordly Anglophile names – Langford
Estates, Hollybrook at Pembroke Pines, The Hermitage at Deer Leap –
where they watch with fascination the lives in "Upstairs Downstairs" or
"Downton Abbey." A poignant version is the half-built Florida exurb
development called Carriage Pointe – the final "e" is the kicker – that
epitomized the 2008 housing-bubble collapse in George Packer's The
Unwinding.

Many encourage their daughters to imagine themselves princesses
and title their sons Master for formal events, and the implied lessons
sometimes stick only too well. They then send those children to prep
schools with a similar cultural signature in their names and rituals, and
then ideally to study amid what's called "collegiate gothic" stone archi-
tecture ("Dorms Like Palaces" is one of the main criteria the Princeton
Review offers for selecting a school). There, if all goes well (I will argue),
the spell used to lure them through the gates will be broken. More often,
as William Deresiewicz complains, elite universities instead put their
students deeper under the spell of neoliberal competition.[3] If those children win places in the 1%, they will probably nonetheless assume that
their work deserves many times the riches of manual laborers, mostly
because of a medieval allocation of status rather than any obviously
superior value in their contribution.

This pattern is weirdly persistent. As early as the late 1500s, it was
sardonically observed by Cervantes, whose Don Quixote fantasized that
he was living in a medieval chivalric romance, leading him into many
ridiculous scrapes with his unromantic contemporary reality. Through
Don Quixote's determination to mistake his life for a formulaic adventure learned from literature, Cervantes also acknowledged another
human tendency this book will emphasize: the need to see one's life as a
well-authored and morally significant narrative.

When futuristic "collectivization" shattered evolved systems of agricultural production and community loyalty in the Soviet Union, leading
to catastrophic famine, the only way the government could recapture
control was to revert to medieval social structures. Workers found

themselves turned essentially back into serfs, "fixed to the land at the pleasure of the kolkhoz *chairman."*[4] *The effort to push past capitalism had revived the feudalism that allowed the proletariat neither to choose their work nor (without the passports they couldn't get) to move around the country.*

The culture of ISIS, in the aftermath of the Arab Spring, similarly offers nostalgia for the Middle Ages to entice people who, for all their professed revolutionary radicalism, could not tolerate a truly new culture, lifted out of history into pure ideology. An article co-authored by a Yale comparative literature professor and a Princeton professor renowned for his expertise on the ideology of ISIS observes that

> The culture of jihad is a culture of romance. It promises adventure and asserts that the codes of medieval heroism and chivalry are still relevant. Having renounced their nationalities, the militants must invent an identity of their own. They are eager to convince themselves that this identity is not really new but extremely old. The knights of jihad style themselves as the only true Muslims, and, while they may be tilting at windmills, the romance seems to be working. ISIS recruits do not imagine they are emigrating to a dusty borderland between two disintegrating states but to a caliphate with more than a millennium of history.[5]

This atavism is reflected in the jihadis' aforementioned dedication to writing poetry in forms from centuries earlier – and also in their fondness for beheadings, despite an ample supply of modern firearms.

Intriguingly, the white supremacists most virulently opposed to Islam make the same kind of historical claims, carrying (as in the notorious 2017 Charlottesville rally) not just torches but shields emblazoned with medieval symbols such as Irish white crosses. A scholar of medieval history has noted the alt-right's "renewal of white nationalist ideologies based on long-discredited versions of ancient and medieval history." That movement's warnings that "'innate' European or 'Western' identities are being threatened by immigration are heavily indebted to false narratives of some preternatural ethnic purity rooted in medieval European soil."[6]

The United States has certainly been less oppressive than the Soviet Union or the ISIS caliphate to most of its citizens over the past century, but in what is structurally an open democracy, we still choose to make the Kennedy, Bush, and Clinton families into royal legacies. Presidential politics reflect this conservative reflex in other ways also. The self-proclaimed "freaks" of 1960s counterculture in the United States produced a ferocious backlash, effectively exploited not only by Presidents Nixon and Reagan, who rode it into the White House, but even by President George W. Bush, whose resentment of it within his own generation shaped the anti-intellectual tone as well as the repressive right-wing militarism of his administration. The emphasis these candidates placed on "law and order," "values," American exceptionalism, national defense, and religious traditions assured an uneasy electorate that their habits and world-view would be protected from challenge. The hard conservatism of the recently resigned Pope, Benedict XVI, was apparently a reaction to the same traumatic history, which for him would have included the Vatican II reforms as well as the European version of 1960s counterculture. Now his more liberation-minded papal successor, Francis, is arousing both excitement and unease, while much of a fiercely knowledge-phobic American electorate welcomes a nostalgic "Make America Great Again" campaign. We cannot manage these culture wars unless we understand the natural functions of cultures.

2 Agency in the Human Hive

It is absurd to suppose that purpose is not present [merely] because we do not observe the agent deliberating.
—Aristotle, *Physics*, 2.8, on the functions of nature

... to have Intelligence means no more than this: to do on one's own, by one's own means and entirely at one's own risk, everything that animals have assigned to them beforehand ....The vacuum represents a threat, but also a chance: to survive, you have filled it with cultures. Culture is an unusual instrument in that it constitutes a discovery which, in order to function, must be *hidden* from its creators.
—Lecture by the military supercomputer Golem XIV, in Stanislaw Lem, *Imaginary Magnitude*[1]

Protestantism was largely a protest against aspects of Catholicism that had evolved into a corrupting and self-perpetuating memeplex. Reform-minded theologians in Early Modern Europe analyzed the way institutional Christianity had, in their opinion, gone badly astray, but vast numbers of their followers settled for demonizing the Pope. Hating a person came much more naturally than critiquing a systemic malfunction. Even once Darwin's perspective became available three centuries later, few even considered applying it to the competitive replication and modification of cultures rather than to living creatures. When Nazism and the Holocaust provoked questions about the persistence of anti-Semitism in the mid-20th century, and the depredations of Soviet and Chinese governments raised similarly dire questions about Communism, and even now as climate-change and income-inequality raise troubling questions about consumer capitalism, people have tended to focus on stories of open or covert personal villainy – Hitler, Stalin, Mao, "the 1%" on Wall Street or in the executive suites of fossil-fuel companies – rather than analyzing larger structures and processes.

These individual targets of blame were very far from innocent, but they were symptomatic carriers rather than the diseases that needed

curing. Excessive focus on individual malefactors reflects two evolutionary legacies. First, our ancestors who assumed any noise or motion was
a predator until proven otherwise tended to survive and therefore out-
reproduced those inclined to wait for proof. So the suspicion of widespread and conscious sinister plots can be attributed less to pathological
paranoia than to the "hyperactive agent detection device" that causes
some people – and some animals also – to overestimate the presence of
dangerous intentions around us.[2] We concoct a scary narrative to match
our suspicions, so we can avoid a tragic ending. As Brian Boyd writes,

> it is safer to mistake a twig for a snake than vice versa. And we
> will interpret something as story if we can. Babies and adults alike
> cannot help seeing a sequence of moving dots in terms of animate
> causality.[3]

Second, *Homo sapiens* evolved in small communities where understanding the personal strengths, weaknesses, and intentions of one's immediate
neighbors was far more important than understanding multiculturalism
or macroeconomics or calcium sequestration. People are seldom eager to
wrestle with large, abstract, and complicated questions anyway, when
they can simply compile a list of friends and enemies, behaving in ways
considered self-evidently right or wrong. The arbitrary aspects of those
norms remain largely invisible because of the evolutionary advantages of
camouflage for the memeplex and because of the cognitive advantages of
shared blind-spots for members of a community.

Now, however, it is becoming both more feasible and more urgent to
ask questions about systemic malfunctions. I am writing this book because, looking at my children and my students and all the other delicate,
striving, fascinating lives around me, I am haunted by the likely costs
of failing to confront the bigger picture. To put it another way, I am
haunted by the waste of our precious ethical reflexes on what are really
secondary effects of cultural evolution – effects we can control if we are
willing to sustain our alertness and accept an awkward combination of
indeterminacy and responsibility, rather than complacently buying the
comforts of simple certainties at such a high cost. Historically contingent systems such as liberal democracy and neoliberal economics serve
their own perpetuation neatly by convincing their human carriers that
(as Francis Fukuyama famously asserted 25 years ago) those systems
constitute *The End of History*. But history is still here to be made.

* * * * * * * * * * * *

If we don't quite see our culture, what do we imagine we are seeing
when we encounter its imprint? In recent decades, literary scholarship has been focused primarily in the area broadly defined as cultural

studies, which was an expansive outgrowth of New Historicism, which combined Geertzian anthropology with leftist politics. Long before the Occupy Wall Street movement, New Historicists focused primarily on exposing the elaborate conspiracies of misrepresentation by which the elites protect their privileges. From this leftist perspective, those privileged elites make social hierarchies (especially the demonic trinity of gender, class, and race) nearly invisible, or disguise the hierarchies as a congruent shadow of the laws of nature, or associate them with a higher cause (such as God's will). Elite culture also cleverly creates manageable little subversions which (like a controlled burn or killed-virus vaccine) can be easily contained and thus protect the body-politic from truly dangerous conflagrations. The pattern is acknowledged in Neal Shusterman's popular 2016 young-adult novel *Scythe*, where the benevolent artificial–intelligence "Thundercloud" governing the society, knowing that some people like being counterculture even when the culture is ideal, establishes an "unsavory" class such citizens can join, with its own norms of dress and diction.

What always troubled me about these readings of history was the problem of agency. How, in the absence of some supercomputer overlord, were all these magnificently complex strategies of deceit on behalf of the propertied few really organized and maintained – strategies that even now can be brought only flickeringly into comprehension, and then only by a tiny group of topflight scholars trained for exactly this kind of reading? Was there ever really a Moriarty for these Sherlocks to pursue back through time, a venomous villain lurking at the center of the web attached to all evils? Or was there only the web: a blind iteration of various algorithms in the biosphere? The history of Western medical practice shows that the defenses evolution has designed within our bodies have usually been better than our deliberate interventions. Why shouldn't the same be true of the evolved defense mechanisms of a sociocultural order?

New Historicist conspiracy theories are easy to question rhetorically. Was the literary genre called pastoral really revived at a level of deliberation comparable to the way corporate lobbyists craft tax-policy proposals advantageous to their paymasters? What would have made all the middle managers willing and able to play that game? Did men in Elizabethan ruffs regularly gather in the back of a Guild Hall where Sir Somebody whispered to the Earl of Somewhere that they should hire some poets to mystify the maldistribution of wealth and naturalize gender-hierarchy?

Such scenarios look like a 1590s version of a notorious 1960s fantasy: the CIA, or the Trilateral Commission, or another "Deep State" agency operating so covertly that we do not even know its name, engaged in a terrifyingly shrewd, epistemologically profound, and utterly encompassing program of puppet-mastery. It makes sense that the leading scholars who have been hunting down these elusive perpetrators of social injustice tend to emerge from a generation that came of age amid that period's battles against what Paul Potter taught the New Left to call "the System," with a revealingly personalizing upper-case S. These scholars naturally feel obliged to try to fight (or pretend to fight) those wars in another venue and with other weapons than the misfired explosives abandoned when the New Left broke up in the early 1970s.

President Nixon's tape-recordings seemed to refute such high-flown suspicions: the information and planning in the White House were even cruder than the notorious deleted-expletive language. But the heated, paranoid-masochistic fantasies survived such revelations, and survived parodies ranging from James Bond movies through the "Get Smart" sitcom to Thomas Pynchon's early novels. They persisted through the rest of the century in the "X-Files" TV series and Oliver Stone's feverish movie *JFK* (which revived some of the earliest and most vivid 1960s conspiracy theories). More recently, similar fantasies have shaped and fueled popular TV series such as "Lost," "24," and "Torchwood," as well as films such as *Minority Report* and the Bourne series. Purveyors of paranoia – as in dire warnings about the Illuminati in the 18th century and Freemasons in the 19th century–never lack for customers.

In fact, the evidence of some such conspiracies – or, rather, some such reactionary conspiratorial functions – seems compelling. Consider, for example, the swarm of books and movies about maternally neglectful or otherwise wicked career-women, some of whose demonic nannies destroy their families, that appeared at a sociological moment near the end of the 20th century when women began acquiring more meaningful rights and executive opportunities in the workplace.[4] Somehow, we seem collectively to warn ourselves, discipline ourselves, and confess ourselves, through what look like mere fictional entertainments.

How does such a mechanism of control work? When governments censor some artworks while commissioning others, it is usually easy to trace the ends and the means; the Kremlin programmed Soviet art, and the CIA actively promoted anti-Communism through many indirect channels.[5] But the private creative side is murkier. The banal if plausible explanation – that aspiring writers and publishers and movie producers are inclined to repeat whatever has been selling – does not erase the broader mystery of why these things sold so widely in their times, and why there seems to be so little evidence that anyone explicitly planned the cultural interventions. The only plausible explanations therefore involve attributing such trends to a *Zeitgeist* or unconscious collective.[6] By some kind of tacit agreement, the essentially conservative human creature exerts itself tribally against fears of change. Despite recent discoveries by the Nobel-winning economist Daniel Kahneman and his "freakonomics" offspring, we cling proudly to our self-image as fully autonomous individuals making free, conscious, and rational choices.

That self-image makes it even harder to imagine how, in the absence of some Peter Quince distributing scrolls to his actors (in Shakespeare's *Midsummer Night's Dream*, 2.1), individuals are recruited for their different roles, including the villainous ones, and taught their lines. If all the world's a stage, we need to ponder what auditions us and directs us: the way we together assemble our castes and their scripts.

As human beings in a society, we each play roles; in the political body, we each do the duty of a differentiated cell under the guidance of a culture that has co-evolved with us symbiotically. That culture functions something like an endocrine system, telling a certain proportion of its sub-entities what to be over the long term (as they change from stem-cell status) and what to do in the short term (in response to threats to overall equilibrium), depending on their immediate environments. I am therefore suspicious of this politicized application of the "hermeneutics of suspicion," the determination to read for a disguised and sinister agenda. Proverbially, it isn't paranoia if they really are out to get you; but what if they aren't doing so deliberately, and what if you are part of the they?

What I am proposing is an evolutionary model of social systems, to replace the Intelligent Design explanation that deduces consciously malign human creators behind our ethically faulty socioeconomic structure. According to the famous Watchmaker argument for the existence of God, believing that such a complex and balanced living world emerged without a controlling superhuman intelligence is like finding an intricate clockwork and believing that the parts had fallen together randomly, but the Watchmaker argument faded in the face of Darwinian insights. Perhaps the assumption that maldistribution of wealth and privilege was entirely engineered and then disguised by evil overlords will also fade when confronted by a Darwinian reading of cultural evolution, aided now by Thomas Picketty's analysis of the inherent tendency of capitalism to increase inequality.[7] This analogy does not preclude our having both the ability and the obligation to change such injustices. In fact, we will have a better chance of doing so if we understand the forces that protect them.

An evolutionary model helps to explain not only how a society generates its commonly held beliefs, but also how the authority of such "common sense" situates people in various roles and hierarchies, allowing a social order to keep reproducing itself. To adopt the terminology of the social-science theorist Pierre Bourdieu, the *doxa* of a society underlie the *habitus* of its citizens and hence perpetuate its inequalities. Instead of anthropomorphizing "the System," and attributing to it conscious intentions, I want to posit a system that defends itself in some of the same ways DNA does. That is to say, the existing socio-cultural structure (being one that has survived) acts as if it were striving to survive, an impression which encourages anthropomorphizing. That adaptive cognitive bias toward attributing malicious purpose in a competitive world makes people imagine conniving human secret-agents behind seemingly evil socio-cultural developments.

There surely are such colluders, and they may deserve to be despised as traitors for selling out the human project to enslavement by the unproductive aspects of memeplexes such as money and bureaucracy. Like the disposable minor villains in many stories, these quislings betray the hero to the evil mastermind under the short-lived illusion that they will benefit from the mastermind's promised favors. A case in point is the revelation that, as early as the 1980s, Exxon scientists and executives were busily working in secret to minimize damage to the corporation's Arctic facilities from the climate-change they knew their fuels were causing, and to maximize the profits as disappearing permafrost made drilling there easier.[8] Nonetheless, they continued for many years denying publicly that any such cause and effect were evident, thus putting their species at risk in order to protect the wealth of their corporation.

It is worth noticing that, for every hundred such narrow-visioned functionaries who are under the illusion that they are serving themselves, there will also be a dozen liberals caught in an unexamined contradiction between their desire to support economic justice and their assumptions about the rights of capital. In both cases, the likeliest path to redemption begins by making people aware of their complicity, and also of why they may feel that their complicity is advantageous for themselves or necessary for the society, when in fact it may benefit only the currently dominant memeplexes.

Plenty of social theorists have proposed structural rather than conspiratorial models to explain social injustice.[9] I want to explore the evolutionary dynamics of such structures, and then offer an adaptationist reading of humanistic scholarship, intellectualism, and creative artistry as devices with which many human societies have willingly co-evolved. We have done so because those devices defend our peculiar human identity and preferred human traits against forces that might contrive to overpower them or, even more effectively, make us forget about them. Both the historical and the imaginative portions of the written archive help us remember what we are as creatures, by looking at what we have been and what we could be.

Insect Intentions

Cultural evolution may provide a useful supplementary hypothesis to our understanding of social injustice. Brilliant and ugly conspiracies have certainly existed, but not always because anybody exactly planned them. They exist because any such system lacking these ingenious ways of exploiting human gullibility and regulating human volatility would not have survived so long. Both the old "great man" theory of history and the paranoid style of New Historicism may thus yield some ground to cognitive science and evolutionary anthropology, with helpful footnotes to entomology and ornithology. Schemes of hegemonic cultural control seem to exist, and they may have developed a symbiotic alliance with more overtly forcible forms of imperialism. But the hegemony is not simply a trick deployed by deliberate strategists of empire.

There is, instead, a machine in the ghost. As Daniel Dennett observes about religions and other competing cultural (rather than biological) reproducers, *"without anybody's realizing it, or intending it,* this relatively mindless process over long periods of time can shape designs to an exquisite degree, optimizing them for local conditions."[10] Thus, I can accept Michel Foucault's argument (with the panopticon prison as the famous instance[11]) that subjugated persons discipline themselves into various roles required by the society without the direct threat of punishment by authorities, or even the immediate presence of such authorities. I do not, however, see this as fundamentally a ruse employed by human monopolists of power, as some followers of Foucault assume.

Instead, the hive-like arrangements of the panopticon prison look to me very much like the self-organizing functions of other communities, such as ants and honeybees, where evolutionary pressures have caused individuals to assume differentiated roles without anyone's conscious choice. Entomologists call it "recruitment," and it is worth pausing to consider the anthropological and sociological implications of the metaphor.[12] For all its political and psychological discomforts, that similarity may have some lessons to teach. These include cautionary lessons about "stochastic terrorism," in which mass-media agitprop is used to weaponize susceptible individuals, who are like the hypnotized agents in political thrillers from *The 39 Steps* through *The Manchurian Candidate*, but are actually just a statistically probable set of the population. That function allows the propagandists to deny responsibility for the assassinations (of doctors such as George Tiller who performed abortions, for example) that their hate-mongering produces. A larger-scale example is the role of Georges Ruggiu's radio shows in provoking the genocide of the Tutsi population in Rwanda. As social networking opens up broader and faster new channels for this type of collective consciousness (a term I borrow from Émile Durkheim, a founding father of sociology), we need to be especially alert to its constructive and destructive potential.

The classical and Renaissance ideas of persons as microcosms of the world and societies as macrocosms of an individual person are helpful here. Human beings are organisms, largely made up of other, smaller organisms. Evolutionary biologists have estimated that our bodies contain as many bacterial cells as eukaryotic cells (the large animal cells that carry our DNA). So "we might more accurately be described as a series of linked and densely populated ecosystems, each a rich mixture"[13]; the symbiont prokaryotic cells are non-self, but indispensable to the self. I believe it can also be useful to recognize ourselves as in some ways resembling differentiated parts of a larger human superorganism. That term was popularized by E. O. Wilson's study of insect colonies, and Wilson was vigorously attacked because of what the theory might imply if applied to human societies. Yet, when I came across Wilson's work (especially his collaboration with Bert Hölldobler), parts of it seemed startlingly apt for describing some phenomena I was tracing.

Let me clarify what I do and do not intend by this comparison. I am not claiming that people are finally indistinguishable from ants, let alone that I endorse the intellectually faulty and ethically disastrous history of applied Social Darwinism. For one thing, since permission to reproduce is not limited to a small monarchical group, we could be defined as semi-social rather than eusocial creatures; mole rats are the only mammal species that seems truly eusocial, because they live in a colony with a single maternal queen and many sterile workers. The human race is therefore not susceptible in evolutionary terms to "strong altruism" in its blind, automatic form. That is, we will often take actions that aid others more than ourselves and our close kin, but seldom actions that actually reduce our own overall reproductive future – unless culture hides that consequence from us, which can make us either saints or suckers. And we have important forms of consciousness not present in these insects. Our superorganism does not wholly determine the actions of its component creatures.[14] This book will insist that individual human choices can be of immense importance.

We are also, however, "the most cooperative of vertebrates,"[15] and should not blind ourselves to the homologies our collaborative functions create between us and species whose communities are more closely related genetically. Clearly, one critical function of nationalism and religion – key sources of violent division in human history, though religion is a more ambivalent case[16] – is to provide a version of kinship within societies much too large to be committed to mutual support by genetics as hunter-gatherer tribes once were. Unified societies therefore outcompete others, and in return reward the memeplex that united them by expanding its presence in the world. For example, "Mutual aid led to substantially lower mortality rates during epidemics, and a norm against infanticide led to substantially higher population growth among Christians" as the Roman Empire fragmented and declined.[17] Believing in a moralistic deity also helps overcome that limitation on altruistic behavior in a large society, which is presumably one reason such beliefs (though various in many other regards) have become so widely dominant: the cultures that believed them had significant competitive advantages. The long and mostly dishonorable history of human exceptionalism is marked by disdain for any cross-species comparisons, a disdain that allies large parts of the scientific and the progressive-political communities with conservative religious traditions. To me it seems foolish pride to pretend that we can gain little perspective on ourselves by seeing how other forms of life function.[18]

I certainly wouldn't compress my point into a formula as simplistic as ants + arts = us; there are far too many steps and degrees crammed into that plus-sign. Yet each individual and each society is an uneasy blend of deterministic potential and volitional imaginative plasticity. Perhaps it is no mere coincidence that, in the Indiana Jones film, one crucial function of the crystal skull is to repel a massive, horrifying swarm of driver ants that consume the Communist enemy. The little enclave that skull creates corresponds to the enclave of academic freedom that tries but fails to protect Professor Jones from the Red Scare functionaries. These zones of resistance to the era's blind conformity – whether it is Soviet or American conformity, enforced by the KGB or the FBI – represent the sanctuary function of high human civilization, wrapped like a skull around the delicate evolutionary experiment of individualized consciousness, to protect it from a biosphere that is otherwise simply playing out the unselfconscious mathematics of survival and reproduction. The skull there represents the cluster of associated categories by which humanity (with its expanded cranium as the key anatomical marker) has long claimed to be unique: in our possession of souls, self-consciousness, free will, and rationality.

Our complex and flexible mental capacities take the place of mass reproduction. No human female extrudes thousands of fertilized eggs, as some sea turtles or insects do, but we do invest a lot in the physical, psychological, and educational nurturing of our few offspring.[19] The creative and communicative faculties of the human mind provide an alternative to the mass production and algorithmic feedback functions of eusocial insect colonies. Instead of instinctively treading a path toward whichever fellow-creatures return with calories, and away from the paths from which no travelers have returned, we imagine realistic narratives up each branch of the decision-trees we encounter. We then decide – not always rationally – which stories seem likeliest to produce a convincingly happy ending, for ourselves as individuals and (through utopian and dystopian genres) for our societies and our species. That process is visible in miniature when our smartphones offer us crowd-sourced information on traffic patterns that allows us to choose the fastest route. Instead of boosting the survival chances of our DNA by raising many offspring, who in our species are quite labor-intensive and resource-hungry, we can use imaginary but verisimilar future selves – sometimes in the form of literary characters – to choose the best paths.

Consider the similarities between the evolved functions of the human collective as I have been describing them, and Hölldobler and Wilson's description of ants:

> Conditioned by the ongoing simultaneous decisions of other colony members, the colony as a whole creates emergent patterns of adaptive response that are difficult and perhaps even impossible to predict from the observed behavior of individuals alone …. Through the combined sense and brains of its members, the colony operates as an information-processing system. The environment challenges it with problems: the workers must locate an adequate nest site, find the right food items and bring them home, establish home ranges and territories, defend against enemies, and care for the helpless young.[20]

Let me reiterate: I am not saying, by invoking a comparison to the ways ant or bee communities distribute their roles, that some persons are simply born to be privileged leaders and others to be common manual laborers. Nor am I suggesting that we would have no choice about letting them be so distinguished if they were so born. Wilson, often accused of being the archetype of such Social-Darwinistic determinism, does not say that either. He does not even say that about ants: he shows that they are often divided into castes by contingent circumstances, and that they can be shifted nimbly in role and status to meet the current needs of the collective. Potential monarchs become drones, and vice versa. "The genes, in other words, determine not castes but caste plasticity: in response to environmental conditions, they either turn on or turn off growth" that "leads the individual to maturity as a queen or as a worker."[21]

The prevailing culture of Shakespeare's time assumed that the admired efficiency of eusocial insects derived from the controlling conscious intelligence of a single leader. Charles Butler's 1609 tract on *The Feminine Monarchie* asserts that "the Bees aborre [abhor] as well polyarchie, as anarchie," preferring "a perfect monarchie, the most natural and absolute form of government." Perhaps these observers, in the Jacobean era of Divine Right kingship, rightly sensed a parallel, but wrongly assessed what the parallel was: they assumed that insects were also primarily ruled by the conscious choices of a few powerful individuals, rather than by evolutionary algorithms. I suspect we still overestimate the role of conscious choices by political leaders in managing our societies. After all, the division of labor and the hierarchy of lineal privilege that even our best-educated conspiracy theorists attribute to contingent political decisions do seem to exist all over the world in social situations where no such consciousness is apparently in control. Indiana Jones's nemesis Dr. Spalko asserts that the 13 crystal skulls "are a hive mind: one being, physically separate, but with a collective consciousness. More powerful together than they can ever be apart." But this is a symptomatic Communist half-truth: it is not even completely right about hive-insects, and is not compatible (as Spalko discovers to her horror) with the human need for delimited consciousness.

Shakespeare himself, in *Henry V*, gives his Archbishop of Canterbury a lengthy exposition of this insect metaphor that suggests that not even the monarch really invents the system (in fact, Shakespeare's plays often make audiences wonder why men are so driven to become monarchs when kingship is mostly just a well-decorated misery). The monarch is instead one more thing invented by the system:

> so work the honey-bees,
> Creatures that by a rule in nature teach
> The act of order to a peopled kingdom.
> They have a king and officers of sorts;
> Where some, like magistrates, correct at home,
> Others, like merchants, venture trade abroad,
> Others, like soldiers, armed in their stings,
> Make boot upon the summer's velvet buds,
> Which pillage they with merry march bring home
> To the tent-royal of their emperor;
> Who, busied in his majesty, surveys
> The singing masons building roofs of gold,
> The civil citizens kneading up the honey,
> The poor mechanic porters crowding in
> Their heavy burdens at his narrow gate,
> The sad-eyed justice, with his surly hum,
> Delivering o'er to executors pale
> The lazy yawning drone. I this infer,
> That many things, having full reference
> To one consent, may work contrariously:
> ....
> So may a thousand actions, once afoot,
> End in one purpose.
>
> (*Henry V*, 1.2.187–212)

This speech anticipates, by four centuries, Wilson's explanation for the differentiations within an insect hive – down even to the idea that the "one purpose" is merely survival of the collective, since the Archbishop is mainly talking about the defense of England and its race.

In 1813 – almost exactly halfway between the moment of Shakespeare's version and the moment of Wilson's – Percy Shelley's "Queen Mab" offered its own comparison:

> The thronging thousands, to a passing view,
>   Seemed like an ant-hill's citizens.

How wonderful! that even
  The passions, prejudices, interests,
That sway the meanest being – the weak touch
    That moves the finest nerve
    And in one human brain
  Causes the faintest thought, becomes a link
    In the great chain of Nature!

(lines 100–108)

Human thought and feeling are parts of a natural network, not exempt from it.

According to Wilson, "The most profitable food source will eventually be selected by foragers as a whole," despite the fact that "no individual makes comparative evaluations of food source quality."[22] Queen honeybees

> regulate the activities of workers by ... a primer pheromone released from the queen's mandibular gland and distributed throughout the colony by grooming and the exchange of regurgitated food among the workers. The pheromone transiently regulates expression in the workers of several hundred genes and persistently regulates the expression of 19 genes.

The pheromone also adjusts "the shift as workers age from nursing tasks in the hive to foraging for food."[23]

Precisely because no agent of the human sovereign bustles around our colonies, scraping class-determinative pheromones on the shells of various citizens to meet the changing needs of the collective, we have developed other ways of differentiating within our superorganism. The power of a flood of hormones to dictate exact behaviors and hierarchies is largely baffled in human beings, freeing us to explore, even if our psychic terrain is still shaped by the channels such floods established. For the human collective as (I have been claiming) for the human individual, culture must take over the extraordinarily complicated task of control, choosing an optimal version for the survival of its carriers, among countless combinative options. That differentiation is likely to resemble the programmed scatter of other species – and in the instance of the intensely collectivist Hutterites, the configurations and severity of the controls do look remarkably like those of some eusocial insects. But our species has to achieve its balance through a radically different mechanism. Again, culture is the agent of management, telling people what they are required to be; no wonder it needs to be so multiple, so attuned to feedback and overload, and so diligent in checking the web for urgent security updates.

Obviously the control exercised by an ant queen differs in many ways from a human monarchy; but must we cling so tightly to an assumption of complete and unique human volition, entirely conscious and free, that we ignore the similarities? Neither a deterministic nor a free-will philosophy actually erases its opposite, instead merely imposing one frame rather than another. Yet many people who understand that balance are nonetheless quick to assume that acknowledging these biochemical and probabilistic models implies the absolute surrender of (some ideally posited) human freedom, in favor of enslavement.

Human beings are not born with genes or later marked with biochemicals dividing us into the 1% of wealthy investment bankers and Silicon Valley inventors, set against (if present trends continue) the mass of struggling manual laborers, service workers, and subsistence farmers. Much of the decision-making work that most species perform automatically – under the guidance of relatively simple and consistent responses to biochemical traces or visual clues, without what we call consciousness – has been transferred to culture by *Homo sapiens*: how we cover our bodies, for example, and how we navigate toward foods, and when to defer and when instead to insist. This may also be true of our class and caste distinctions, which to some extent mimic the hive or colony function of differentiating tasks and reproductive roles.

Subjects who had just been obliged to make a decision showed "less physical stamina, [less] task persistence in the face of failure, more procrastination, and less quality and quantity of arithmetic calculations" than those who had studied the same choices without being forced to decide.[24] If the work of sorting experience is too difficult for any individual human mind to master – too intricate and multiple to avoid dangerous errors and sheer exhaustion, despite the occasional superior insight – so too is the work of optimizing the algorithm for survival of the collective. As Stanza IV of the Stevens poem puts it,

> A million people on one string?
> And all their manner in the thing,
>
> And all their manner, right and wrong,
> And all their manner, weak and strong?
>
> The feelings crazily, craftily call,
> Like a buzzing of flies in autumn air,
>
> And that's life, then: things as they are,
> This buzzing of the blue guitar.

Yet, humanity's niche is as formers and reformers of our environment. That role may have started with clothing and hand-tools, but has since become farther-reaching, especially through agriculture – which may be the most powerful and yet also least recognizable memeplex that uses human beings to perpetuate itself, neglectful of the costs it imposes on human and environmental health.[25] In a world that we have made so much more volatile, and in which our bodies are so slow to evolve, the ability to make deliberate adjustments of our culture has become precious. For practical as well as ethical reasons, we need to nurture our ability to update and overrule the dysfunctions of programming that was transferred from genetic structures to socio-cultural ones.

It also seems noteworthy that wild honey bees seem to be surviving the recent epidemic of colony collapse better than domesticated bees, as if our homogenizing cultural control were detrimental, not only directly in our continued use of neonicotinoid pesticides (one speculative culprit), but also indirectly in transmitting our tendency to homogenize for the sake of efficiency, which limits adaptability during environmental crises.

Perhaps the most illuminating fact to be derived from comparing human and insect societies is that the human version entails distinctly more dysfunctional elements. The distinguished entomologist Thomas Seeley concludes his 1995 book on *The Wisdom of the Hive* by observing that "the system of control devices found in a honey bee colony is extremely sophisticated and endows a colony with exquisite powers of adaptive response, both to internal changes and to external contingencies," and that while

> all biologists are keenly aware of the amazing adaptive responses of cells and organisms .... few biologists recognize that evolution has likewise endowed certain animal societies with impressive abilities and has fashioned elaborate mechanisms of communication and control inside these societies to produce their remarkable group-level skills .... recognition of the ingenuity of natural selection in devising mechanisms of social coordination strikes me as the quintessence of the knowledge generated by these studies of the bees.[26]

That knowledge may be usefully applied to the social coordination of human beings – especially by asking why we endure inefficiencies the insect communities would long since have overridden.

Bees select sites for a new hive by a collective meditation that appears more reliable, efficient, and cooperative than human legislative deliberation. Seeley's wonderful 2010 book *Honeybee Democracy* extols the hive as a model of democratic practice, but I have two reservations about that. First, the hive mind is an excellent mind if, but only if, there are no goals or ideals beyond the survival of that hive. Second, the decision about locating a new hive is not really democracy, since only a few percent of the bees – a few hundred scouts from a swarm of ten thousand – actually control the decision. It is therefore more like a university: those decision-makers are the ones who have conducted carefully calibrated field research and then consulted each other in a system of peer-review. If a finding looks promising, another scout goes out to verify the report independently, and others become interested when positive results are confirmed. The group thus weighs all the evidence and neither leaps to a hasty conclusion nor dithers unproductively awaiting absolute certainty. They then communicate their consensus, telling all their clustering hive-mates where to go next: what their safest and most productive next move will be.

Still, if the question is whether to be or not to be bees, the answer is probably no: we don't aspire to become programmed insects. As Freud writes in *Civilization and its Discontents*, "It does not seem as though any influence could induce a man to change his nature into a termite's. No doubt he will always defend his claim to individual liberty against the will of the group."[27] So the next question becomes, which of our inefficiencies have a positive correlation with something that we value in our species, and which ones appear instead to be memeplexes that perpetuate themselves at the expense of our potential? To put it another way, what aspects of our culture, to the extent we can distinguish it from our nature, are symbionts with our higher aspirations, and which ones are merely parasites that enter through our flaws? How do we differentiate, in deciding which egg to nurture, between the one that the cuckoo bird slipped into our nest to displace our true offspring, and the one that arises from our essence and will promote the survival of that essence in our evolving habitat?

In 1998, two different big-budget Hollywood films were released that seemed to wrestle with these questions. The protagonist of *A Bug's Life* is an individualistic ant whose wild inventions repeatedly create problems for his colony; by the end, however, his individualism has inspired the colony to mount an ecologically clever defense that rescues them from generations of subjugation by grasshoppers. In *Antz* – arguably a family-friendly adaptation of *Brave New World* – the yearning of a worker-ant named Z-4195 to express his individuality eventually breaks down all the barriers separating queen, worker, and soldier ants in the colony, turning a military dictatorship (after an uneasy interregnum) into a thriving multicultural community.

Insects are not Prince Hamlet, nor were they meant to be: "An evolutionary trade-off exists in the properties of the algorithms between simplicity and quickness on the one side and calculation and delay on the other side ... small brain size has tipped the social insects to the simple and quick."[28] Very little of their decision-making runs expensive software. These cinematic fantasies about insects liberated from blind conformism imply that human society is not altogether different in its regimentation. But they also imply that if an ant (given highly individualized human traits in these films) can transform its colony by resisting the arbitrary recruitment to roles, in ways that at first seem merely disruptive but prove salutary as conditions shift, perhaps the human individual can achieve the same transformation.

By 2007, however, ecological anxieties seem to have taken precedence over traditional liberal concerns about top-down social control: in *Bee*

Movie, the protagonist tries to escape the strict rules and roles of insect life, but ends up having to rebuild the ecosystem.

****

The question that the renowned 19th-century philosopher John Stuart Mill and George W. Bush – not the likeliest duo – have both asked is: efficiency to what end, prosperity to what purpose? It's no wonder we don't know, if it isn't finally for us, as Richard Dawkins has controversially suggested.[29] From the perspective of evolutionary genetics – as opposed to a Christian teleology like that of *Paradise Lost*, where procreation offers a bridge to ultimate vindication and immortality – human beings are the means to a meaningless end, just as bees or ants are. To the extent that we aspire beyond merely delaying the extinction of our species, we have to invent our purpose – or, from some theological and philosophical perspectives, discover it. That invention is as much the project of creative artists as inventing optimal machines is the project of mechanical engineers. Otherwise our purpose will be chosen for us by evolving memeplexes, leaving us miserably half-aware of our enslavement.

Like the smooth aristocratic apologist Menenius addressing the mutinous plebian masses at the beginning of Shakespeare's *Coriolanus*, evolutionary psychologists often urge us to recognize that resistance is futile: that we need to know ourselves and accept our programmed roles in the collective. They talk us back from rebellion into the cozy embrace of the overlords who really have no interest in our personal thriving at all. They are right, I believe, to defend the study of evolutionary psychology against the widespread dismissiveness of other social scientists who believe we make free choices guided only by our societies, and not by universal mental heuristics that were adaptive during the lengthy hunter-gatherer experience of our species. Consciousness would be intolerably confusing without some prior evolved structures of cognition, and forms of cooperation indispensable for our species would too often have failed without some default rules of interaction that led to evolutionary success.

I believe, however, that even evolutionary psychologists often underrate the intricacy of human experience. As the ubiquity and durability of cultural structures suggest, the psychological patterns are necessary but not sufficient to overcome the potential chaos. And while those patterns serve consciousness by offering relative simplicity and stability, the same attributes mean we also need culture as a prosthesis that enables us to adapt to the very different and always changing circumstances of our far-flung and highly innovative species. Infants have a sense of morality, as recent work (especially by Karen Wynn and Paul Bloom) at Yale University's Infant Cognition Center has demonstrated, but how to apply and adjust that moral reflex for more complex human interactions later in life has been a central question across a range of humanistic disciplines for centuries, and remains central to countless novels and movies.

Many sophisticated social theorists impose a paradigm that is finally as grimly deterministic as that of the reductive evolutionary psychologists. Foucault's conception of pervasive power has led many social theorists to conclude that change is nearly impossible, or at least inexplicable, because the enveloping culture renders change literally inconceivable to the subjects who would have to enact the change. No one, they argue, can stand far enough outside the system to exert leverage on it.

Yet (as mentioned in Chapter 1) the oppressed can hardly help noticing that the self-idealizing systems of power are not what they claim to be, and an evolutionary model of social organization, including its cultural aspects, offers an explanation of how change can occur and why it meets resistance. During the collective organism's adaptation to new circumstances (including its own success, which manifests itself as growth of population and knowledge), new or recovered cultural ideas can thrive, if their human advocates have enough rhetorical skill to deceive the watchdogs of the status quo, or if material and political circumstances support direct action. Understanding transformative individuals as both effect and cause of mutations usefully hedges the question of whether history is made by persons, or persons by historical inevitabilities that choose their puppets.[30] A fatal cancer usually begins with a single mutant cell – and a seeing eye must have begun with only a few cells sensitive to a wavelength that others could not know even existed.

Social constructivists emphasize the limitations of the notion that human history is essentially the work of autonomous heroic or villainous individuals. The same warning can be derived from zero-player computer-game experiments with cellular automata – grids that sort themselves guided by a few basic rules followed over many iterations. These experiments generate patterns strikingly reminiscent of human social structures and economic behavior. A relatively simple simulation shows that even a population consisting entirely of individuals quite satisfied to be mostly – as long as not entirely – surrounded by individuals of another skin color would eventually produce a pattern of extreme segregation.[31] Each agent in that situation "would no doubt regard itself as a model of tolerance and, noticing the formation of color clusters, might conclude that a lot of other agents must be racists." Slight prejudices can, after multiple iterations, produce stark divisions. Another simple artificial-society simulation called Sugarscape

> produced a skewed distribution of sugar that looked very much like the skewed distribution of wealth in human societies, even though

> nothing about the agents' simple behavioral rules pointed to any such outcome .... simple rules could produce complex social phenomena that mimicked migrations, epidemics, trade.[32]

The patterns produced by the cellular automata and other general modeling systems confirm that the role of sinister centralized intent in these social ills is easily overestimated. Certainly active, conscious racism by both governments and individuals persists in modern Western society – creating segregation through red-lining, for example.[33] Crony capitalism and legalized bribery distort supposedly free markets to favor the already wealthy. But the sinister schemers' power is multiplied by an algorithmic function that is not a conspiracy.

This patterning certainly doesn't excuse us from making an effort to resist what deserves resisting. On the contrary, a key use of agent-based modeling is finding patterns similar to social patterns, in order to determine where to intervene to ameliorate them most efficiently. Furthermore, such computer simulations demonstrate that changing the character of even relatively few individual units or slightly altering even a single rule of reaction can radically change the outcome. Social science has shown that a few honest officials can tip a society from a vicious cycle of increasing corruption to a virtuous cycle of increasing honesty.[34] An occasional glimpse of forgiveness that mitigates the revenge-instinct can over time steer an entire society away from genocide, as even Ariel's brief, second-hand, conditional reminder of human sympathy causes Prospero to revise his revenge tragedy into a comedy of dynastic marriage at the start of Act Five of Shakespeare's *The Tempest*. Portia in *The Merchant of Venice* exclaims, "How far that little candle throws his beams! / So shines a good deed in a naughty world" (5.1.90–91) – an idea Wallace Stevens echoes in Stanza XV of "The Man with the Blue Guitar": "A Candle is enough to light the world." This phenomenon, sometimes called "disproportionate causality," suggests that a Kantian or Existential morality can also be a good political strategy. What matters finally is that each individual make a good-faith choice to follow what that person believes reflects a human ideal and constitutes rightful conduct for all, and that such choices be made without denying either love or death.

Literature and humanistic education are ideally suited to inform and support these kinds of choices. Kim Lane Scheppele summarizes one advantage nicely:

> In regimes that infringe on human rights, we can see the centrality of what I will call humanistic tactics among those who resist .... They stand in the interpretive space between the power of the State and its effects. Resisters often comply with repression but with an asterisk or an ellipsis, a message that reads differently in different

interpretive communities. Knowledge of literature – of strategies of reading, of cultures of interpretation – are crucial to self-authorship in this context, particularly when other resources are unavailable. In general, but especially in regimes where human rights are scarce on the ground, humanistic tactics may be the last refuge of dignity ... 'in the Soviet Union ... where it was very difficult to criticize the State openly, people quoted the law of the State back at it ...'. A legal system cannot figure out what to do with this. The law has no sense of irony ....[35]

Such gestures may seem trivial, even defeatist. Yet the opening pages of this book describe an archeologist using allusions to T.S. Eliot and John Milton to sneak a crucial early warning to Indiana Jones that the Soviet military cannot recognize. A comparable tactic was the way slaves in the United States sometimes used the singing of Christian spirituals to conduct forbidden communications through seemingly innocent channels. Scott demonstrates that most resistance to top-down injustice tends to be small and negative: the "infrapolitics" of foot-dragging, petty theft, vandalism, and wry slanders of the oppressors.[36] Gertrude Stein's novel *Mrs. Reynolds*, written in Vichy France, records the resistance to Nazi occupation that consisted not of Resistance assassinations but instead consisted of ongoing circumlocutions and other indirect little signals among a community that sustained their psychological solidarity against what was being imposed on them.[37] As Michel de Certeau argues in *The Practice of Everyday Life* (1980), daily life teems with instances of individual resistance to a society's dictates – resistance that (like jaywalking) opens up new pathways.

Many destructive social tendencies that become robust once they are settled in as economic and political systems are highly susceptible to even tiny changes at transitional moments. Cultural paradigm-shifts offer a renewed opportunity to intervene – before attitudes again clump into partisan institutions – with those who would rather serve a regulating meme than endure an open mind. Genetic drift, which derives from seemingly random events rather than the competitive selection emphasized by Darwin, is most active in small populations in insular settings. Sometimes, "biological evolution ... proceeds much more quickly than the mechanisms available imply that it should" through "small groups of organisms, in particular, peripheral isolates," because "Once a species is sufficiently well established, sheer numbers make change excruciatingly slow."[38] The same may be said of cultural evolution, which is one reason (as the second half of this book will argue) that scholars and artists partly insulated from popular opinion are so important. They won't always be right, especially as viewed from the norms of the community as a whole, but they supply a set of experimental alternatives. Their work escapes the ruthless logic of the evolving memeplexes of the society at large, and has mechanisms to weed out counterproductive mutations before they are disseminated.

This value of individual consciousness, traveling askew to the cadre of shared beliefs or practical advantage (like the Renaissance poet John Donne at the end of "Goodfriday, 1613, Riding Westward"), has clear analogues in the epidemiology of medical diseases. The superb science writer David Quammen reports that Greg Dwyer, Professor of Ecology at the University of Chicago "had studied all the famous mathematical models proposed to explain disease outbreaks in humans," and "had noted the crucial effect of individual behavior on rate of transmission," including the transmission of HIV/AIDS "among American gay men, among the general populace of Uganda, or among sex workers in Thailand." As Quammen observes, "Dwyer's models have shown that heterogeneity of behavior, even among forest insects, let alone among humans, can be very important in damping the spread of infectious disease," which means that

> individual effort, individual discernment, individual choice can have huge effects in averting the catastrophes that might otherwise sweep through a herd .... "Any tiny little thing that people do," Dwyer said, if it makes them different from one another, from the idealized standard of herd behavior, "is going to reduce infection rates ... There's only so many ways gypsy moths can differ ... But the number of ways that humans can differ is really, really huge .... How much does it matter that humans are smart? ... I'm actually going to say that it matters a whole lot."[39]

It's not easy being the dissenter, as the ant heroes of *A Bug's Life* and *Antz* find out. Assent is social glue, and dissent is explosive. Studies show that differing memories are an acute cause of conflict among siblings, and that couples often unconsciously align their recollections while happily together, then diverge sharply (even on matters of fact irrelevant to their relationship) when they become hostile. Other studies show that "experimental subjects are willing to go against the clear evidence of their senses when all the other people around them are making sensory judgments that are off-target."[40] Peer pressure – or prince pressure, in the case of obsequious Osric yielding even his sense of hot and cold to Hamlet's shifting claims (5.2.94–101) – can make cowards of us all.

But the same research showed "that if even one dissenter was present, the subject was able to voice his or her own independent judgment." That is the function of Abdiel in *Paradise Lost*, the one seraph who heroically resists Satan's recruitment. In John Milton's expository strategy, Abdiel thus frees the reader from taking Satan's side as well, or at least from rationalizing a surrender to sin as inevitable. With the Puritan revolutionary cause in tatters, and a corrupt aristocracy back in power, Milton may well have seen himself as Abdiel. Perhaps humanities professors can be forgiven for also sometimes feeling kinship with Abdiel, when they show their students that they need not bow before the plutocracy in hopes of sharing its gilded blandishments.

Exemplary resistance can work against fear as well as against greed, and can work in real-world settings as well as in psychology labs and theological poems: consider the example of Hajji Abdul Wudood, whose refusal to surrender his son to Taliban officials "triggered a revolt against the Taliban that has spread to a dozen villages in a region that has been among the nation's most formidable Taliban strongholds."[41] Or the example of Malala Yousafzai's courageous feminist refusal to submit to the same forces, which, while she was still a teenager, won her a Nobel Peace Prize and established her as one of *Time* magazine's hundred most influential persons. As at so many crucial moments of human history, a seemingly isolated act of resistance may achieve what thousands of soldiers and millions of dollars and megatons of explosives could not. The eminent historian Timothy Snyder's 2017 book *On Tyranny* traces the importance of a single young Polish woman, as well as (on a larger scale) of Churchill's stubborn Britain, in foiling the Nazis. Hannah Arendt – who warns in *Eichmann in Jerusalem* (1963) about "the banality of evil," whereby normal conformism can enable monstrous behavior – makes a similar observation in her philosophical overview of the history of political action: "the smallest act in the most limited circumstances bears the seed of the same boundlessness, because one deed, and sometimes one word, suffices to change every constellation."[42] The famous play and movie called *Twelve Angry Men* shows how a single alert and conscientious dissenter can defeat injustice and expose the hatred behind it.

Jesus himself can be seen as such a dissenter, rejecting the overbearing memeplex of Pentateuchal law and its priests in favor of a more tolerant system of culture. He was perhaps aware that (as this book has argued) unsettling all authorities at once would be counterproductive – hence, "render unto Caesar the things that are Caesar's" (Matthew 22:21) – but he did argue for a more empathic view, open to multiple perspectives and conveyed often through parables rather than literal, legalistic reading of the Books of Moses. The Roman coin was stamped with Caesar's image, but humanity is (according to Genesis) stamped with the image of God, and so is answerable to itself and its Creator rather than to any social governing system.

This does not mean we can automatically endorse individual resistance to local norms; exceptional behavior can damage rather than heal. Game theory confirms what was sadly obvious to anyone watching soberly the hippie utopia in San Francisco half a century ago:

> free-riders will have an obvious fitness advantage: they benefit from the altruism of others, but do not incur any of the costs. So even if a group is composed exclusively of altruists, all behaving nicely

towards each other, it only takes a single selfish mutant to bring an end to this happy idyll.[43]

The Haight-Ashbury cultural revolution was particularly poorly arranged to deal with a problem that limits generosity in so many evolutionary settings, but seldom arises in a beehive.

In human society, goodness still matters, even in its least political forms. As George Eliot wrote about the heroine at the end of her classic novel *Middlemarch*,

> the effect of her being on those around her was incalculably diffusive: for the growing good of the world is partly dependent on unhistoric acts; and that things are not so ill with you and me as they might have been, is half owing to the number who lived faithfully a hidden life, and rest in unvisited tombs.[44]

To the extent that the cultural system is a self-regulating organism, change is difficult. But to the extent that cultural change is what is called an "emergent phenomenon," even small changes (such as the humanistic interventions this book is urging) may, if suitably placed and directed, have massive effects. The eminent Harvard legal scholar Cass Sunstein observes that "norms can be far more fragile than they appear: hence 'norm entrepreneurs' can help solve collective action problems, and hence 'norm bandwagons' and cascades are common."[45] A few innovators can produce large-scale shifts. Choose your evolution is therefore my condensed message to the next generation. Instead of adapting yourself to minimize conflict with the dominant memeplex, maximize the presence of your best potential self, as you would wish others to do. The influence of memeplexes is neither good nor bad inherently, any more than other evolutionary shifts are. But, as a species – unlike insects – with some range of autonomous choice, some rational consciousness for making that choice, and the tools to make such choices widely consequential, we need to become advocates for what we believe to be good, rather than passively playing out the games offered for our regulation and amusement by a system that has evolved to resist our resistance.

For human behaviors and social systems to endure – and we generally need them to, for our physical and psychic survival – they must function as what chaos theory terms "strange attractors," emerging from the infinite possibilities of an original situation and drawing outcomes increasingly toward themselves. They must have a talent for what the Situationists called "recuperating": a way of steering countless wayward tendencies back into their own sustaining outcomes, of recapturing (to adapt a favorite New Historicist formulation) "subversion as containment." Thus, the Beatles' song "Revolution" eventually resurfaced as an advertising jingle, wrapping an aura of hip resistance around a sales pitch for high-priced footwear created for the profit of a mega-corporation that exploits non-white workers in the Third World. "The Hanging Tree," the grim anthem of the uprising of the underclass against their disco-glitzy oppressors in the *Hunger Games* books and movies, was remixed into a finger-snapping, bass-backbeat disco-dance-party number that sold over a million copies. Many other instances of co-optation have followed a similar pattern.

The study of complex systems allows some middle ground between the understanding of reality, and hence of social structures, as either inevitable or random. If the reality we confront is an evolutionary phenomenon, then it is very likely to be some instance among all the possible realities that has a particularly high tolerance for absorbing oblique impacts, with no more than a temporary wobble in its stance. In other words, those portions of an outcome unlikely to be changed by minor perturbations – the stroke of a butterfly's wing that (in Edward Lorenz's famous speculation) causes a hurricane weeks later and continents away – will endure much longer, which is why mountains stay in about the same shape much longer than clouds do. Thinking in evolutionary-theorist rather than the more familiar conspiracy-theorist mode suggests that a cultural and economic attribute that endures is likely to be one that (like the capitalism of the revolutionary moments of the 19th century as understood by Antonio Gramsci, and like "late capitalism" as understood by Fredric Jameson) has the ability to assimilate change within itself, acting in effect like a stable equilibrium solution.

From this perspective (retreating from abstract speculation toward on-the-ground realities), the Occupy Wall Street collective may have done the right thing by bearing witness to the arbitrary and parasitic character of the current plutocracy, rather than formulating specific policy demands that a money-driven legislative system would never accept. The same point may apply to the Bernie Sanders insurgency in the 2016 Democratic primaries. Since that system would not have endured if it could not delude most people into thinking it benign and/or inevitable, the Occupy movement provoked (while it lasted) intense anxiety among the worshippers of high finance: investment bankers and their loyal allies in politics and the media. The self-sustaining myth of the so-called free market as the foundational test of valid undertakings and the epitome of justice, with consumer capitalism as the only road to happiness, must be challenged as a premise rather than merely in its practices. Otherwise the bulls and bears will have their aspiring tamers for lunch, and put any cost on their tax-deductible expense accounts. This far into the evolution of the pattern, marginal regulation is unlikely to unsettle the concentration of outcomes, or the concentration of wealth. The self-perpetuating allure of the strange attractor itself must be dispersed by humane disruptions.

The poet Walt Whitman saw that imperative when the Gilded Age began to eclipse the sense of moral mission that, for some, drove the US Civil War:

> The eager and often inconsiderate appeals of reformers and revolutionists are indispensable, to counterbalance the inertness and fossilism making so large a part of human institutions. The latter will always take care of themselves – the danger being that they rapidly tend to ossify us. The former is to be treated with indulgence, and even with respect. As circulation to air, so is agitation and a plentiful degree of speculative license to political and moral sanity.[46]

Interchapter: Software is Hard on Humanity

There's a downside to a care-free system. Consider the example of the SAP (Systemanalyse und Programmentwicklung) system, which advertises itself as "the world's largest inter-enterprise software company." Its software now manages and integrates supply-chains and other key functions both within and among countless major business operations worldwide. SAP produces a self-repairing, virtually self-conscious dendritic structure – one characterized by "ability to learn, autonomy, self-organization ... and coevolution"[1] *– that allies itself with a powerful model of consumer capitalism and sustains and rewards the corporate entities that harbor it (as several of its allied systems do) by sanitizing human consequences into statistics. It thereby disguises its depredations, and those of its corporate users, as simply the inevitable deference to a bottom line – the efficiency-measure to which everything in the universe must self-evidently (despite the resistance of the naïve and the sentimental) submit itself.*

It may therefore be important to recognize SAP as a co-evolving me-meplex: a creation in service of humanity that has (like the "technological singularity" of much dystopian science fiction) developed to the point that its preserves itself at a cost to the species that invented it. It allows human managers to disown responsibility for the brutality of our economic system. Throughout late 2017, SAP ran an expensive ad campaign featuring a slogan that promised large businesses what cultures promise human minds: to "Make all this make sense." The ad starred a grey-suited Clive Owen asking of a big production facility, "Is this thing thinking? This thing is thinking!" What it isn't doing is caring – at least not about anything but quantifiable efficiencies, and in no verb tense but the continuous present. That epitomizes the systems increasingly running the global economy. Corporations have accomplished amazing things under capitalism. But squint your eyes just a little and it looks like a particularly dreary revival of human sacrifice, on a massive scale.

3   The Evolution of
Memeplexes

It can be asserted that the community, too, evolves a super-ego under whose influence cultural development proceeds. It would be a tempting task for anyone who has a knowledge of human civilizations to follow out this analogy in detail.
        —Sigmund Freud, *Civilization and its Discontents* (1930)[1]

Do cultures evolve, because some survive over time while others, less talented at sustaining their own structures and finding new carriers, go extinct? They certainly seem to. The ones that can groom a nurturing environment for themselves, defend themselves against rivals, and reproduce themselves across generations will be the ones that remain.

Does this process work exactly like the more familiar form of evolution that depends on the genetic reproduction of DNA? Of course it doesn't.

Some geneticists dismiss the study of cultural evolution as pointless non-science, yet there are many questions worth asking and uncharted areas worth exploring in this field. Genetics offers homologies as well as illustrative analogies, but genetics are not foundational to the way differential reproduction works in various settings on various entities.[2] Any system that produces variation and heritability, and links variation to different rates of survival and replication, can generate evolution.

Darwin himself appears to have recognized that cultural formations co-evolve with human beings:

> It must not be forgotten that, although a high standard of morality gives but a slight or no advantage to each individual man and his children over the other men of the same tribe, yet that an increase in the number of well-endowed men and an advancement in the standard of morality will certainly give an immense advantage to one tribe over another. A tribe including many members who, from possessing in a high degree the spirit of patriotism, fidelity, obedience, courage, and sympathy, were always ready to give aid to each other and to sacrifice themselves for the common good, would be

victorious over most other tribes; and this would be natural selection. At all times throughout the world tribes have supplanted other tribes; and as morality is one important element in their success, the standard of morality and the number of well-endowed men will thus everywhere tend to rise and increase.[3]

If we recognize "a standard of morality" as a cultural formation or memeplex – that is, a self-replicating grouping of ideas, behaviors, and institutions – then according to Darwin a certain such standard would be selected by the reproductive success of its carriers. But "morality" implies a presumptively desirable set of tendencies. Militarism and tribalism are no less natural co-evolutionary phenomena than altruism. The question is which products of nature we choose to nurture as fruits and which we eradicate as weeds.

Invisible Tyrants

This book has explored why human beings are vulnerable to cognitive overload, and why that makes us dependent on cultures, which provide a kind of external prosthesis that protects us from overload by helping a community agree on certain right ways to think and behave. Now I want to explain how that dependency allows cultures to evolve into entities that serve their own reproduction rather than humanity's best interests.

Evolutionary biology suggests that a species survives because its cluster of core attributes, variously incarnated, has the ability to protect and replicate itself, often including the ability to convert potential enemies in its environment to its own advantage. Cultures function in similar ways. Whether a memeplex is mutualistic or parasitic – in other words, whether it thrives by benefitting its believers or instead by exploiting them – it has to insinuate itself into the functions of a human community. The symbiosis between cultural forms and *Homo sapiens* verges on the "obligate" form, where the linked entities don't merely aid each other, but depend on each other for their very survival.

It is inconvenient for the trumpet flower to build a blossom deep enough to force the hummingbird to pollinate it before taking its nectar; building that extended structure consumes energy and discourages other pollinators. It is similarly inconvenient for the hummingbird to have to build such a long beak to get at that nectar. But evolution has forced them into what biologists call an "arms race" that left them both with inefficiencies, whereas a diplomatic truce might have offered the same neutral outcome at a lower cost to both sides. Many creatures could save energy through a trade pact or nonaggression treaty with others in their environment. That may not be an option for trumpet flowers or hummingbirds, but it is for human beings, who have rationality and language that should enable us to look at history, plan for the future, and work out solutions together: what Hamlet calls "such large discourse, looking before and after," which shouldn't rot away "in us unused" (4.4.36–39). Collaborating life-forms will naturally always be seeking to cheat for advantages, but if we are fooled by neoliberalism and militarism into thinking there is no realistic way for human societies to function apart from brutal competition, we waste an essential advantage of our human capacities.

Blind evolution doesn't care about the future. The only defense that most species have against problems yet to come – no matter how imminent and catastrophic – is the variability that has enabled their population to adapt to environmental changes in the past. The classic example is the peppered moth, which is either light or dark in its coloration. When the Industrial Revolution coated surfaces with soot, the dark moths predominated, presumably because their camouflage was advantageous. As modern environmental controls allowed those surfaces to lighten, the species was able to adapt, because the recessive allele for light coloration was still around to generate moths that could take advantage of the changed camouflage.[4] Human beings can do much more, but it doesn't exactly come naturally. To fight climate-change and mass extinctions requires that we favor scientific intelligence and forward-looking altruism over the alliance between the evolved bias of animal brains toward immediate advantage and the corporate-capitalist function that emphasizes short-term monetary profits and demands endless growth.

* *

Let me pause to clarify that, when I say that a system grooms an environment, or that it is seeking to cheat, that is shorthand for the way nearly all evolutionary entities act *as if* they had a desire and a plan to succeed. They don't – not in our sense. Human beings and a few other species do such things consciously, but evolution causes countless other things – living creatures and (I am arguing) memeplexes – to appear to strategize, because those that behave in ways that favor the spread of their own type tend to persist in the world.

Some memeplexes run a protection-racket, creating problems and sustaining tensions so that we become ever more dependent on them to manage those problems and tensions, while also forbidding (by declaring them inherently immoral) alternative means of self-soothing such as casual sexual release, the ingestion of pleasurably relaxing drugs, and the simple pleasures of idleness.

Brown-headed cowbirds leave their eggs in the nests of other types of birds, who then accept the burden of tending the eggs and feeding the alien hatchlings. Why? Probably because the cowbirds periodically check on the nests, and if the hosts have harmed or neglected the cowbird eggs, the cowbirds earn their nickname of "mafia birds" by destroying the host's eggs. Presumably each individual cowbird doesn't calculate that this behavior will benefit its kind overall, but the cowbird population has evolved to carry out the protection-racket instinctively. Nor, presumably, have the host warblers read in *The Warbler Times* about this pattern of revenge; probably the reason they usually nurture the cowbird offspring is because the ones that meekly accepted that imposition were the ones likelier to have surviving offspring, who were then genetically likelier to have that more accepting tendency. The complications of brood-parasitism go beyond that transaction, but it is certainly part of the explanation. In many other cases, "laymen are often dumbfounded by how nature could have given rise to parasitic manipulations in the first place; some stratagems seem so clever and cunning that only a human or an omniscient god could have dreamed them up."[5] As parasites were long under-attended in biology, so the parasitic functions of cultural evolution have gone under-recognized.

Creatures don't even need to have brains to develop what look like strategies. If one strain of gut bacteria can trick us into preferring the food that allows it to outcompete other gut bacteria, even when that food is unhealthy for us,[6] why couldn't ideologies develop an ability to exploit us without having any conscious intention? Such connivers don't even need to have bodies. Some scientists dismiss the idea of cultural evolution because cultures essentially consist of mere information. But so does DNA. And so do viruses, which ingeniously commandeer bodies and energies to spread that information – as anyone who has received and/or transmitted a cold or flu by sneezing should know.

* * * * * * * * * * * *

Any surviving socio-cultural order – a type of government, a religion, a system regulating sexuality, or social class – will likely be one that has survived by aligning itself with persistent human psychological tendencies and exploiting convenient gaps in the firewall of our psychological independence. The gaps that presumably developed to permit children's necessary reliance on parents and on the warnings of elders empower memes that play on fear as well as trust. The balance seems to have tilted toward fear in 21st-century US politics, where the right-wing depicts the threat from big-government control as second only to the threat from immigrants and (other?) barbaric infidels. Militarism and nationalism – which play the parental roles of disciplinarian, protector, and validator of narcissistic identity – are contagious across borders, and thus propagate themselves easily through the world, even though they clearly seem harmful to both the biological survival and the moral stature of the human race (Einstein called nationalism "an infantile disease ... the measles of mankind"[7]). In a remarkably monstrous alliance of memeplexes that harmed both human populations and human morality, Nazi and

Soviet atrocities continued unabated from 1933 to 1945, partly because they allowed these ideologies to collaborate in promoting each other toward absolute power. Each provided a demonic Other which had to be fought regardless of cost.[8]

Something similar could be said about Sunni and Shiite Muslims, and Hamas and Israeli militants, in the Middle East. Yascha Mounk's well-regarded 2018 book *The People Versus Democracy* sees a similar dynamic now arising dangerously between "illiberal democracies" and "undemocratic liberalism"; the former is a force of reactionary populism, the latter a force of progressive elitism, each providing the other with something to scorn rather than understand.[9] White Supremacist and Antifa groups may have done the same thing for each other in a small way in the past few years – giving each other publicity and credibility while pressuring moderates to choose between defending one or the other. Obviously, advocates of genocide and opponents of genocide are very far from morally equivalent, but the dynamic is worth recognizing. A rash descent into the comments section of politically themed websites reveals only too vividly how memeplexes feed off their ability to form us into tribes that caricature and enrage each other, with each tribe protecting itself from the obligation to consider more nuanced views and excluding the enemy from the category of the human. All the while, the websites – and the Internet is itself a marauding memeplex – thrive on our bile.

A more recent case of such collaboration, as observed by William Connolly,

> is the formation of a distinctive evangelical-capitalist resonance machine in the United States in which constituencies in very different subject positions have amplified bellicose dispositions in each other. As each exacerbates complementary tendencies in the other, through the definition of shared projects and enemies, an aggressive theo-econo machine emerges larger and more intense than the sum of its separate parts.[10]

Put more simply, Christian fundamentalism has entered an unholy alliance with the structures of business in America so that they not only support each other (under the umbrella of conservatism) but sometimes even reinforce the aspects of the other that are least humane.

Sweet Sorrow

The Darwinian aspect of memeplexes sometimes leads them to align themselves with peculiarities of our biological evolution – advantageously for them, destructively for us. The sugar industry thrives partly because that industry exploits our evolutionary adaptations. We inherit strong appetites for salt and especially sugar (mine are Olympic-level for both) because those substances were rare and precious in the hunter-gatherer diet through most of human history. Now those appetites collaborate with the structures of the modern food industry – and also with certain opportunistic, manipulative gut bacteria, and also with greedy opportunistic people – to produce epidemics of high blood pressure, obesity, and Type 2 diabetes that are spreading worldwide. That collaboration reveals something important: in this and many other instances, no bright line separates the evils knowingly produced by unethical human selfishness from the systematic dysfunctions caused by co-evolutionary dynamics. The systems steer human selfishness into particular channels and amplify its impact, while themselves benefiting from harnessing human selfishness to their own.

The history of Big Sugar (as the larger entities in that business are sometimes called), right up to the present, makes clear how various powerful cultural formations – colonialism, racism, capitalism, advertising, and globalization – have empowered each other and protected each other from any humane misgivings. Those formations have also protected this hugely profitable industry from the medical evidence that would otherwise presumably have reined in its runaway force.

Powerful agricultural interests use large campaign contributions to induce legislators to make the government (and hence taxpayers) pay the costs of cleaning up their pollutants; this transaction has been starkly evident in the damage the phosphorous runoff from the sugar industry has done to the Everglades. The same kind of legalized bribery sustains price-supports and import tariffs on sugar that are costing the United States nearly two billion dollars a year. It also sustains massive subsidies (structured, incidentally, to favor large farming corporations) on the production of high-fructose corn syrup, which makes products sweetened with that syrup an attractively cheap but unhealthy source of calories for people in poverty. In fact, the entire history of the large-scale sugar industry has been characterized by corruption of government officials, and by alliances with extreme versions of capitalist functions such as wage-slavery. The hacienda system under Spanish rule took the Morelos region from subsistence maize to sugar produced by landless peasantry. The sugar plantations in Hispaniola were a major destination of enslaved Africans in earlier centuries, and the situation of Haitian workers in the Dominican Republic still bears some shocking resemblances to its ancestor there and elsewhere in the Caribbean. The system has improved its efficiency and its publicity, but it is hardly more just or humane.

Big Sugar has also evolved so it could continue to thrive in a changing cultural environment. To sustain their profits in the more foodie, health-conscious consumer environment of the 21st century, the industry had to adapt. It did so by disguising extremely sugar-intensive foods (such as flavored yogurts, granola energy bars, and fruit-juice smooth-ies) as health foods. Meanwhile, the agents of Big Sugar have actively campaigned – like the tobacco industry in previous decades – to sup-press information that would allow us to confront this addiction. That corruption seeps down into the practices of science: research funded by Coca-Cola has deliberately distorted governmental guidelines since the 1960s, deflecting the blame for sugar's ravages onto other less guilty culprits such as dietary fat.

To the extent that independent science makes itself heard, the sugar-pushers shout it down as an attack on liberties and the American way of life. When the mayor of New York City tried, with a solid basis in sociological and medical research, to limit the sale of sugary sodas in cups larger than 16 ounces, he was vilified and ridiculed in well-funded campaigns as an elitist (and, without quite saying it, a know-it-all New York Jew) who was attacking the freedom to choose.

Public education budgets are cut so severely that schools can't refuse of-fers from the Coca-Cola and Pepsi corporations to pay for the placement of their alluring vending machines. Soda thus becomes the normal default snack for students: a profoundly unhealthy habit that continues through life. Early learning is served with a side of sugar addiction. A horrifying number of Americans in the conservative southeast and Appalachian re-gions are practically drowning in Mountain Dew – their teeth rotting away, their livers and pancreases driven to surrender. These epidemics are spreading in Central and South America even faster than in the United States. Australian Aborigine populations have been similarly devastated by the arrival of the Pepsi Corporation. The Nestle Corporation has been saturating Brazil with traveling carts of their high-calorie, low-nutrition processed foods – carts pushed by people who can't make a decent living otherwise, selling on credit in poor neighborhoods with few alternatives. Would these populations really choose short, sickly lives for themselves and their children if they were free from the sway of self-protective me-meplexes that conspire with self-protective but outdated gene-complexes that crave all the salt and sweets they can get? We can't gain true freedom until we come to recognize our nearly invisible chains.

Skillful and expensive marketing has persuaded many Americans to equate the empowerment of for-profit corporations with personal free-dom. Left-wing populists think people may be awakening from that fantasy, but right-wing populists seem to be clinging to it, even when their own families are clearly being exploited and even fatally poisoned by industries near their homes.[11] The self-perpetuating empowerment of these corporate "persons" means that we're now effectively ruled by entities that (according to what a Distinguished Professor of Corporate and Business Law at Cornell argues is a convenient myth[12]) have a fi-duciary duty to focus only on accumulating wealth, lest they illegally betray their shareholders.

As a result, they then have more money available to convince people of their necessity and even their goodness. They can buy, not just biased versions of science to deny the damage they do, but also ever more profitable favors from legislators. They can hire skillful attorneys to circumvent any inconvenient legislation that slips through, threatening lawsuits and filing appeals until no public-interested entity has the standing, legal skill, and financial means to finish the fight. The notorious Citizens United ruling by the Republican-appointed majority on the Supreme Court took the fiction that corporations are persons, which was useful for enabling contracts and litigation, and extended it into considering them citizens with a right to unlimited political speech, so there are no limits on what corporations can spend, and no meaningful limits on how stealthily they can spend it, to choose our public executives and legislators, who then appoint judges who say all this is as it should and must be.

But obviously it should not, and this book denies that it must. The good news is that American voters seem to be developing some immunity to massive campaigns of political advertising on television, and the success of some soda-tax initiatives in 2016 suggests that honest health science is beginning to reach a society that is much more thoughtful about food than it was a few decades ago. The bad news is the same old news: it would be naïve to doubt that these interests, which adapted to the age of television so successfully, will evolve new ways to make their money persuasive.

The *New York Times* reports that, in 2010,

> a coalition of Brazilian food and beverage companies torpedoed a raft of measures that sought to limit junk food ads aimed at children. The latest challenge has come from the country's president, Michel Temer, a business-friendly centrist whose conservative allies in Congress are now seeking to chip away at the handful of regulations and laws intended to encourage healthy eating.[13]

Even more recently – in fact, the day before this manuscript is due in for copy-editing in late June of 2018 – the soda industry got California's state legislature to rush through a bill making it illegal for any city or county in the state to impose any tax on sodas for the next 12 years. The industry extorted this protection by creating a ballot initiative, backed by more than $7,000,000 of their money, which would have blocked cities or counties from raising any kind of taxes or the state from raising fees without super-majority votes. Given anti-tax reflexes and that massive backing, that initiative could have passed, making it impossible for communities to fund basic services or deal with crises even if a clear majority favored doing so. The legislature therefore gave the soda industry its special protection, in exchange for the industry withdrawing the ballot initiative. Bad people doing bad things? You won't hear me disagree – but I would add that the systematic functions of a memeplex reward them for doing so. The jerks shall always be with us, but we don't need to help them rule us.

Anyway, the ability of large for-profit corporations to shape policy in their favor already resides far more in lobbying than in direct campaign contributions. Money is abetted by what political scientists call "agency capture" – a revolving door between government regulators and the far-better-paying industries they are supposed to regulate.[14] Public bureaucracy is corrupted away from its supposed service to the society at large because that bureaucracy and private corporate profiteering are each able to gain more power by conspiring with each other. A recent study demonstrated that "economic elites and organized groups representing business interests have substantial independent impacts on U.S. government policy, while average citizens and mass-based interest groups have little or no independent influence."[15] That may reflect the expertise corporate lobbyists can offer legislators on many complex issues, but it is not quite democracy, any more than a system that prevents any but the wealthy from making their arguments audible to the electorate is truly "free speech."

What turned the biochemical sweetness of fructose and sucrose that was so delicious to our ancestors so sour for today's *Homo sapiens* was a confluence of co-evolving entities – some biological, some socio-cultural. Corn and sugarcane are around because corn's ability to make polyploids made it easy to domesticate, and sugarcane's ability to resist pests and tolerate a wide variety of soils made it easy to grow, while both produced enough sugars to make people farm them. Agriculture is around because, by decreasing uncertainty and eventually increasing the supply of calories, it produced a greater population of agriculturalists – a population too large to revert successfully to the old hunter-gatherer ways, even if those were in several ways better. The post-slavery plantation system is around because abolitionism – a rare but precious intervention of humane consciousness that built an alliance with Christianity against racism – obliged the exploitation of both workers and the environment to take new forms. Capitalism was around to drive that process because it had enabled the parts of Europe that ran on credit to overcome the parts of Europe that were run by traditional monarchy. Capitalism then out-competed Communism, for reasons I will explore later, and is proving as depressingly effective as Communism was in disabling capitalism's most recent rival, environmentalism.

Corporations are around to extend and exploit those triumphs because they have structural advantages in a capitalist system, especially in insatiable capitalism's symbiotic alliance with consumerism. Advertising is around to disguise all these depredations, and a lobbying industry exists to protect them from the law because corporations have the wealth to hire publicists with expertise in manipulating consumers' psyches as well as lobbyists with inside access to regulatory agencies. And we are around because our ancestors were the ones who developed a taste for salt and sweet that gave them useful nutrients and energy, and were clever and patient enough eventually to farm and trade rather than just forage for such sources, even though that achievement has now put several of the organs that regulate our digestion under siege.

The human race will thrive only if we make intelligent, conscious choices that override those ancient appetites and these modern institutions, which have both programmed us to obey them. That requires not only medical-scientific knowledge but also a new social-scientific perspective – one that looks for a malfunction rather than a villain. We may hate the Fanjul family of sugar-barons for its lucrative but brutal impact on its field-hands, public health, and mangrove swamps, but the system will keep producing similar agents if we imagine that condemning the bad guys will win the war.

The corporations that have evolved to dominance are generally the ones that neatly circumvent the social conscience of their executives. The current system not only obliges those employees to the interests of investors, measured in money, but also isolates ethical responsibility between layers of management, each meeting quantitative targets, while mostly protecting the managers from personal criminal liability. In the kind of unregulated market that conservatives advocate, success depends on ruthlessness.

Other current financial memeplexes unproductive for the commonwealth – say, flash-trading and heavily debt-leveraged corporate acquisitions on Wall Street, or flipping houses on Main Street, or payday loans on Desolation Row – are like cleaner-fish. They attach themselves subserviently to the shark-like money-meme not only because it feeds them, but also because its immense power over the American psyche and political system defends them also. Try to attack such practices and the silent predator – the invisible monster haunting the financial horror story *The Big Short* – shows its shiny rows of teeth.

The similarity to predatory behavior in the animal kingdom extends to the way profiteering private equity (as Naomi Klein showed in *The Shock Doctrine*) quickly moves in whenever a public system is wounded by a disaster, seizing its territory for further depredations. So the cycle of money for money's sake spins faster and faster. Jane Mayer's 2016 book *Dark Money* masterfully exposes the Koch brothers' patient, elaborate schemes for controlling public opinion and policy, at least partly so that their huge fortune can become an even huger fortune: proof enough that sometimes there really is a conscious human conspiracy that allies itself with capitalism's control of the American political process.[16]

Capital is drawn to capital, as workers' wages stagnate and their pensions disappear, while large corporations and their executives and investors accumulate more and more cash. Only by looking back half a millennium or more can we realize how strange it would once have seemed to rent out one's body – its time and its labor – for nothing more grounded than a salary,[17] especially when that recompense comes as a number from a distant abstraction called a corporation. Nor is it easy, from within contemporary culture, to notice how peculiar it is then to rebuild the self by purchasing brand-name products and mimicking the types of happiness the ads for those products show them generating. That compensation is part of a diversion of our reflexive love of the good into "goods" to be bought and then displayed for an impersonal kind of personal prestige. The consolations of consumerism ultimately feed energy back into the system that erased the workers' humanity to begin with. Granted, this has become a tired and tiresome list of complaints from liberal intellectuals (who make their own set of identity-affirming purchases), but it may be worth revisiting if we can analyze the underlying functions instead of just disdaining their manifestations.

There are two leading theories about why human beings would obey cultures that have significant maladaptive traits. "The big-mistake hypothesis attributes maladaption to *individuals* misusing antique rules in modern novel environments"; the aforementioned appetites for sugar and salt fit that explanation. "The costly information hypothesis attributes maladaption to *population-level* evolutionary trade-offs that are intrinsic to cultural adaptation"[18]; sometimes the costs of inventing and testing new behaviors outweigh the benefits of merely imitating the established behaviors. What I am proposing is a conjunction of these two hypotheses: individuals often use outdated rules because it spares mental struggle, and because it is in the evolved nature of successful cultural systems to preserve themselves in a population even if they are no longer adaptive.

These memeplexes are, in the body-politic, the equivalent of host-manipulating parasites such as *Toxoplasma gondii* – a parasite which apparently tricks the brains of rats into being attracted to house-cats instead of fleeing them, thus (at the cost of the rats' lives) winning its way into the gullets of cats, who are its main carrier and transmitter to human carriers.[19] The lancet liver fluke sends an agent into the ant's brain which makes the ant sit atop blades of grass so it will be eaten by cattle or sheep, the parasite's ultimate host.[20] Other parasites perform similarly exploitative – and often highly elaborate – tricks on snails, birds, roaches, and spiders, turning them into weird little robots that give their lives over to helping the parasites thrive.

To shift the scale of the metaphor for a moment, memeplexes sometimes resemble what geneticists call "segregation distorters": genes that "cheat" by increasing their own replication without serving the propagation of the creature more generally. This kind of "gene drive" seems considerably more likely in cultural than in biological evolution. Those genes thrive in evolutionary terms not by adding to communal survival, but instead by tilting the normal balance in cell division (meiosis) from the normal 50-50 probability of either parental gene variant (allele) being reproduced at a certain place in the chromosome. They just have to make sure not to damage their carriers so fast and so fatally that (like the Ebola virus, as compared to the flu virus) they actually limit their own ability to spread.

None of this means that cultural formations are inherently bad; they just aren't necessarily good either. Human Behavioral Ecologists attempt to explain cultural variations as adaptive responses to various environments – and clearly many are. Memeplexes are often benign symbionts with our species. The evidence seems strong that human beings have been cyborgs (of a sort) from the early phases of our emergence as a species, extending our physical capacities with abilities – transmitted by teaching rather than purely by genetics – to manufacture tools. *Homo sapiens* lack the powerful jaws and other musculature of the Australopithecines but developed the ability to make weapons. There is even reason to suspect that our main ancestors lacked the individual intelligence of Neanderthals,[21] but made up for it by passing along knowledge about tool-making and other survival skills more elaborately within our communities. Now we have massive technology to supplement our powers of memory and calculation. These cultural inventions serve as prosthetics for our limited minds and bodies.

Being beneficial to our species is not, however, the only reason a trait might spread in our cultures. A cough "represents both your body's effort to expel the germ *and* the parasite's determination to spread itself,"[22] and human behavior is often clearly sub-optimal, even in the narrow terms of genetic evolutionary survival. Many examples confirm Gillian R. Brown and Peter J. Richerson's observation that

> The social learning strategies that are studied by Cultural Evolutionists could lead to the acquisition of maladaptive information (i.e., information that fails to enhance genetic reproductive success) in some instances, as long as the learning strategies themselves are favoured by selection.

Furthermore, "the risk of acquiring maladaptive information might have increased substantially in modern environments, for example because mass media exposes us to many attractively packaged cultural variants designed by advertisers to increase their sales, not the recipients' fitness."[23]

Because memeplexes often spread horizontally across populations, rather than vertically by sequential generations of inheritance, their propagation is not limited by whether they increase the evolutionary fitness of their human carriers. They don't have to be beneficial, just alluring – especially in a world where young people are receiving such an unprecedentedly high percentage of their information from sources other than their parents and related elders. Sophisticated marketing doesn't hard-sell a product but – more insidiously – sells cultural norms that are conducive to sale of the product, or uses the over-imitation and what anthropologists and archeological psychologists call the "prestige bias" bred in us by evolution to make us mimic the consumer behaviors of famous actors or athletes, even when the product is irrelevant to the area of their achievements.[24] And even if these cultural forces didn't damage fitness narrowly conceived as rates of genetic reproduction, they might still damage humanity's higher-order goals. Buy a tube of something that doesn't really help, and you have wasted a few dollars; buy from movies a hyped formula of how a woman should look or how a man should drive, and you may waste your love and your life, and toxify the environment for all around you.

Many human activities continue even though they appear to be net losses for both the species and the individual. Chain letters get human beings to reproduce them, despite their zero-sum or net-negative value, through some mixture of threat and promise. Addictive gambling is a more consequential example, with Las Vegas and other casinos as the visible precipitate of a memeplex that exploits a vulnerability in our mental construction: fast-thinking distortions of probability, augmented by a narcissistic belief that one's own special destiny outweighs the odds.

Fervor for a college or professional sports team seems illogical in similar ways, considering the vast amounts of time, energy, and human capital sports consume while producing far more losers than champions and no useful lasting product. Rooting for a team can be defended as a useful and ingenious adaptation that diverts us from the even more costly phenomenon of actual internecine warfare, but a less admiring view would see sports not as diverting tribal violence, but instead as channeling courage and loyalty into meaningless nonproductive heroics.[25] The now-massive supply of televised sports may lure transformative virtues into isolated, apolitical cul-de-sacs. From that perspective, such contests resemble other forms of distraction and controlled release that an unjust status quo has evolved to divert people from righteous collective revolutionary action, with anger focused on the decisions of erring referees rather than the decisions of corrupt political representatives. This has proven a durable function: nearly 2,000 years ago, the satirist Juvenal was already complaining that Roman citizens were surrendering their control over government in return for the "bread and circuses" that government provided them – especially the gladiator battles, then at their peak.

Who Wins Culture Wars, and How

Religions of longstanding influence have generally armed themselves against falsifying exposure. A dominant strain of Christianity says that the Lord – though all-powerful, omnipresent, and benevolent – moves in mysterious ways, and the reward for your covenant with Him occurs in an afterlife invisible from the earth. Blind faith is the best kind, followers are told, and the more convincing any outsider is in provoking doubt about this theology, the more obviously that outsider is the disguised and seductive demon that the theology prudently warned against.[26] A similar Chinese finger-trap for dissent sustained the Cold War (as Chapter 5 will explain): any questioning of Stalinist Communism on one side of the Iron Curtain was treated as a symptom of either mental illness or pro-Western enmity to the people, while on the other side of the Iron Curtain, any complaints about runaway corporate and plutocratic power were deemed a sure sign of treasonous pro-Soviet fellow-traveling.

Scott Atran has made a strong case for understanding religion as an accidental byproduct of several interacting, genetically powerful modules of interpretation, belief, and behavior;[27] but that does not preclude religions evolving into memeplexes with defensive and expansionist habits. Atran himself has shown, no less convincingly, that "Terrorists, for the most part, are not nihilists but extreme moralists – altruists fastened to a hope gone haywire."[28] That is the kind of malfunction this book aspires to explain.

Brilliant observers of cultural history from Friedrich Schiller in the 18th century to Max Weber in the 20th have seen the modern world as "disenchanted" – moved, that is, from traditional supernatural beliefs toward pure scientific rationality. From my perspective, however, much of this change has been merely the transition from one set of memeplexes to others that may seem more rationalistic but still have internal assumptions biased toward their own survival and seeded (as an evolutionary model would predict, and as Weber himself perceives) with legacies of their religious ancestors. These systems immunize themselves against challenge: objections to psychoanalysis, identity politics, or Marxism, for example, are deemed symptoms of exactly the truth that psychoanalysis, identity politics, or Marxism reveals. To ease the pain of a complex human brain encountering an under-defined reality, believers must perceive a foundational and transcendent truth in these systems, rather than mere self-affirming premises, which explains the dangerous drift that the distinguished anthropologist Ernest Gellner and others have noted toward "re-enchantment": the empowering of other, secular memeplexes to defend people from raw reality.

Communism is certainly one of the most important secular meme-plexes of the past century. The irony is that it became a leading instance of what Marx hoped Communism would erase:

> This fixation of social activity, this consolidation of what we our-selves produce into an objective power above us, growing out of our control, thwarting our expectations, bringing to naught our calcu-lations, is one of the chief factors in historical development up till now. And out of this very contradiction between the interest of the individual and that of the community the latter takes an independent form as the *State*, divorced from the real interests of individual and community, and at the same time as an illusory communal life …. The social power, i.e., the multiplied productive force, which arises through the co-operation of different individuals as it is determined by the division of labour, appears to these individuals, since their co-operation is not voluntary but has come about naturally, not as their own united power, but as an alien force existing outside them, of the origin and goal of which they are ignorant, which they thus cannot control, which on the contrary passes through a peculiar series of phases and stages independent of the will and the action of man, nay even being the prime governor of these.[29]

I might dispute the implication that these arrangements are "illusory," since I believe they become real forces. But the specific observations fit well with my understanding of such socio-cultural formations – including capitalism – as external forces produced by us but not identical or even sympathetic to us. They "come about naturally," creating hive-like systems we can escape only by recognizing them as contingencies not optimized for human fulfillment.

Nothing could demonstrate more emphatically the relevance and ur-gency of recognizing anti-humane cultural evolution than the recent rise of right-wing populist nativist movements across Europe, beginning in France and Hungary, and now prominent from the United Kingdom to the former USSR and (most recently) Brazil and even Sweden, as well as in the United States. What the stunning British vote to exit the European Union and the even more surprising rise of Donald Trump to the US Presidency show is how easy it is to deflect the blame for a blameworthy system onto stock villains such as elites and foreigners – especially since intellectuals and immigrants offend the craving for traditional cultural consensus that I have argued is a fundamental human desire. As Karl Popper observed as he stared down the dual tyrannies of Fascism and Communism in the mid-20th century,

> civilization has not yet fully recovered from the shock of its birth – the transition from the tribal or 'closed society', with its submission

to magical forces, to the 'open society' which sets free the critical powers of man .... the shock of this transition is one of the factors that have made possible the rise of those reactionary movements which have tried, and still try, to overthrow civilization and to return to tribalism.[30]

That backlash is augmented by the decadence of the institutional alternatives. The European Union was originally envisioned by many as an instrument of peace, fairness, environmental prudence, and shared prosperity. While it retains some such functions to a degree rare elsewhere in the world, its functions as a peacekeeper have been eclipsed by its functions as an economic regulator, and its economic policies have largely been co-opted by the technocracy of neoliberalism, which (like globalization in general) disempowers workers to the benefit of multinational corporations and creates debt traps while claiming priority over other forms of communitarian thinking.

If people cannot be brought to contemplate the grinding machinery of neoliberalism, or the way the super-rich have tilted its output toward their own bank accounts, or the broader spiritual and environmental costs of a consumerist ethos generally, they will find scapegoats. When things aren't the way they used to be for the lighter-skinned passengers on the supposedly good ship Empire, those passengers grab crosses and torches and come for the Muslims; and then (if there aren't enough witches to burn) the next likely targets include the Jews, the dark complexioned, the intellectuals, and the lesbian, gay, bisexual, and transgender (LGBT) communities. Again, people choose to see a conspiracy of evil others deliberately undermining the integrity and health of this socio-cultural body (Trump has clearly implied as much about Barack Obama and even about the FBI), and they turn toward nationalist and even racist dictators who promise to make the changes disappear, rather than trying to choose something better. They sense a need to rise critically against the system, but can only manage to rage tribally on behalf of ideas of purity and security.

Within the United States today, the globalizing neoliberal memeplex and the ascendency of a Silicon Valley economy have been especially cruel to rural and smaller old-industrial communities, which are generally the least prepared to take a skeptical look at established elements of culture. Obama controversially commented that "they get bitter, they cling to their guns and religion." Or, as the popular new-country singer Brandy Clark puts it, more sympathetically, "we pray to Jesus and we play the Lotto / 'Cause there ain't but two ways we can change tomorrow." Since those are seldom the communities where fresh alternatives are being generated, in forms of culture or forms of employment, they aren't the ones that the emerging alternatives are designed to serve – which only amplifies their resentment toward the highly visible and mostly big-city campaigns to rescue other, more visible minorities, asylum-seekers, and those who have immigrated without legal authority. To be told they are victimizers rather than victims has to be especially galling.

Their cultural system is not working, because its economic viability – never robust in many of the more conservative regions of the United States – has been wrecked by a bigger system. So, these communities face a choice between recognizing that their culture is (like most) both arbitrary and outdated, and therefore trying to change it, or instead seeking scapegoats to punish for the decline of American privilege, Christian privilege, white privilege, and male privilege. It serves the interests of wealth and big business, dependent on that global economic model, to encourage the latter response: shame converted into wrath and thence into reactionary politics. Efforts to change the existing model are likely to come from humanistic and artistic elites, so conservative politicians preemptively encourage their constituents to focus on the patronizing aspects of those proposed interventions (and they don't lack for valid examples). The rise of Trumpism in 2016 suggests that, forced to choose between being thoughtful about the problem or being angry about the problem, and between undertaking the uncomfortable task of accommodating change or believing a strongman can magically make the problems and even decades of history disappear, many Americans crave leaders who endorse the latter responses. The very bald-facedness of the lying, which moderates assumed would discredit and disqualify Trump, seems to be a source of satisfaction to his loyalists. The promise that no fact need ever be allowed to disturb the security of your tribe's belief-system can be very alluring.

The massive opioid epidemic in these declining working-class communities certainly looks like another effort to make those problems disappear, or at least to evade the pain of challenging the traditional culture and wrestling with the powerful, complex forces that have overwhelmed it. The comparably massive problems of alcoholism in the English slums of another urbanizing era – the earlier 19th century (as chronicled by Daniel Defoe and Henry Fielding among the great early novelists) – offer further evidence that, in order to subjugate a community, the deleterious substance needs an alliance with an economic force disrupting that community's cultural traditions.[31]

The reactionaries in America's rural areas and small cities whose factories and small businesses have closed may blame the government and hate the intellectuals and urban centers that are better adapted to the 21st-century economic environment. Yet – thanks in large part to those supposed enemies – those reactionaries who say they voted for Trump because things could not get any worse in their communities have conveniences, liberties, health care, and food and entertainment options that most human beings – probably even most monarchs – who have ever lived on earth would have envied. They are struggling but they are not actually starving.

Or at least not starving physically: an underrated insight from Postcolonial studies is the violence done to a society by breaking the integrity of its culture, alongside the more direct and exploitative colonial brutalities. Across a wide range of cultures, people care not just about being alive, but also, deeply, about their life-stories, which must be a meaningful part of some larger positive narrative to make a conscious life tolerable. As one addict in opioid-ravaged West Virginia described it, "the constant hunt for heroin imposed a kind of order on life's confounding open-endedness. Addiction told you what every day was for, when otherwise you may not have known."[32] Recognition of the deep desire for cultural stability, and of the importance of guiding that desire through narratives rather than through disapproval backed by force, will be essential for dealing successfully with depressed Appalachia – and with displaced ISIS/ISIL jihadis as well.[33]

The right wing in American politics insists we are enduring a culture war, but refuses to recognize the nation's traditional systems of control as anything but freedom. Conservatives see the government as a parasitic memeplex, but won't acknowledge that their own belief system and the consumer-capitalist economic systems might also have evolved into parasites. Meanwhile their liberal opponents insist that there is no need for cultural conflict: that we can all just get along, and government programs can produce happy equality. Together, they discourage people from thinking hard (never a hard thing to discourage) about the systematic problems produced by cultural evolution and the runaway memeplexes it produces. This book aspires to help both factions recognize a common enemy.

We may still eventually and justly conclude that many of our political opponents are stupid, evil, or both: guilty of the evil of choosing stupidity to avoid acknowledging truths that would challenge their narrow self-interest and its accompanying rationalizations and blind-spots. Yet, our communities would benefit if we all initially tried to understand our political opponents as something other than bad people deliberately doing wrong. My theory acknowledges that reactionaries are a necessary element in the regulation of mutation, serving the system by conserving it, conserving the system by serving it. This recognition is cognate with Edmund Burke's justly admired 18th-century defenses of conservatism: that the presumptive wisdom of established human arrangements, such as common law, exceeds the ability of any enthusiastic theories of the moment to outguess it – a version of the algorithmic wisdom of the collective distributed over time rather than space.

* *

Right after the deadly attack on the anti-fascist demonstrators in Charlottesville in late 2017, a lead writer for the prominent neo-Nazi "Daily Stormer" website boasted that their movement is thriving because "People realize they are not atomized individuals. They are part of a larger whole because we have been spreading our memes." Any intelligent resistance needs to recognize not only the allure of all-consuming commitment to a culture that claims ancient roots, but also the importance of actively propagating healthier memes that can fill the same psychological receptors.

If the left – especially a Democratic party establishment that doth protest too much, to cover its guilty complicity with neoliberal economics and its wealthy beneficiaries – is eager to narrow politics into identity-politics and a competition of grievances within that rubric, then aggrieved white people may choose to play the same game. Stokely Carmichael's "Black Power" slogan was easily misrepresented and deployed by regressive forces to turn fearful reactionaries against the Civil Rights movement of the 1960s. When, half a century later, people who hear about the Black Lives Matter movement are censured for saying that all lives matter, they may be direly and even willfully naïve about past and present racism, but they can do subtraction, and the bottom line matches a message they have been hearing for years. There is enough evidence of compensatory efforts – sometimes showy, sometimes stealthy – toward historically disadvantaged groups on campus and in some hiring situations to confirm the suspicions of people who believe those groups are now unfairly advantaged. These is also more than enough evidence of pervasive bias against such groups (from small but cumulative indignities to life-limiting and even life-ending events) to confirm a belief that those compensatory efforts are still far from enough, but that evidence often comes from social-science research that right-leaning people can dismiss as just a function of the academy's liberalism.

"Whitelash" voters may be either sneaky or oblivious about their collusion with a destructive but longstanding memeplex, but their votes still count. Add in the inherent distress and resentment of multiculturalism among people who depend on the cognitive cocoon of their traditional culture as much as on other longstanding privileges. Combine that with the bias of the Electoral College toward rural and hence whiter and more conservative voters, and the demographics that by 2040 will likely allow those same voters, though comprising only a quarter of the US electorate, to choose a super-majority of the Senate. Factor in the gerrymandering that makes a further mockery of the fundamental "one person, one vote" principle, and the "voter-fraud" fraud and cynical voter-roll purges designed to depress the voting of students, racial minorities, and the poor: polling-place extensions of racism that are intensifying, with the connivance of a Republican Supreme Court majority that seems to care more about partisan advantage than about democracy. The bottom line shows that the rainbow-chasing left has a serious practical problem, admirable causes notwithstanding.

That problem becomes all the less tractable when politics are reduced to identity politics, because every political difference becomes a personal affront; and while it is difficult to convince people to change their politics, it is still a lot easier than getting them to change their identities. Social-justice movements have often succeeded when their project is clearly seeking the rights, and accepting the responsibilities, of full citizenship, as in the instance of same-sex marriage and in renewed progress toward the long-stalled Equal Rights Amendment to the US Constitution. Martin Luther King stated his goals as "full citizenship rights" and "real equality" for all Americans, including whites in poverty; he spoke of "militarism" as an American disease, and brought a unifying spiritual component into these political causes.

Citizenship seems to be a category that can retain a balance of individual rights and community support, and sustains the hope of an *e pluribus unum* nation. If human societies that have a sense of unity tend to thrive and squeeze out others, as extensive evidence as well as common sense suggest, then it seems imperative that we find modes of unity that are less toxic than fascist and Communist and racist ones have proven. A lot more people will audition for a role that casts them as heroes of a recovering community than for a role as irredeemable villains who barely make it onto the stage; and demographics suggest that, if the under-30 generation had exercised their duty and privilege of voting as often as the over-50 generation did in 2016, the United States would be on a very different track.

Recent immigration controversies, however, have caused the left to devalue that category of citizenship (along with many forms of patriotism). There are plenty of inhumane, unjust, and hypocritical aspects of nativist politics; the United States has a responsibility toward those our support of oligarchical dictatorships has endangered and impoverished; and the Trump administration's treatment of refugees is heartless and demagogic. But the implication that any policy to control immigration is a moral outrage is far from self-evident, though many progressives treat it as such.

From this perspective, the anxiety driving the resistance of many Trump voters in the United States and comparable nativist movements in Europe cannot legitimately be dismissed – as social-justice activists like to do – as merely hate. That anxiety may focus on a fear of foreign terrorists, which seems statistically indefensible enough to look like merely an excuse for dehumanizing other races and religions; the danger to any individual is minuscule, and the perpetrators of terrorism within the United States are usually white American men. The fixation, in Sweden, Germany, and elsewhere on the idea that non-white men are violating white women is an ugly symptom, and growing economies and shrinking crime-rates cannot cure it. Yet the underlying discomfort entails a question the globalizing world needs to take very seriously. The next few chapters will argue that artistic communication that reconciles novelty with tradition in ways that illuminate our common humanity, and education that enables people to accept and even appreciate complexity, are imperative, because otherwise – to me, a terrifying prospect – multicultural societies may be both inevitable and impossible. As current debates about immigration make clear, the elite left focuses on the inevitability while the populist right focuses on the intolerability. Both have a point, but each thrives on ignoring the other.

That has to stop. When a population becomes obsessed with culture-wars and racial rivalries, a system whose premise is ruthless competition for wealth will gratefully go about the business of business (for an effectively condensed description of that process, listen to the early Bob Dylan song "Only a Pawn in their Game"). As for any master illusionist, the key is misdirection. If immigrants and even refugees can be made the main target of resentments spurred by cultural collision and the declining compensation of labor, what might be an effective economic revolution will be absorbed into a reactionary memeplex. Whatever progressive potential exists in the Trumpist wave of resistance will be identified by the left as mere gullibility and racism, thereby providing the right every opportunity to offer the disaffected a more gratifying way of understanding their own resentment: they would be "Great Again" if they weren't being cheated by left-leaning liberalism and its pet causes.

Anxiety about mass immigration is understandably amplified in a system premised on competition producing the lowest possible pay for employees. When globalization arrives in the form of alien persons supposedly diluting whatever opportunities remain for classes whose limited privileges were already in decline, then racism and nationalism become a mutualist alliance. That alliance, usually abetted by sexism, is the prime mover of what Columbia and UCLA Law professor Kimberlé Williams Crenshaw – looking from the point of view of persons enduring overlapping and mutually reinforcing categories of disadvantage – has influentially termed "intersectionality."[34] This book is interested in the other side of that coin: the way dominant forces overlap and reinforce each other. The axis of patriarchy, pornography, and the Internet is one example in recent decades; the mutually reinforcing function of homophobia and the HIV virus is another; the prison-industrial complex and its symbionts in the urban educational system may be a third. Such systems often subordinate the inconvenient humanity of their carriers, and they need vigilant taming lest they consume that humanity. Meanwhile, the labor movement that advocated solidarity and constituted the main counter-force to industrial capitalism between the two World Wars has withered. Literature can model resistance that avoids the dire problems of outright political revolution while offering a more positive vision of other ways to live, as individuals and as communities. The novels of Ursula Le Guin, for example, provide compelling re-imaginations of gender, marriage, and economics.

The recent shift from emphasizing "diversity" (which many hear as a euphemism for race and gender quotas) toward "inclusion" seems promising; pluralism is a struggle, but it can be toward the common goal of a just society. Advocates for long-oppressed groups may justly ask why blindness to race and gender in the cause of national unity is suddenly imperative in the few areas where those groups are finally receiving protections and reparations, when for so many centuries in so many areas of life, the white male Christian establishment had enforced and celebrated its biases largely unchallenged. All I can say is that, if activists keep feeding the forces of backlash so that the legislatures and courts are packed with self-perpetuating reactionary forces, the chances for peaceful progress look terribly slim.

Nor is any of this is to deny that racial prejudice and jingoism are dire problems that abet each other, as history has so often shown they can be. But they are impossible to subdue effectively unless we recognize them as "Darwin machines": entities that are, by sheer algorithms of selective survival, well attuned to control the mindset of human beings.[35] I don't claim to know exactly how to weigh the competing values (and I do know how tiresome the tireless one-upmanship of leftist critique can be), but I am convinced it is important to recognize that race, class, and gender do not only intersect; they can at times be obliged to compete. Hard-won opportunities for women to hold paying jobs outside the home have often devolved into an obligation to do so because a stagnated single wage can no longer support a family.[36] Admitting a student from a successful, well-educated African-American family to an elite university might do less for social mobility, equal justice, and diverse perspectives than admitting another white student from more impoverished circumstances. If neoliberalism can get its enemies to fight over its table-scraps, it weakens the opposition. It also reinforces its premise that everything in human life is finally about fierce competition.

Doesn't the intense and nearly universal condemnation of genocide reflect a recognition that evolutionary competition – the free market of genetics – can produce terrible violations of human values: crimes against both body and spirit? Shouldn't that be enough to unsettle the assumption that such competition is both necessary and good in most other areas of human interaction? Shouldn't it also be a warning that it is extremely dangerous to subject ourselves to self-affirming systems of collective belief and behavior – runaway memeplexes – without some kind of conscientious circuit-breaker informed by history and empathy?

Charles Taylor's magisterial 1989 book *Sources of the Self* shows that modern Western identity is woven together from many legacies. The ideal characteristics of this model of selfhood include freedom and benevolence, as well as unfathomable individual interiority that can lead to aesthetic self-expression and to authentic life-stories. That fabric of values may be fading or fraying, or simply put up for sale as a remnant, but we should not trash it without asking first what will take its place in civilizing the naked wildness of the human mind. The drive that Taylor admires toward "hypergoods" through "strong evaluation" – choosing by feeling and principle, rather than by habit, convention, and immediate expediency – is close kin to the drive this book advocates toward the best of human potential through recognition of parasitic memeplexes.

The neoliberal corporate culture that counts nothing except monetary profit deftly joins with consumerism to tell us that the world is ours to use for our pleasure and glory. But if the unspoken mission-statement of that alliance were audible, it would say, "Let your species (and countless others) suffer in servitude so that I can rule as widely and live as long as possible." In that sense, it is not so different from what the villains of countless fantasy and science-fiction stories say. Yet our governing villains come in very alluring disguises: as comfort, safety, status, piety, patriotic tradition, common sense, and an absolute bottom-line truth about what naturally must rule the world. So, like the Trojans in *The Iliad*, we let the secretly weaponized gift-horse through our gates, and it won't go back out without a fight.

Iron Fists in Velvet Gloves

George Orwell's essay "Notes on Nationalism" was first published in *Polemic* in May of 1945 – the same month the Germans surrendered in World War II. It strikes me as a perceptive warning that the war underlying that War was far from over, because human beings tend to replace their capacity for open-minded rationality, their love of others, and even their care for their own thriving, with a fierce devotion to what I have been calling a memeplex. Orwell calls it nationalism, but he emphasizes that "the emotion I am speaking about does not always attach itself to what is called a nation – that is, a single race or a geographical area. It can attach itself to a church or a class, or it may work in a merely negative sense, against something or other and without the need for any positive object of loyalty." It is "the habit of identifying oneself with a single nation or other unit, placing it beyond good and evil and recognising no other duty than that of advancing its interests." "The abiding purpose of every nationalist," Orwell warns, "is to secure more power and more prestige, *not* for himself but for the nation or other unit in which he has chosen to sink his own individuality." These units include "such movements and tendencies as Communism, political Catholicism, Zionism, Antisemitism, Trotskyism and Pacifism."

One key symptom Orwell observes is a determination to exclude from consciousness facts or ideas that conflict with the favored perspective.

That observation fits well with my belief that people subjugate themselves to memeplexes to avoid the burden of fresh and complex thought:

> The nationalist not only does not disapprove of atrocities committed by his own side, but he has a remarkable capacity for not even hearing about them .... When one considers the elaborate forgeries that have been committed in order to show that Trotsky did not play a valuable part in the Russian civil war, it is difficult to feel that the people responsible are merely lying. More probably they feel that their own version *was* what happened in the sight of God, and that one is justified in rearranging the records accordingly. Indifference to objective truth is encouraged by the sealing-off of one part of the world from another.

Orwell's observation also fits only too well with the breakdown of productive debate in the Trump era of "alternative facts" and "fake news." This comforting flight from the world's ambiguities damages not only the functions of politics but also the functions of art that (this book argues) can help control political malfunctions: Orwell comments that "aesthetic judgements, especially literary judgements, are often corrupted in the same way as political ones," because attributing any virtue or owing any sympathy to a contrary viewpoint is unbearable. It is a warning some activist schools of literary criticism should consider.

The fanatics among us, Orwell concedes,

> each of them simply an enormous mouth bellowing the same lie over and over again, are obviously extreme cases, but we deceive ourselves if we do not realise that we can all resemble them in unguarded moments. Let a certain note be struck, let this or that corn be trodden on – and it may be corn whose very existence has been unsuspected hitherto – and the most fair-minded and sweet-tempered person may suddenly be transformed into a vicious partisan, anxious only to 'score' over his adversary and indifferent as to how many lies he tells or how many logical errors he commits in doing so.

Yet, for Orwell as for me, it would be a terrible mistake to abandon the quest to improve this world simply because these evolved entities are powerful and their interaction is complex:

> If one follows up this train of thought, one is in danger of being led into a species of Conservatism, or into political quietism. It can be plausibly argued, for instance – it is even possibly true – that patriotism is an inoculation against nationalism, that monarchy is a guard against dictatorship, and that organised religion is a guard against superstition. Or again, it can be argued that no unbiased outlook is

possible, that all creeds and causes involve the same lies, follies, and barbarities; and this is often advanced as a reason for keeping out of politics altogether. I do not accept this argument, if only because in the modern world no one describable as an intellectual can keep out of politics in the sense of not caring about them. I think one must engage in politics – using the word in a wide sense – and that one must have preferences: that is, one must recognise that some causes are objectively better than others, even if they are advanced by equally bad means. As for the nationalistic loves and hatreds that I have spoken of, they are part of the make-up of most of us, whether we like it or not. Whether it is possible to get rid of them I do not know, but I do believe that it is possible to struggle against them, and that this is essentially a *moral* effort. It is a question first of all of discovering what one really is, what one's own feelings really are, and then of making allowance for the inevitable bias.

That captures nicely the main ethical exhortation of the book you are reading now.

In his more famous work, *Nineteen Eighty-Four*, Orwell's protagonist Winston Smith assumes that O'Brien – the agent of the Thought Police who is torturing Smith for insufficient loyalty to the ruling Party – will defend the Party's repressive tactics as a necessary protection of the delicate human psyche. They exerted control "because men in the mass were frail, cowardly creatures who could not endure liberty or face the truth, and must be ruled over and systematically deceived by others who were stronger than themselves." That matches my explanation for why we grant cultures the power to restrict our thoughts and behavior.

What O'Brien tells Smith is something quite different, however: "The Party seeks power entirely for its own sake. We are not interested in the good of others; we are interested solely in power." That darker truth corresponds to my warning that the institutionalized forces to which we have granted authority in hope of protection are Darwin-machines whose evolution narrows their motives to their own perpetuation.

It is essential to remember that imposing pain on dissidents and erasing history (as in *Nineteen Eighty-Four*) is not the only technique by which such systems can erase the attributes of humanity that are inconvenient for them. They can also do so, more subtly and more sustainably, by narrowing our definitions of pleasure and excusing us from the burdens of historical thinking. As Neil Postman – one of my favorite commentators on American life in the late 20th century – wrote in praise of Aldous Huxley's classic 1931 novel *Brave New World*,

> What Orwell feared were those who would ban books. What Huxley feared was that there would be no reason to ban a book, for there would be no one who wanted to read one. Orwell feared those who

would deprive us of information. Huxley feared those who would give us so much that we would be reduced to passivity and egotism. Orwell feared that the truth would be concealed from us. Huxley feared the truth would be drowned in a sea of irrelevance ... It is not necessary to conceal anything from a public insensible to contradiction and narcotized by technological diversions.[37]

In 2017, with the Soviet Union long defunct and a Reality TV celebrity strewing obvious lies elected to lead the United States, it seems hard to doubt that Huxley's was the shrewder prophecy.

Some aspects of modern cultural stabilization are benign, but others are oppressive in the subtle ways that Alexis de Tocqueville anticipated almost two centuries ago in his famous analysis of *Democracy in America*: unlike the ancient tyrannies that "fell most heavily on some few ... if a despotism should be established among the democratic nations of our day, it would probably have a different character. It would be more widespread and milder; it would degrade men rather than torment them."[38]

The Irish literary genius Oscar Wilde's 1891 essay "The Soul of Man under Socialism" offered a similar warning: when authority

> is used with a certain amount of kindness, and accompanied by prizes and rewards, it is dreadfully demoralising. People, in that case are less conscious of the horrible pressure that is being put on them, and so go through their lives in a sort of coarse comfort, like petted animals, without ever realising that they are probably thinking other people's thoughts, living by other people's standards, wearing practically what one may call other people's second-hand clothes, and never being themselves for a single moment.[39]

Lives are spoiled by parasitic cultures, and not only in multiply oppressed classes, although most brutally there (as in the punishment of Wilde's own homosexuality). Watch the young people in classic novels by Edith Wharton or Henry James who see the follies and corruption of high society and vow to live freer, more spontaneous, more truthful lives, yet are always somehow drawn back into the same emotional hollows. Or, in a different genre of masterpiece, watch Michael Corleone drawn back – though no one wanted that to happen – into the Mafia life that he was on a path to escaping, in Coppola's first *Godfather* movie. Sensitive artists, unpleasable practitioners of social critique, and protest-happy college students are dismissive cultural clichés, but in the absence of obvious pain, someone must diagnose this insidious kind of malignancy before it becomes inoperable.

Herbert Marcuse's justly renowned reading of First World societies at the start of the 1960s performs that kind of diagnosis, depicting consumers as unaware of their own entrapment into a kind of flatland.

He begins with the assertion that "a comfortable, smooth, reasonable, democratic unfreedom prevails in advanced industrial civilization," reducing opposition, he says, "to the discussion and promotion of alternative policies *within* the status quo." For Marcuse, this is another form of totalitarianism, all the more dangerous because the subjects cannot identify the tyrant, and cannot even feel the tyranny.

Having lost track of real needs in favor of manufactured ones, people experience what Marcuse calls "euphoria in unhappiness" – a great phrase. Social critique in the 21st century has, no less deftly, called this epidemic disease "affluenza." The system needs the waste that lets us feel indulgently free. It keeps us stupefied, Marcuse writes, with "such deceptive liberties as … free choice between brands and gadgets," but "Free election of masters does not abolish the masters or the slaves."

Nor does religion offer a way out anymore. Avant-garde belief systems had become no more revolutionary than standard modern Christian groupthink: "Zen, existentialism, and beat ways of life" struck Marcuse as "no longer contradictory to the status quo and no longer negative. They are rather the ceremonial part of practical behaviorism … and are quickly digested by the status quo as part of its healthy diet."[40] Marcuse's food metaphor here is a version of the body-politic metaphor I have been using: a culture must not only defeat competitors, but must also develop enzymes that allow it to break down those rival bodies and convert them to its own energizing purposes. If, in the genetic competition among life-forms, "any increase in Machiavellian skill by one 'player in the game' will select for enhanced skill in the other,"[41] why wouldn't something similar happen between competing memeplexes? A fresh look at our world suggests they have become very good at that game, but are not making us good in the deeper and broader sense of that word.

Presumably no email has gone out from plutocrats@neoliberalism. com to a listserv of all the world's retailers and advertisers saying, "Keep distracting the multitudes with small comforts, sexual titillation, and status cues, so we can continue exploiting workers and the biosphere unimpeded, and we will cut you a small share of our nearly infinite riches." But the system did manage to send out that message – or to send out some equivalent of a hormone to provoke that function, which a feedback system indicated was necessary for the body-politic to maintain stasis. Not that the system cares whether it stays alive – again, it is a mistake to project intention – but it behaves the way a consciously self-protective being would, as people are (from one perspective) made of DNA clusters that behave as if they care, in convincing us to care about things that favor them. The version of our social system that has survived is, predictably, the version that was arrayed so that it would deploy this tactic. Many parasites, from viruses up to large complex organisms, depend on their ability to make their host-victims passive without making them quite dead.[42] Television seems often to have that effect, and so is a valued ally of many memeplexes.

If that seems surprisingly clever for something without a brain as such, especially when it requires controlling such clever creatures as we are, consider not only the seemingly fiendish exploitative ingenuity of viruses and parasites, but also the best-selling popular science writer Michael Pollan's demonstration that corn has used the human race (to our detriment) to spread its DNA.[43] Even more obviously, harmful products such as alcohol and tobacco convince us to reproduce them: they affect our brains and nervous systems in ways that cause us to brew and grow them on a massive scale.

So do more thoroughly artificial products. A century ago, the poet William Carlos Williams wrote of the telephone,

> Each time it rings
> I think it is for
> me but it is
> not for me nor for
>
> anyone it merely
> rings and we
> serve it bitterly
> together, they and I[44]

Many today feel themselves no less bitterly servile to their email servers and ubiquitous semi-urgent text messages. And many parents endure a daily struggle for the hearts and minds of their children, against video games that are constructed to offer the human mind the same kind of instant, instinctive, addictively intermittent gratifications that junk food offers the human body. The dealers don't have to buy and resell dope while at physical and legal risk; they just sell our youngsters the dopamine already stored in their brains, which was evolutionarily designed to guide them toward healthy outcomes. As I write this paragraph, fantasizing I can help liberate whole human societies from such skillful manipulators, I hear that very argument going on for the umpteenth time in our kitchen.

Looming in the data-cloud over all of us are vast and growing machine-learning programs that exist only because they can detect and direct our tendencies as consumers. Software that reads our web-surfing tendencies and offers us advertising targeted to our particular appetites mostly operates with no intervening human decision. The better a version of that software is at controlling us, the more marketers (whom it feeds) will build it, feed it with energy, provide it with protection, replicate it, deploy it, and help it teach itself how to get even better at controlling us. As I will explore in Chapter 7, it is not surprising that so many science fiction stories lately worry about the moment when machines unite into a conscious entity to which our human traits are merely an annoying inefficiency. But engineering our own escapes is difficult when we fail to recognize that our servants are really the prison guards – that the devices we use are also using us.

Technology gives so many of us a superficial feeling of personal power: it enables us to pursue our desires (in travel, diet, entertainment, and the quest for information) instantly, and broadcast our views just as fast. Yet technology is allied with the neoliberal money-meme in ways that, from the perspective of traditional humanistic values, look practically diabolical. In the creative arts and journalism, electronic reproduction has made it nearly impossible for most creators (of writing, images, or music) to make a living from their products. Digital technology makes it easier for financial institutions to skim off the wealth produced by other workers as well, and easier for large corporations to increase their profits by eliminating jobs, distributing the few remaining jobs to the lowest bidder worldwide, and policing the efficiency of those low-paid workers mercilessly. It seems increasingly clear that utopian predictions of a benign liberation from work by new technologies and free trade were either naïve or propagandistic.

The established nexus of social, cultural, and economic forces is so strongly presumed to be true and necessary that whatever dystopic outcomes the system generates are shrugged off as simply a cost of doing business, which is all there is to do. The means – the memes – are presumed to justify the ends. In some cases, our best hope may be to sustain a balance of power between opposing memeplexes competing for our loyalty – for example, setting globalizing capital against nationalistic rivalry – so we can move more freely where their fields of sway cancel each other out.

Despite all the complaints about various consequences of the system currently ruling the human world, the only real challenges to its fundamental premises arise from an emerging alliance of traditionalists and futurist visionaries. The traditionalists include cranky Luddites, people with sentimental memories of less crass times, and Catholics following Pope Francis's reboot of the Christian project of blending care for the needy with spiritual aspirations. The futurists are typified by groups like the anti-consumerist Adbusters organization, which defines itself as "a global network of culture jammers and creatives working to change the way information flows, the way corporations wield power, and the way meaning is produced in our society."

The traditionalist and futurist forms of resistance converge in the work of Jaron Lanier, one of the original visionaries of Virtual Reality. His 2010 manifesto *You Are Not a Gadget* pleads for the preservation of the wholeness of complex individual minds: a traditional humanistic project that Marxists might dismiss as bourgeois sentimentality. The dangers of the Internet that Lanier warns against make it seem a clear instance of the dangers of memeplexes: the Internet had been developing self-perpetuating and self-expanding functions not intended by its idealistic original inventors. Lanier further warns that until we recognize how these functions make themselves seem natural and inevitable, we can't intervene or make ourselves other than their servants. What Lanier and other engineers see as the problem of technological "lock-in" (the QWERTY keyboard is a notorious example) matches the competitive function I see in the memeplexes that survive. Along the lines of both Marcuse's warnings and my insect comparisons, Lanier asserts that, even while thinking the Internet was a liberating, generative novelty, "We had instead entered a persistent somnolence, and I have come to believe that we will only escape it when we kill the hive."[45]

These fundamental challenges will strike many people as silly, naive indulgences, or else as the hopeless task of Sisyphus in Greek myth, up against the relentlessness of gravity. But it is hard to know where to start – where to restart – without arts and humanistic thought, which have always combined a reverence toward the past with an idealism about possible futures. Creative artists and scholar-teachers have a central – and time-proven – role in enabling resistance to the evils produced by cultural evolution.

Debating Cultural Evolution

Each particular socio-cultural system seems an improbable survivor, considering all the complicated, resource-expensive, and sometimes destructive routines it obliges its body-politic to run and maintain. Yet it persists, usually because it has evolved the ability to invade its hosts almost unnoticed, assimilate the potentially disruptive foreign objects it encounters, turn them into sources of its own energy, and retain its ability to reproduce itself nearly identically over time.

The last category should not be underrated, despite the fact that we are no longer dealing with a primarily biological entity. Although memes – pieces of cultural information of various sizes, in overlapping combinations – are often transmitted by social rather than directly by sexual intercourse, they require carriers as much as viruses do. Compare the distribution of Catholic Christianity (which fiercely opposes birth control) with the distribution of Shaker Christianity (which fiercely advocated celibacy) over the past two centuries to see the point. The same function is visible in the rise of early Christianity, which encouraged large families (the Bible has God tell Adam and Eve to "Be fruitful and multiply" only 28 verses into its first book), in a society that often did not. Differential rates of durable replication determine the survival of ideas as well as of biological creatures.

Furthermore, Christianity has turned its wrath especially against abortion and homosexuality – by no means the sins the Bible or Jesus himself most actively condemned, but sins that directly limit the pro-creative fitness of the belief-system's carriers. When the president of the United States Conference of Catholic Bishops suggested considering humane exceptions to the church's strict ban on contraception, the Vatican not only refused, but began systematically limiting his authority.[46] In late 2017, conservative theologians at the Catholic University of America cancelled the scheduled speech of a well-known and widely popular Jesuit priest because he had written a book called *Building a Bridge: How the Catholic Church and the LGBT Community Can Enter into a Relationship of Respect, Compassion, and Sensitivity.* Catholicism again appears to have acted as if it were a creature determined to preserve its reproductive share in the memetic economy by preserving its advantages in the genetic economy.[47] Many sects within Orthodox Judaism appear to do the same.

From the perspective of a religious memeplex, wiping out carriers of rival beliefs is a useful supplement to breeding more of your own. Even religions whose original leaders and sacred texts seem to advocate love and tolerance toward those with other beliefs seem to evolve into religions demanding that such "infidels" be converted or killed. The 2017 massacres of Rohingya Muslims by a Buddhist majority, led by a Nobel Peace Prize winner, is only the latest of some painfully stark examples. Why would that keep happening unless the belief-systems that survive tend to be the ones that exploit their followers' craving for undisputed certainties and use those followers to suppress competing belief-systems?

Eminent anthropologists have noticed what appears to be a surprising paradox: religions that impose more severe demands on the time, wealth, comfort, and even safety of their members often out-compete religions that let their followers live more efficiently.

> Analyses show that religious groups with more costly rituals were more likely to survive over time than religious groups with fewer or less costly rituals .... greater ritual attendance predicts both declared willingness to die for one's god, or gods, and belief that other religions are responsible for problems in the world.

The same scholars observe that "Since natural selection tends to filter out behaviors and beliefs which do not contribute to an organism's fitness, it is difficult to see how costly religious behaviors ... could have originated, spread, and endured in so many societies."[48]

That all becomes much easier to explain, however, if we recognize the parasitic durability of belief-systems themselves, and their evolved fitness for the environment they inhabit, which is human consciousness in social situations. The resulting explanation is threefold. First, people who make such sacrifices feel more strictly guided by their memeplex, which we have seen is something the overloaded human mind craves.

Second, people who have sacrificed for their belief-system are therefore more invested in it, making them more willing to believe that "other religions are responsible for problems in the world" and are therefore worth fighting to the death.[49] Third, people who make major sacrifices are far more convincingly devoted to the greatness of their cause, which thereby gains credibility with onlookers because it has elicited more than a casual or feigned allegiance.

The survival of cultural systems is even easier to explain when their relationship to the members of their communities is mutualist rather than exploitative. Some cultural rituals promoted behavior that helped stabilize the natural environment that communities depended on, even though the practitioners did not recognize that purpose. A Nuer tribe thrived partly because their different culture allowed them to dominate their close kin, the Dinka.[50] Mutually reinforcing cultural and genetic evolution interact to shape everything from Tibetan marriage to the social contexts of the lactase enzyme.[51]

Lactase offers a classic instance of the co-evolutionary cycle that is at the heart of most "dual-inheritance" theories linking human genetic and cultural systems. Most human adults have trouble digesting milk because they lack the enzyme that turns lactose into glucose. Milk is food for baby mammals, and most of them stop producing that enzyme once they finish breastfeeding. In parts of the world that raise animals for their milk, however, most people have a dominant allele that lets them continue producing it. That genetic variant has developed unusually quickly, becoming widespread in Northern Europe over the past 5,000 to 9,000 years, evidently because of the variant's cyclical interaction with the cultural variant called dairy farming.[52]

Dairy-farming apparently came first, but it gave a reproductive advantage to those who could continue to feed on milk when necessary. As more and more such people appeared in the population, there was more and more reason to tend more cows. And the more cows there were making milk as a primary food for the community, the more people with the gene out-survived and out-reproduced those without it. That lactose-processing trait also arises in populations (such as some in India) conquered by foreigners who practiced dairy farming, and has apparently developed independently in six separate populations of dairy farmers, while Mediterranean people have mostly worked around the problem in a different way, literally culturing milk into lactose-free products such as yogurt and cheese.[53] Changes in human cultures and changes in human genes can thus reinforce each other rapidly and cyclically – and cultures can make a population increasingly dependent on them, dictating the shape and rhythms of a society's very way of life.

A larger scale version of the autocatalytic cycle that promoted lactase seems to have produced a genetic innovation in the hominid brain that enabled cultural learning and complexity, which gave a reproductive advantage to minds capable of managing them: education, cooperation, and detailed communication through language have surely been primary factors in the competitive success of our species.[54] Those upgraded brains, in turn, enabled further cultural refinements, which rewarded even more brain-power – at least, as long as the cultural forms kept that brain-power in productive channels, reducing the burdens of decision-making and occasions for intra-group conflict.

Some geneticists nonetheless question whether there is any mechanism of inheritance in the realm of memes. But parents obviously transmit cultural as well as genetic information, and teachers and books also transmit a cultural heritage. Furthermore, cooperating in the tribe's mutually re-assuring system of belief and symbolization improves the odds of bodily and psychic survival, as well as the odds of mating and having one's offspring valued by the tribe. So cultural systems tend to conserve their identities.[55] As Ernest Gellner remarks, "any single theoretical innovation is most unlikely to be successful. On top of this, the innovation will constitute (at best) a social solecism, or possibly some worse kind of transgression."[56] Consider the fate of antinomians such as Anne Hutchinson, whose dissenting theology caused her to be driven out of the New England colonies into the wilderness, where all but one of her hard-raised household of 16 were massacred in 1643 by Siwanoy when that tribe's feud with the Dutch exploded. An established meme and its loyalists can radically improve each other's likelihood of survival and reproduction.

In the world of academia, the memeplex of biological sciences naturally competes with the memeplex of social sciences. The great paleontologist and popular science writer Stephen Jay Gould refused, and other evolutionary biologists still refuse, to treat the scenarios offered by cultural evolutionists as hypotheses, insisting instead on calling them "just-so stories." That, however, is an overly dismissive term for abductive reasoning: the inference of the likeliest explanation from a range of instances, which is the intent of this book.[57] The only fair measure is whether the explanatory story being offered fits the available evidence better than other stories. DNA and other evidence assures us that the first armadillos were not (as Rudyard Kipling's *Just-So Stories* playfully assert) a combination of hedgehog and turtle, and that leopard spots are not the fingerprints of an Ethiopian man. But what explanation for the dominion of various religious, political, economic, and symbolic systems makes more sense than that they have evolved opportunistically in their changing environments? And that those which – lovely though they may have been – could neither reproduce themselves efficiently nor adapt in a competitive universe have gone extinct?

In the *New Yorker* magazine a few years ago, the distinguished polymath Anthony Gottlieb scoffed at David Barash's *Homo Mysterious:*

Evolutionary Puzzles of Human Nature for concluding "that it is 'highly likely' that religion owes its origin to natural selection." Gottlieb rejected that conclusion as an unjustified "article of faith."[58] But what alternative explanation for the near ubiquity of religions, nearly all of them mutually exclusive, in human cultures across time and geographies, is so persuasive as to render an evolutionary basis unlikely? Gottlieb finally dismissed the entire project of trying to understand how the human mind has evolved:

> To confirm any story about how the mind has been shaped, you need (among other things) to determine how people today actually think and behave, and to test rival accounts of how these traits function. Once you have done that, you will, in effect, have finished the job of explaining how the mind works.[59]

Concern for the well-being of my readers obliges me to recommend against holding our breaths awaiting the completion of that job; instead, I intend to continue a conversation that, in this as in many fields, may get us closer to some useful truths by pondering how things have come to be as they are. There is something remarkably anti-humanistic and even anti-intellectual about assuming that imperfect knowledge is no knowledge, and that we can simply chart the present and skip the fool's errand of speculating about the past and its implications for the future. Does a snapshot always tell us more than a story?

Certainly it is possible to recognize, not only in religion but also in jingoism and its accompanying hard ideologies all over the world, evidence that (as the eminent philosopher of cognitive evolution Daniel Dennett puts it),

> Memes that are fortunate enough to have stewards, people who will work hard and use their intelligence to foster their propagation and protect them from their enemies, are relieved of much of the burden of keeping their own lineages going.[60]

That so many Christian priests and missionaries have believed propagating and protecting the Word to be even more important than doing the same for their own genetic offspring seems strong evidence that memeplexes can sometimes compete successfully against other evolutionary drives. So does the plea "Give me liberty, or give me death!" that is often attributed to Patrick Henry as a foundational moment of the American Revolution. That plea recurs in a degraded form in the slogan "Better dead than Red" that epitomized American resistance to Communism during the Cold War, and has settled comfortably into the motto of New Hampshire: "Live Free or Die." It matters, of course, who gets to define freedom.

The Cold War provides an interesting, large-scale, contemporary instance of competition between memeplexes. The opposition between Communism and capitalism goes beyond economic policy and geopolitics. Where capitalism strives to mystify its own ideological character and conceal its nature as an evolving memeplex, Communism announces itself as one. The USSR attempted to do consciously, at a central administrative level, what the human collective evolves to do anyway: invest in the maximum survival of its membership as the ultimate moral imperative. The value of altruism to the genetic community of a species presumably helps establish that imperative in *Homo sapiens*, which does not mean that morality is merely illusory, nor that it is inherently good.[61] The Soviet Communist giant staggered and fell, partly because (as with other utopian movements) that deliberate version of the human conspiracy is at once too complicated and too simplified, like trying to walk by issuing a sequence of conscious commands to the relevant sequence of muscle groups, rather than allowing unselfconscious habits to take their course. Muscle-memory, which is a kind of accumulated personal tradition, is more efficient than a flurry of bureaucratic memos from the conscious mind.[62]

Furthermore, the Communist ideology was so close to the fundamental self-replicating mission of our genes and the pervasive community-consensus mission of a culture that it left no room for intellectual dissent or seemingly frivolous (rather than programmatically instrumental) artistic creativity. On a practical level, bureaucratic functions metastasized, while their supposed functionaries were still humanly capable of craving and holding old-fashioned power, status, and material benefits for themselves and their families. The very fact that cultural systems so maladaptive for their human populations can develop and spread seems to be evidence that these systems are, to some extent, independent agents.[63]

* * * * * * * * * * * *

My argument for this phenomenon is speculative and discursive. I am not producing the rigorous taxonomy and quantification of the quasi-evolutionary processes of cultural change that some geneticists, linguists, and anthropologists might offer. Fortunately for me, those more technical approaches have been pursued masterfully in recent books such as Alex Mesoudi's *Cultural Evolution: How Darwinian Theory Can Explain Human Culture & Synthesize the Social Sciences.*[64] Reviewers have been duly impressed with the evidence Mesoudi has gathered. Their reservations have focused on the book's project of uniting all social science around cultural evolution, on its reluctance to "treat culture as a *system*" or ask "how the dynamic stability of the system comes about,"[65] and on its tendency to see cultural evolution as fundamentally benign and progressive. While building on the work of Mesoudi and others, I am making no such imperial claims within social science, only asking (no small request, I admit) that cognitive neuroscience, evolutionary biology, cultural anthropology, and the arts and humanities notice one way their fields may interact. And what I am arguing such interaction reveals is precisely how the development of cultural systems toward stability can do us damage while camouflaging that effect, and how that damage can be recognized and mitigated.

Despite that book, despite many relevant scientific findings, despite a range of important scholarly studies of the role of the arts in the evolutionary process,[66] and despite a spike of books within just the past few years analyzing that process, the notion that cultures evolve at all continues to be brushed off as folly by some biologists. Perhaps the most prominent voices of that dismissiveness have been the brilliant and combative geneticist Richard Lewontin and his collaborator Joseph Fracchia, a theory-minded historian.[67] They claim that culture cannot evolve because a society is not an organism, and that it is not an organism because persons exercise will, whereas cells do not. That claim relies on an assumption that human individuals are basically autonomous, which has been widely refuted by major social theorists, and also relies on an oddly narrow definition of the forms of interaction possible within an organism, despite overwhelming evidence of mixed competition and cooperation within the microbiome of any given person. In general, non-malignant cells respond to their local biochemical milieu, as more elaborate life-forms do. So, people do not make wholly free choices, and cells make choices based on the balance of information they receive.

Fracchia and Lewontin see no point in trying to trace evolutionary aspects of (for example) language or technology, because the mechanisms by which a memeplex would evolve do not look exactly like the ones by which an animal would. We may observe a process of selection and reproduction by which an old cultural entity changed into a new one better fitted to its changing environment (which is not merely a biological or atmospheric environment). Yet, because their standard rule and technology cannot measure it quantitatively, Fracchia and Lewontin deny that cultural evolution exists: "for a variational theory, it must be possible to count up the number of times each variant is represented." That is surely not how all valuable observations about human societies begin, nor is it where many of them end. To the common warning that someone equipped only with a hammer is likely to see every problem as a nail, I would add that someone equipped only with an excellent Philips screwdriver may be tempted to insist that a slotted screw is not a screw at all, and therefore not worth turning.

Even if we accept Fracchia and Lewontin's narrow definitions, the work of Russell Gray and Mark Pagel in historical linguistics suggests that it is possible to identify and quantify the spread of variants of the same word and thereby to reconstruct the evolution of language using phylogenetic methods. Linguistic cultural transmission closely matches genetic models.[68] A 2008 study in the journal *Behavioural and Brain Sciences* concludes that language functions as "a complex and interdependent 'organism', which evolves under selectional pressures."[69] Charles Darwin himself wrote,

> The formation of different languages and of distinct species, and the proofs that both have been developed through a gradual process, are curiously parallel .... Dominant languages and dialects spread widely, and lead to the gradual extinction of other tongues. A language, like a species, when once extinct, never, as Sir C. Lyell remarks, reappears .... We see variability in every tongue, and new words are continually cropping up; but as there is a limit to the powers of the memory, single words, like whole languages, gradually become extinct. As Max Muller has well remarked: "A struggle for life is constantly going on amongst the words and grammatical forms in each language. The better, the shorter, the easier forms are constantly gaining the upper hand, and they owe their success to their own inherent virtue." ... The survival or preservation of certain favoured words in the struggle for existence is natural selection.[70]

The critical moment for the long-term survival of neologisms occurs about 40 years after their emergence, presumably because a next generation either does or doesn't sustain and transmit the verbal usages they learned from their parents during childhood.[71]

My own research has shown that Shakespeare's impact on the English language doesn't result (as widely supposed) from a prodigiously large vocabulary. It results instead from his talent for making his neologisms "sticky." Shakespeare consistently framed the new words with contextual definitions so they could be understood and utilized by those who heard or read them. And his environment made these novel locutions valuable for listeners and readers: in the unprecedented melting-pot of languages and dialects as well as social classes that was Elizabethan London, the ability to speak and understand the very latest (and hence coolest) products of linguistic evolution was essential for status (and hence survival).[72] Shakespeare engineered his offspring to thrive in their environment. As Gary Taylor, a leading editor of Renaissance drama, has demonstrated, lasting masterpieces have a talent for making themselves memorable in multiple situations, so they can continue to compete successfully for carriers.[73] So, while I am grateful to Lewontin and Fracchia for their eloquent defense of literary study and the humanities in general against reductive approaches from the sciences, I believe there are important insights to be gained by positive dialogue along that disciplinary border.

Fracchia and Lewontin further complain that "a fundamental problem results from the assumption that these cultural units, say, the idea of monotheism ... somehow spread or disappear from human populations, namely, no theory of cultural evolution has provided the elementary properties of these abstract units." So, unless their taxonomy fits, unless there is an allele to be tracked, they would forbid us to assume that religions develop and either propagate or go extinct – despite the fact that they obviously do. Was Darwin's theory baseless and worthless because he couldn't identify or quantify the exact mechanisms and "elementary properties" of genetic replication? Would they insist that Mendel never did genetics and should be ignored, since he had not mapped the genome of the pea plants he studied, only looked at patterns among the outcomes? Fracchia and Lewontin accuse memeticists of ignoring the fact that

> there must be some mechanism by which a new generation of successors retains some vestige of the changes that occurred in a previous time .... Theorists of cultural evolution, ... do not even know whether an actor-to-actor, not to speak of a parent-to-offspring, model of the passage of culture has any general applicability.[74]

It is as if they had never heard of a scholarly book, or a debate developing over time, even though they were participating in both as they said so.

Insisting that, if some phenomenon is difficult to measure exactly, it must not exist, seems rash. Yet Fracchia and Lewontin dismiss any study of what certainly looks like "descent with modification" (to use Darwin's term) as non-science, rather than just not a particular kind of science at this point in its development. Furthermore, they persistently attack explorers of cultural evolution for claiming that such evolution explains everything (a claim few serious scholars in the field would ever make), or for failing to explain everything. Fracchia and Lewontin set up memeticist straw-men who do not and cannot recognize the importance of historical particulars, among which they repeatedly and tendentiously list outrages such as "Nazi persecution of Jews" and "the genocide of Native Americans," as if those crimes were an inevitable side-effect of any sociobiological hypothesis, and as if those horrors had nothing to do with aspects of cultures that make them thrive or expire under particular circumstances. Would they say that genetic science is useless because it doesn't by itself explain the decline in Jewish-ancestry DNA in Europe in the decade beginning in 1939, or of Native American-ancestry DNA in the United States in the century beginning in 1830?

Proposing causal explanations can be useful, even when (as Fracchia and Lewontin complain) that information is insufficient to predict exactly what will happen next in a highly complex system of emergent phenomena. Too narrow an insistence on a genetic model may, Michael

Carrithers has warned, wrongly preclude a theory of memeplexes that could "help in clarifying the possibility of sociocultural diversity." So, as the eminent and versatile biologist David L. Hull also urged,[75] I am resisting the tendency to insist on a complete and completely satisfactory theoretical explanation for memes and their evolution, and instead testing whether some illuminating ideas can be achieved by recognizing that something like reproductive fitness works on cultural practices shared by a number of people, as well as on genes similarly shared.

The reluctance to recognize Darwinian evolution shaping cultures has been eroding. Shennan offers his readers a helpfully tangible and specific instance, though one that evades some of the complications of evolution for entities such as cultural systems that are more multiple in their functions and more overlapping in their instances. The replacement of snowshoes by snowmobiles "*is* an evolutionary process, not just some more or less plausible analogy to genetics."[76] There have been generations of each device, transmitted with modifications and selectively multiplied according to their fitness to their niche (Cree hunters who make or buy such things to get around northern Canada). As the efficiency of snowmobiles improved, snowshoes are decreasingly produced, and as the old ones fall apart, snowshoes head toward extinction. More broadly, Shennan concludes that

> The fact that cultural transmission operates through social learning does not make it less Darwinian than genetic transmission. Both are specific instances, with their own properties, of a more general category of information transfer processes that lead to the production of heritable variation and its modifications through time.[77]

Peter J. Richerson and Robert Boyd "urge great care with loose analogies to mutation and selection because several distinct processes" influence cultural developments, "and none exactly like natural selection,"[78] but they end up finding many places where the similarities are illuminating. For example, "Religious innovations are a lot like mutations, and successful religions are adapted in sophisticated ways beyond the ken of individual innovators."[79]

The further objection has often been two-pronged: that memes, as Richard Dawkins initially proposed them, are too particulate to be meaningfully traced, while larger cultural entities (including what I am calling memeplexes) are not consistently enough grouped to be shaped by evolutionary processes. On the first point, however, Richerson and Boyd argue that "A Darwinian account of culture does not imply that culture must be divisible into tiny, independent genelike bits that are faithfully replicated."[80] On the second point, they note that functions such as "moralistic punishment and conformist bias" keep cultures different enough from each other, and integral enough to themselves, to produce group selection.[81] Their analysis on these points does not seem one-sided. I would add that a closely related competitive process could govern the selection of a region's cultural norms and structures. If a group excelled as warriors, or as farmers, and thereby dominated, assimilated and/or eliminated lots of otherwise competing groups, presumably a set of warrior or farmer cultural values would spread.

Cultural evolutionists have not ignored questions about the validity of a Darwinian model. Dan Sperber has performed a perceptive epidemiology of representations (resembling what others call memes) that emphasizes the combination of suitability to human cognition and suitability to the functions of a local environment. He doubts that memes undergo Darwinian evolution, since there is more transformation than replication in their transmission, though he believes that the psychological mechanisms shaping these anthropological phenomena are themselves Darwinian.[82]

Joseph Carroll's otherwise helpful summary of the field he calls "Literary Darwinism" rejects any "supposed parallel" because "No idea or cultural practice contains a molecular mechanism adapted by natural selection to replicate itself."[83] Take out the word "molecular," however – that is, think about Darwinism rather than the technical neo-Darwinian focus on genes – and the objection disappears. Carroll further objects that, because memes have to exist in human carriers, "Memes could thus not be 'autonomous' in the way that genes are autonomous." But genes can hardly thrive outside their carriers, and evolution cannot work on genes alone: it works on the bio-physical expression of those genes as they create an "ism" known as an organism. Anyway, just because memeplexes are shaped by the psychological structures of the human mind does not preclude them evolving in self-preserving ways as they interact with those structures. Most forms of life would not count as examples of natural selection if we eliminated all instances that co-evolve with other forms of life and are shaped by the requirements of their environment.

Even those who believe cultures could evolve competitively have tended to assume that the survivors would be adaptive for their population, but that assumption, too, has begun to erode. Richerson and Boyd have noticed that "rogue cultural variants evolve devious strategies to evade the effects" of their negative attributes, and that "Because the rate of cultural adaptation is rapid compared with genetic evolution, rogue variants will often win arms races with genes." They later write that in "a simulation of a Darwinian system using imitation instead of genes, natural selection created conditions that allow selfish cultural variants to spread," and that "moralistic punishment can stabilize *any* arbitrary behavior – wearing a tie, being kind to animals, or eating the brains of dead relatives .... moralistic punishment can stabilize cooperation, but it can also stabilize anything else."[84] Another leading figure in this field,

Joseph Henrich, concludes that "social norms will tend to remain stable even when they help neither the group nor the individual," as in cases such as female genital cutting.[85]

Schopenhauer's encompassing "will to life" – which is not a property only of individuals – may help to explain the seeming life-force within even seemingly inanimate creatures such as cultural memes, including political systems. Schopenhauer's heir Nietzsche attributes an organismic drive to social orders as well as individuals:

> Even the body within which individuals treat each other as equals, as suggested before – and this happens in every healthy aristocracy – if it is a living and not a dying body, has to do to other bodies what the individuals within it refrain from doing to each other: it will have to be an incarnate will to power, it will strive to grow, spread, seize, become predominant – not from any morality or immorality but because it is *living* and because life simply *is* will to power.[86]

The role of this idea in the ascendancy of Nazism does not discredit it, since that horror epitomizes the way such an entity can disable humane reflexes.

The notion that ideas have a real existence independent of any specific human thinker is hardly a radically new one. It was prominent as early as Plato's theory of Forms. The Averroists of the mid-13th century maintained that ideas exist apart from the individual persons who may hold them at any time. A belief in monopsychism – that our minds and souls only seem individual, but are in fact part of some larger whole – runs through many ancient and modern mystic traditions, including some Kabbalist and Rastafarian cults that have rebounded in recent decades. Even mainstream Christian theology has frequently maintained that the essential ideas have their real existence in the mind of God, where our mind-souls can draw on them. I am merely proposing a more distributed model.

My claim requires only an acknowledgment that beliefs can function in a way not wholly subordinate to the individuals who hold them, but can instead travel through history and evolve through varying reproductive success as conditions around them develop. In the 19th and 20th centuries, in response not only to Darwin but also to social trauma (especially the US Civil War) other major modern intellectuals such as William James, Oliver Wendell Holmes, Jr., and John Dewey came to believe

> that ideas are produced not by individuals, but by groups of individuals – that ideas are social. They believed that ideas do not develop according to some inner logic of their own, but are entirely dependent, like germs, on their human carriers and environment. And they believed that since ideas are provisional responses to

particular and unreproducible circumstances, their survival depends not on their immutability but on their adaptability.[87]

What I am suggesting is that, as human evolution led to cognitive overload, which, in turn, necessitated culture (as my first chapter explained), cultures themselves have evolved into forces with a life of their own. We therefore need to be prepared to train them while they are training us.

Human beings and their cultures have survived in each other, and been perpetually reshaped by each other – by their need for each other – since the early days of our species. Ideas cannot thrive if they require receptors that would not at some point have benefited human beings to develop, and human minds are remarkably bad at forming, maintaining, and transmitting ideas about things such as consciousness, free will, and mirror reflections – all things that require us to see ourselves without quite being ourselves. These kinds of ideas are evidently subject to what Colin McGinn calls "cognitive closure";[88] my belief is that cognition *is* largely closure, or at least that cognition is impossible without culture's assistance in closing down unsettling questions and closing out most possibilities.

As Freud's super-ego constitutes the internalization of a culture's moral rules, so culture constitutes an externalization of the top-down aspect of the cognitive process, which applies templates and memorial contexts to the bottom-up supply of potentially chaotic sense-data. Culture offers a society what heuristics offer the individual: short-cuts for answering potentially exhausting mental problems, usually good enough to replace exact analysis, but subject to patterns of error that allow us to be foolish and systematically exploitable.

This defensive taming of reality can be costly for individuals as well as for groups. Freud asserts that "hysterics are undoubtedly imaginative artists" and that "the ceremonials and prohibitions of obsessional neurotics drive us to suppose that they have created a private religion of their own," leading him to conclude that

> these patients are, in an *asocial* fashion, making the very attempts at solving their conflicts and appeasing their pressing needs which, when those attempts are carried out in a fashion that is acceptable to the majority, are known as poetry, religion, and philosophy.[89]

These neurotic defenses are failed artworks, however; not only because they are private rather than communal in the liberation they attempt but also because what they attempt may not be liberation at all, but instead the appeasement of a neurosis. The failure of private mental defenses should alert us to the possibility that public versions can perform a similarly self-empowering entrapment on their cultural constituencies.

Stephen Jay Gould convincingly argued against imposing a teleology – a meaningful purpose or ultimate goal – on biological evolution. Viewing cultural change as necessarily improvement may be wrong for similar reasons. Evolution is a survival of what fits – and what thrives in Chicago might die out quickly in Beijing, and what thrived in Chicago in 1920 may fail in Chicago in 2020. Marxist and Soviet theory sometimes overlooked this fact because its "dialectical materialism" wanted to describe all of human social history as a series of battles between contradictory systems leading toward the ideal justice of communism. Naturally the Marxist Soviet leaders liked to believe their dominance to be both inevitable and beneficial. But that belief mistakes social evolution for social progress – the survival of the fittest leading to some eternal best.

This book aspires to correct a common version of that mistake: the assumption that cultures are a freely chosen reflection of a human community's developing wisdom. Correcting that assumption is not a risk-free project in an era when, at least on some elite campuses, the critique of cultural formations is presumptively outrageous if those forms belong primarily to historically oppressed groups and the critic does not. But my point is far from imperialist: the dire mistake that so many arrogant colonial invaders made was assuming, first, that conquest was proof of virtue, and, second, that what worked in the conqueror's home physical and social environment would also be helpful in the world of the conquered.

Social systems usually evolve toward stability, despite the challenges imposed as technologies increase interactions with alternative systems – or maybe because of those collisions. If the question is whether globalization is an expansion or a narrowing, the answer may be that the former provokes the latter. Multinational corporations co-evolve with consumer capitalism, taming cultural conflict by putting the same mass retailers in malls worldwide, and logos provide what local tribalism no longer can. Individuals reflexively support that stability and homogenization, because peace of mind depends on believing that the culture is optimal or inevitable, and on having clear channels for pursuing designated objects of desire.

The intensely capitalist character of Vietnam in the 21st century shows that the seductive powers of consumer culture, even over quite a modest span of time, can overpower brute military force; the Communists won the war, but lost the culture-war, which proved more consequential. On a broader scale of time and space, "Over the millennia, small, simple cultures gradually coalesce into bigger and more complex civilisations, so that the world contains fewer and fewer mega-cultures, each of which is bigger and more complex"[90] – another suggestive correspondence between biological and cultural evolution.

How can we use the recognition that culture has taken over some of the work of genetics? The influential media-theorist Marshall McLuhan moved from the idea of a perpetually conflicted "global village" to the idea of an encompassing human-technological culture that "ends 'Nature' and turns the globe into a repertory theater to be programmed."[91] A related observation is evident in the title of the admirable environmental advocate Bill McKibben's meditations: *The End of Nature*. That book and McKibben's subsequent book *Eaarth* suggest that human beings have become, however clumsily and at times unwittingly, the drivers of nature rather than just its subjects.[92] That change is analogous to my claim that we struggle with the complications of managing for ourselves (through individual deliberation and collective culture) many functions that basic biology has managed for most creatures. Francis Bacon's dream of humanity ruling nature instead of being ruled by it has seemingly come true. That dream seems increasingly like a nightmare, however: not only because we evidently lack the wisdom or self-discipline to manage something as big and complex as the biosphere but also because we cannot assume our culture will be programmed with any real ethical and prudential intelligence.

If we are in the repertory theater posited by McLuhan, we need to ask whether we can become its open-minded, open-hearted playwrights rather than its scripted actors. Fortunately, if we recognize the globe as a theater and want it to become a drama that evokes the deepest qualities of human beings, we do have the example of Shakespeare, whose Globe theater bore the motto, *totus mundus agit histrionem*: the whole world acts in plays.

Mutation, Dissent, and the Agents of Social Change

If cultures evolve, then some of their functions will resemble the functions of other evolving entities. People often enlist in the defense-mechanism of their socio-cultural systems. Reactionaries during crises of conformism may resemble white blood-cells, rushing to the rescue of the self-identity of the collective body-politic. Gossip, for example, has long been a key element in a culture's immune system, attacking behavioral variants – a system intensified by social media and the mass shaming it encourages.[93] But an immune system needs to be good at recognizing the difference between invaders and what are really parts of the healthy self, lest it generate an autoimmune illness such as Type 1 diabetes, lupus, multiple sclerosis, or rheumatoid arthritis. In confronting invaders, it also needs to distinguish between energizing mutualists – some of whom we need to survive – and parasitical rivals, including viral hijackers of the cell's normal program. Even if these are only metaphors for the functions and malfunctions of cultures – and I suspect they are more than that – they helpfully describe a complicated phenomenon that may otherwise be hard to see.

Could these memeplexes really have evolved into deft manipulators of the human groups that serve as their carriers? It seems more plausible if we recognize that such cultural formations were created partly to control our dangerously open and complex consciousness by offering an integrated world-view that is shared by a community. If channeling our thinking is something they are made for, then that is something they will be good at – and better after ceaseless iterations of consequential trial and error in competition with other variants.

For similar reasons, tracing the exact relationship between a memeplex and the behavioral phenotype it produces may actually be easier than parallel efforts with genes. The eye-catching reports in popular media that scientists have "found the gene for" formerly mysterious aspects of mental life are often excessive and reductive, producing publicity at the cost of nuance.[94] A gene may code for multiple traits, a trait may be controlled by multiple genes, and environmental factors affect what phenotypes emerge.Studies of the fruit-fly *Drosophila*, however, prove that many peculiar details of behavior are consistently associated with genes selected by evolution.

It is fair to wonder whether human social systems have endured enough successive generations to evolve the complex survival tactics I attribute to them. But the key failings I detect in modern Western culture were already underway and under protest in ancient Western culture. "In the sixth century B.C.E., Theognis of Megara was already lamenting the decline of ethics as wealth and individualism rose."[95] With the right agent, Theognis could easily have gotten his lament on many mainstream 21st-century media outlets.

In cultural evolution, dissent is mutation: an offer of a future that is unlikely to gain lasting acceptance. Since a mutation has not been selected by a long history of survival, it is much more likely to be extinguished than passed along over multiple generations. There is a reason our genetic code has gotten so good at copying itself and fixing errors. While most mutations are inconsequential, most of the consequential ones are destructive. In the body as in the body-politic, mutations can be cancerous. In national politics, revolutions are rarely bloodless and always incomplete, even when fundamentally benign, even when driven by what seems enlightened consciousness opposing tyrannous overlords. Look at the French Revolution, the Russian Revolution, the gangsterish aftermath of the overthrow of Soviet Communism, and the nightmarish fall of the Arab Spring. Outside of an improv troupe or a brainstorming session, "no" is often a good default answer to initiatives. Rats evidently find it safer to focus on whatever foods their fellow rats have survived eating.[96] That pattern of diet shows how the natural conservatism of culture can actually produce fads, which are more like a self-limiting virus-driven fever than like a true mutation within the cultural body.

Not all cultural variants are as uncorrelated to the needs to the organism as genetic mutations are, however. Some, such as deeply considered utopian visions, are versions of directed mutation or of horticultural grafting and selective breeding. In both the biological and cultural instances, the collective depends on the presence of variants if it is to adapt to environmental shifts over time. This is a major survival-value of sexual reproduction, which mixes genomes and recombines alleles; the jumble produces the variations that enable evolutionary selection to work on a species, allowing that species survive a changing world through many generations.

A vivid cultural instance of that value is the fact that

> The florescence of art in the Upper Paleolithic ... has been explained as a response to sweeping climatic change. Specifically, these art products are believed to have been used to exchange information requisite to the implementation of novel hunting strategies necessitated by changes in faunal dispersal patterns.[97]

As Brown and Richerson observe, "the Pleistocene was a stunningly variable environment that was statistically quite unpredictable .... glacial environments became increasingly packed with high amplitude noisy variation," and

> social learning would be most useful in environments with lots of unpredictable variation that is concentrated in events with durations too long for adaptation by individual learning but too short for genetic adaptations to evolve, just the sorts of variation that typify the Pleistocene. Human cultural complexity and brain size increases appear to have roughly paralleled this increase in climatic variability.[98]

In other words, the peculiarities of the human brain, including its investment in the strange practice of the arts, apparently emerged from a period where such flexible and creative thinking was a key to surviving changing conditions. The same may be true in the 21st century. More generally,

> when the pace of environmental change becomes too fast and the number of challenges too great, genetically fixed if-then rules break down and must be supplemented by rapid non-genetic evolutionary processes that generate and select new solutions to current problems. As for the immune system, so also for psychological and cultural processes.[99]

It can therefore benefit a collective to have a few outliers of varying kinds and degrees even though it will lose most of them because they fail to reproduce.

The value of mutability greatly increases if a mutation's likely consequences can be evaluated before they must be fully lived, before the mutant diverts significant community resources to its own struggle for survival. Drama deliberately generates variations (of ritual, diction, personal behavior, and the structures of perception) in a safe containment of formal convention and acknowledged fictionality. As we make decisions, we run scenarios through our heads. The tragic tale of Shakespeare's Ophelia, for example, can warn people away from deadly mistakes, whereas an unhealthy mutation in nature's *Drosophila* can be stopped only by the extinction of its carriers. Our species has developed ways of accelerating the evolution of culture, particularly through the hypotheticals of art. We are all – and artists are especially – experimental disrupters in this engineering of human society, and we do it partly by a version of the rapid-prototyping practices now gaining favor among designers of material objects and software programs.

That is part of the value of universities, which convene a group of intellectual mutants and mutagens assigned to cooperate in developing and testing ideas that seem promising. They discard some and propagate others – as even medieval scribes did[100] – while also maintaining a bias toward the accurate preservation of the cultural past in archives, schematics, and analysis of history's lessons. And, as for scribes and other copyists over recent centuries, a fundamental precept remains *lectio difficilior potior:* when faced with a choice, prefer the stranger instance, the more difficult word, and preserve an odd variant rather than what has likely been produced by mere conformism to common sense by some intervening transcriber.

A key virtue of electoral democracy, quite distinct from the ethical argument that people should all have equal shares in determining how they are ruled (which Shakespeare, among many other shrewd observers, seems to have doubted), is simply that it imposes periodic peer-review, whereby the policies of state are tested against the experiences of an electorate that judges how well those policies fit their current needs and beliefs. That makes it harder for tyrants – including tyrannical memeplexes – to stifle dissent against their self-perpetuating project.

Scholarly peer-review and art reviewers are hardly error-proof, any more than elections have been, but they are the redundancy built into this system of cultural engineering to make it more reliable. The adversarial aspect of reviews and the respect for critique in these areas of human endeavor help this system resist becoming itself an exploitative memeplex (although they don't provide immunity against less intellectual forms of exploitation, as many graduate students and adjunct faculty can testify). Arts communities and universities certainly develop some unhealthy collusive functions: trading rave reviews instead of giving honest ones ("log-rolling"), for instance, complacently adopting fashionable new orthodoxies, or even just pretending to understand and admire each other in conference Q&A sessions. Unlike many other sociological phenomena, however, these groups have established defenses to mitigate that tendency. The genres of satire and parody – mock-epic, for example – are partly devices kept handy so literature can explode its own decadent memeplexes.

High-level science is surprisingly similar to great art in this regard. Lacking as much experience on this side, I will quote Bernice Eiduson's remarkable study of top-flight 20th-century scientists at Berkeley. Eiduson found that their "Heightened sensitivity is accompanied in thinking by overalertness to relatively unimportant or tangential aspects of problems," which

> encourages highly individualized and even autistic ways of thinking. Were this thinking not in the framework of scientific work, it would be considered paranoid. In scientific work, creative thinking demands seeing things not seen previously, or in ways not previously imagined; and this necessitates jumping off from "normal" positions, and taking risks by departing from reality. The difference between the thinking of the paranoid patient and the scientist comes from the latter's ability and willingness to test out his fantasies or grandiose conceptualizations through the systems of checks and balances science has established .... Without this structuring, the threat of such unrealistic, illogical, and even bizarre thinking to overall thought and personality organization in general would be too great ....[101]

The next chapter will show how dependent the success of artistic genius is on a similar mixture of norms and deviations, and why both science and art offer promising ways out of the trap of self-perpetuating cultural functions that have become harmful.

Even with this guidance, mutation may be especially advantageous in environments that change very rapidly. But we have created such environments, the Los Angeles of 2018 – my here and now – being a prime example. Densely populated, culturally diverse places where both people and information are constantly in agitated motion produce a feedback loop of accelerating change, at least as measured by technological change.[102] This process is reflected in the emphasis on new and crossover art forms in urban settings, in contrast to the arts and crafts of (say) small and isolated Amazonian tribes, which are almost purely conformist and traditional, with the ideal performance perfectly matching the received songs and steps. In culture as in genetics, small and isolated populations lose diversity: memes, language, and artistic form all show diminished complexity and variation.[103]

The reproduction of cultures includes what Gould and Lewontin call "spandrels" in genetic reproduction: attributes that no longer serve any valuable function, but tag along inside us as side-effects of some inheritance that does, so that their wastefulness goes unnoticed and unpunished. According to the anthropologists Boyd and Richerson, the balance between the efficiency of cultural conservatism and the need for occasional innovations is

> an interesting problem for economists. Traditions often work; when they do, they are useful because they reduce the costs of acquiring information and lower the possibility of making errors. However, if everyone were to depend exclusively on traditional rules, what would cause traditional rules to be modified in response to changes in the environment?[104]

My point is that the same question should interest scholars beyond economics: students of cultural change, especially at the fertile borderlands of sociology and psychology (including cognitive science).

For most evolutionary psychologists, "culture is the manufactured product of evolved psychological mechanisms situated in individuals living in groups."[105] But – as Bradd Shore demonstrated in an earlier effort to connect psychology to sociology[106] – culture is also an evolving, self-replicating entity with many attributes that cannot be easily explained by mechanisms of Pleistocene psychology. Kim Sterelny has made a strong argument that the human mind was formed less to meet any highly specific needs of Pleistocene survival and reproduction than to be adaptable to changing physical and informational regimes.[107] What those mechanisms can partly explain, however, is our extreme vulnerability to the drive of surviving cultures to replicate, even when those cultural forces offer no real compensation. As Brown and Richerson observe,

> recent work in developmental and comparative psychology shows that human culture does in fact transmit information quite accurately by cognitive systems apparently selected for that exact purpose rather than for restricting variation by strongly biasing what can be learned .... young children are much more accurate imitators than are apes. Children quite faithfully replicate the arbitrary, non-functional patterns of behaviour that the experimentalists introduce into their experimental tasks.
>
> Apes largely ignore such actions .... Experiments designed to uncover the cognitive underpinnings of cultural transmission also strongly suggest that our cognition has evolved so that infants and children could acquire the quite complex and often counter-intuitive ideas and practices of their culture.[108]

Homo sapiens tends to preserve the bathwater just in case it conceals a baby.

Henry Plotkin observes that

> whatever adaptive gains derive from copying the behaviours of conspecifics has resulted in the selection of underlying cognitive mechanisms the workings of which spill over into the copying of behaviours that have no effects whatever on increases in individual or inclusive fitness.[109]

What that statement omits is the likelihood that such copying may sometimes have deleterious effects: for example, not just wasteful purchases, but also the spike of suicides that follows celebrity suicides. Both seem to be side-effects of our deep-seated tendency to imitate the actions of seemingly successful persons in our cultures (though perhaps celebrity suicides are contagious because they prevent victims of depression from imagining that fame and fortune might cure them). What was once a solid strategy for obtaining social status can now be an absurd and very costly error.

****

Recent polls suggest that challenging the worst aspects of capitalism is not a mere pipe-dream of leftist intellectuals. Probably because the Cold War and Soviet Communism itself are ancient history to them, and the malfeasance behind the 2008 financial collapse is a vivid memory, "a majority of Millennials now reject capitalism," while socialism is favored by a plurality,[110] and a major 2018 poll finds that they increasingly favor labor unions over corporations.[111] Political movements outside the United States – for example, the rise of the *Podemos* party in Spain and Andrés Manuel López Obrador's candidacy in Mexico – indicate that this shift is widespread. But whether that movement finds its way around the left side of predatory capitalism or (as other recent European elections have indicated) the right side – or whether some opening can be found that does not flirt with dangerous extremes – is an open and all-important question. Here again, partisan memeplexes that demand unquestioning loyalty to a whole cluster of beliefs cannot be allowed to make us disdain useful alliances, and Peter Kolozi's scholarly 2017 book *Conservatives against Capitalism* traces a conservative mistrust of unfettered capitalism through most of US history.

My goal is a social theory that accommodates the insights of classical conservatism while recognizing also the validity and value of ethical progress and of the revolutionary impulses of creative minds. Because the traditions of a culture are prior to any individual, and are often (like crowd-sourced predictions) wiser than the average individual, they will justifiably resist transformation by some whim local in time or space. But dissenting ideas are essential as times change. So is the diffusion of those dissents by intellectuals, who tend to ally with artists as the loyal opposition to any established consensus, cognitive as well as political.

Creative literature is an aesthetic phenomenon that has a particular social value. The makers of artistic fictions often alert us to runaway memeplexes that formerly had successfully disguised themselves as simple truth, natural order, and ultimate justice. As a substance in fluid suspension, its use not yet deterministically crystallized, art seems at times to offer a transparency to reality, but with symmetrical facets offering hints of a higher order: supercooled water in altocumulus clouds becoming snowflakes, or multi-mirrored telescope bringing together different perspectives on the universe. Sometimes stained-glass window, sometimes fun-house mirror – and sometimes a cutting edge. Art negotiates between the vast potential of cognition and its cultural constraints. It also offers a usefully provisional version of experience that includes but also transcends the normal spectrum of complaint and praise, awakening us to full individuality while speaking lovingly toward something valuable in our shared imperfect nature.

Interchapter: The Crow Tribe in Flight

The Crow tribe of the Northern Plains suffered much more than physical deprivations when it became impossible to act within the categories of their culture. The tradition of planting of the coup-stick in battle is another example of a memeplex that seems maladaptive to physical survival. Once a Crow warrior leading an attack put that stick in the ground, he was forbidden to retreat; he must defend that marker – and thereby become a privileged hero – or else die trying, no matter how hopeless the situation.[1] *But when, as Jonathan Lear's* Radical Hope *observes,* "The very acts themselves have ceased to make sense," *the result is a very real threat to the group's psychic survival.*[2] *All that remains (as for the non-metropolitan white communities discussed in the preceding chapter) is the flat-line grey, indifferent universe so common in depression – a disease which can be the result rather than the cause of seeing the obligations and promises of one's culture as lacking any ultimate foundation.*

Betrayed, battered, and displaced by other tribes as well as by the US government, the Crow faced another potentially fatal loss: they "lost the concepts with which they would construct a narrative."[3] *Their chief Plenty Coups (1848–1932) therefore had to become* "a new Crow poet: one who could take up the Crow past and – rather than use it for nostalgia or ersatz mimesis – project it into vibrant new ways for the Crow to live and to be."[4] *So he ostentatiously discarded his coup-stick and war-bonnet, and did what the actual poet Stevens urges in Stanza XXXII of* "The Man with the Blue Guitar": "Throw away the lights, the definitions, / And say of what you see in the dark / That it is this or it is that, / But do not use the rotted names." *Plenty Coups recounted a dream narrative that categorized change – in this case, a tribal shift from nomadic hunting, which was no longer viable, to agriculture – as itself a heroic act, enigmatically recommended by a prophetic chickadee who* "gains successes and avoids failure by learning how others succeeded or failed, and without great trouble to himself."[5] *This education sounds very much like the low-cost prudential function of fiction I have been describing. While the outgunned Sioux, under Sitting Bull, clung to their warrior and dance traditions to fight the white invaders, the Crow have survived better because their leader clung instead to the memory of a dream which left room to reinterpret their cultural norms in ways that enabled a survivable compromise. This is not to claim that the Crow have happily recovered their losses, nor to criticize other tribes for resisting more fiercely. But it does again suggest that imaginative stories provide space for cultural adaptations that aid survival.*

4 The Blue Guitar and the Uses of Art

"With mankind," [Captain Vere] would say, "forms, measured forms, are everything; and that is the import couched in the story of Orpheus with his lyre spellbinding the wild denizens of the wood."

—Herman Melville, *Billy Budd*

Thus far, my analysis has outlined a painful dilemma: to the extent we can choose at all, we can hardly choose happily between the chaos of cognitive overload on the one hand, and on the other hand the lifelessness of merely formulaic perception that subordinates any individual experience to categories, consensus, and collective utility. If unregulated consciousness is intolerable, even without the resulting burden of social ostracism, but accepting regulation is stultifying and conduces to tyranny, what hope is there for the human mind? No one will be surprised to hear that a literature professor thinks that a promising answer lies in artistic creation, and in interpreting poetry and its sister arts under the protection of academic freedom.[1] The second half of this book will focus on the underrated redemptive functions of the arts and humanities, especially in negotiating the conflict between control and freedom.

The human mind resembles a nuclear reactor: amazingly generative within the little containment dome, but always at risk of running fatally amok in a meltdown, and ceaselessly producing toxic waste. Art is a name for the technologies which (like dreaming) allow us to reprocess that seeming waste into fuel for trips whose purpose is both business and pleasure. Art, especially narrative art, allows our brains to do some useful mapping and forecasting, traveling across space and time, while enjoying the reinforcement of patterns by which we feel happily at home in the world, patterns we tend to call beauty.

Two things are crucial to understand here:

1 Fictions – stories or other imaginary entities – are much more powerful and pervasive things in human life than most people realize.
2 Fictions are much more malleable than most powerful and pervasive things in human life.

Fictions are powerful, not just in human minds but in the real world that human minds have shaped. Yuval Noah Harari's wonderfully readable book *Sapiens*, which puts so many aspects and phases of our collective experience into lucid perspective, identifies fiction as the single human invention that has allowed our species to conquer the earth.[2] The more technical work of Ian Tattersall, a distinguished paleoanthropologist and emeritus curator at the American Museum of Natural History, concludes that the key characteristic behind the triumph of our Cro-Magnon ancestors over the Neanderthal branch was that Cro-Magnons "led lives drenched in symbol," creating artworks, decorating the graves of their dead, and inventing human language.[3] Business CEOs and the politicians they fund who together want to chase literature out of higher education (as the new US Common Core pedagogy seems inclined to chase fiction out of reading for younger students) should be aware they are throwing stones in a glass house: the corporations they run are fictions that exist – like the rest of a culture – only because a larger community has agreed to treat them as a reality.

The consequences of corporations in the material world are real, of course: a factory, for example, and what it makes. But in a post-industrial age the fantasy that the imaginary is trivial and the material is all-important stands exposed. When a corporation such as Google, which is a name put on some concepts atop some structures of information, is worth more in the markets than all the world's car manufacturers combined, we should reconsider the supposed ontological superiority of "the real world" that business people tout. Information, the shared imaginary of a culture, and the words (including legal constructs as well as literary ones) by which we shape and stabilize such things, are immensely valuable.

Well over a century before Google even existed, Walt Whitman's *Democratic Vistas* made a comparable point much more magnificently: "the slightest song-tune, the countless ephemera of passions arous'd by orators and tale-tellers, are more dense, more weighty than the engines there in the great factories, or the granite blocks in their foundations." Therefore,

> should some two or three really original American poets, (perhaps artists or lecturers,) arise, mounting the horizon like planets, stars of the first magnitude, that, from their eminence, fusing contributions, races, far localities, &c., together, they would give more compaction and more moral identity, (the quality to-day most needed,) to these States, than all its Constitutions, legislative and judicial ties, and all its hitherto political, warlike, or materialistic experiences.

So, "View'd, to-day, from a point of view sufficiently over-arching, the problem of humanity all over the civilized world is social and religious, and is to be finally met and treated by literature."[4]

Nor should scientists disdain such imaginative flights and the influence of language – and of course most do not. Their abilities fill me with envy and their achievements fill me with awe, but their systems are not reality itself or even a transparent window on reality, though refined enough to be predictive and thereby productive. My spouse briefly majored in electrical engineering, then computer science, then cybernetics, then math, but shifted to a literature major when she noticed that most scientific progress was essentially a step toward the next slightly more apt metaphorical model. She decided to focus on a discipline that took seriously this truth about the nature of human consciousness and sought to make the best use of it.

Harari asks what allowed *Homo sapiens* to shatter the longstanding barriers against a community of more than about 150 individuals,

> eventually founding cities comprising tens of thousands of inhabitants and empires ruling hundreds of millions? The secret was probably the appearance of fiction. Large numbers of strangers can cooperate successfully by believing in common myths.
>
> Any large-scale human cooperation – whether a modern state, a medieval church, an ancient city or an archaic tribe – is rooted in common myths that exist only in people's collective imagination. Churches are rooted in common religious myths. Two Catholics who have never met can nevertheless go together on crusade or pool funds to build a hospital because they both believe that God was incarnated in human flesh and allowed Himself to be crucified to redeem our sins. States are rooted in common national myths. Two Serbs who have never met might risk their lives to save one another because both believe in the existence of the Serbian nation, the Serbian homeland and the Serbian flag.[5]

A memeplex thus protects and propagates itself.

How the Arts Manage Sex, Death, and Knowledge

Notice that the opening of Wallace Stevens' "The Man with the Blue Guitar" depicts the artist less as a generator of material than as one who trims it and refracts it:

> The man bent over his guitar,
> A shearsman of sorts. The day was green.
> They said, "You have a blue guitar,
> You do not play things as they are."
> The man replied, "Things as they are
> Are changed upon the blue guitar."

But, are they? An ancient Indo-European heritage established poets as magical makers and shapers of the world.[6] Literary critics warn that

W. H. Auden must surely have been partly ironic in asserting (in his eulogy to W. B. Yeats) that "poetry makes nothing happen." This could be false modesty, and I suspect Auden was toying with the etymology of *poesis* as "making" and the connotation of "forcing." Perhaps there are two lurking modifiers: "poetry makes nothing *outward* happen *quickly*." Auden goes on to call poetry "a way of happening," and Yeats himself, in "Sailing to Byzantium," claims that art offers stability and beauty that will outlast and outshine even the empires that exalt it – a claim supported by a great deal of history, and only partly retracted in Yeats's wistful "Adam's Curse." Another great Irish poet, Seamus Heaney, has recently written that "In one sense the efficacy of poetry is nil – no lyric has ever stopped a tank. In another sense, it is unlimited."[7] As the cellular-automata and chaos-theory models suggest that small variations and vibrations can eventually generate vast consequences, certain chords that resonate with the human heart and mind can end up changing the real world precisely by inspiring us with imagined worlds.

E. E. Cummings's "much i cannot" makes a similar sly boast, again toying with the question of what a poet "makes": though he admits he "cannot / tear up the world," he insists that "my weakness / makes more than most / strength," and consequently "we'll before / what's death / come(in one bed." The hand that rocks the iamb beds the beloved, eventually, and (zen-like) rules the universe even if it cannot rule the world. The mixing of poetic braggadocio and seduction epitomized by that Cummings poem had been rehearsed more than three centuries earlier, in many of Shakespeare's sonnets and in the love poetry of John Donne, whose "The Canonization" predicts that the self-indulgent, love-indulgent behavior his more practical, politically connected, and money-minded friends criticize will eventually bring them all begging to him as the miracle-worker who – precisely because of what they considered his follies – can bring back "peace" when nothing is left but "rage." The ardent poet will become the patron saint of a love without which the careerists' world (they will have come to realize) is neither tolerable nor sustainable.

Of course, the arc from a self-abnegating opening to a megalomaniacal conclusion recalls the predictable cry from the rejected wooer: "Someday you'll be sorry," as in the song popularized by Louis Armstrong, and in the Beatles' "Someday you'll know I was the one." Donne offers a brilliantly nasty version in "The Visitation." But "The Canonization" directs that warning away from the beloved and toward the entire socio-cultural order that wants to separate them. Donne's "The Sun Rising" turns against the sun for the same reason. It echoes the claim of "The Canonization" on behalf of poetry and love as mutually affirming and preserving agents, and it extends Donne's characteristic exaltation of erotic pair-bonding as a defense against the terrors infinite time and space impose on self-conscious mortal beings.

All of these lyrics set themselves, like gems on a dark foil, against the looming specter of death: the form in which the concept of the infinite and the collapse of insular selfhood threaten many people most fiercely. That is one reason I favor a reading of art as a protective as well as mutative function of collective human culture, rather than the narrower evolutionary reading in Denis Dutton's *The Art Instinct* and Jared Diamond's *The Third Chimpanzee*, which understand art as primarily display-behavior generated by the dynamics of sexual selection. No doubt many of our more striking attributes once served that otherwise counterproductive peacock-feather function and partly still do. But as we co-evolved with our complex culture, particularly through the use of language, those creative behaviors would also have provided new perspectives and generated more nuanced meanings, which would, in turn, have offered opportunities for individuals and for the culture as a whole to adapt to crises produced by, among other things, the expanded brain itself.

The physical expansion of that brain did not necessarily correspond to new levels of consciousness, but the capacity of that larger brain to host interactions among distributed functions seems nonetheless to correspond to an expanded mind, which is closely linked to a more active "theory of the self."[8] If a broader and more multiple view of the world raises the threat of cognitive overload, the coincidence of that view with a stronger sense of selfhood provokes a psychological and spiritual crisis concerning our mortality.

The human species has acquired the ability to contemplate death and eternity, but not – in most of the population through most of recorded history – the ability to tolerate their implications without invoking the aid of some larger entity. Our minds automatically aspire to understand, but as the world often overburdens those minds with possibilities immune to certainty and simplicity, so the same minds overload our spirits with the simple certainty of mortality. I suspect that people attribute omniscience and eternity to a deity partly so that it can take from us the annihilating burden of knowing death (and our relation to it) ourselves. Like a kind parent, God tells his fretting children that some problems should be entrusted to one's elders to handle. Christianity, which counters the prospect of personal annihilation in overdetermined ways – combating, enduring, denying, and also transcending mortality – has predictably thrived in the memetic economy. Not all religions promise a glorious afterlife, but the religions that have become the largest and most widespread – Christianity and Islam – have featured that belief prominently.

Among the many incalculables against which culture must defend us is the perpetuity of death: a peak moment of both certainty and uncertainty, with paths of measureless duration (including none) heading in any direction (including none). As the Christian consensus has weakened in Western culture, especially among the younger generation, other popular narratives have risen to fill the gap, while expressing doubts about their own adequacy and side-effects.

So, it is probably no mere coincidence that the most prominent villains in popular culture over recent decades have become villainous in a futile flight from mortality, a flight that led them toward tyranny. In the *Star Wars* films, Anakin Skywalker is corrupted into becoming Darth Vader by a promise of the power to overcome death itself (specifically, in futile hopes of defeating a prophecy – will they never learn? – of his beloved wife's mortality in childbirth), and has his own dying body replaced with black metal prostheses: the dark side of the transformative force of Yeats's golden Byzantine songbird. Vader oversees the construction of a "Death Star" weapon which, once completed as a sphere, would essentially mark the end of freedom in the universe. In the Harry Potter books, Lord Voldemort's name suggests a flight from death, as "Darth Vader" may suggest "Death Evader," and also recalls Edgar Allan Poe's character Valdemar, who lingers in hypnotic suspension between life and death. Voldermort vainly stores bits of his soul in scattered secret horcruxes to preclude any more absolute form of death. That move again backfires, leaving him not really alive and finally causing him to be annihilated.

The same problem of being unalive as the cost of being immortal pre-occupies the zombie stories that have recently returned to great promi-nence in the youth culture (and across generations in *Game of Thrones*), and in the vampire stories that have remained popular for the past 200 years, most recently in several television series and Stephenie Meyer's *Twilight* books and their movie versions. In Tolkien's fictional universe, recently revived into a half-dozen movies, Morgoth shares the deadly syllable with Voldemort. Morgoth's heir in evil, Sauron, later called the Dark Lord of Mordor, goes through a vampire phase in his quest for ultimate knowledge and power. The ring functions much as Voldemort's horcruxes do, and the benign wisdom of Gandalf matches that of Dumbledore – and Christ – in emphasizing that accepting death can be a crucial virtue. In the big-budget 2016 *Doctor Strange* movie, the villain Kaecilius relies on forbidden knowledge in an obsessive quest for immor-tality, and is opposed by a character named Mordo. A similar pattern emerges in the perpetually back-from-the-dead slashers in several series of movies that have been widely popular in the past half-century.

Sauron's quest also reflects the links between cognitive irritability and overachieving memeplexes: as Tolkein put it in his explanatory notes, Sauron "loved order and coordination, and disliked all confusion and wasteful friction."[9] The craving for total control over the elusive quo-tient of human life, expressed in these stories as a furious and ruthless quest for ubiquitous surveillance and secret knowledge, seems to be (ac-cording to the warnings that pervade popular culture) part of the same fatal error as the pursuit of eternal life: the refusal to accept the partial, the limited, and the approximate, which are humanity's destiny in both comic and tragic modes.

Epistemological overreach is the equivalent, in a moment of time, of refusing mortality across the span of time: knowing the present completely feels like an eternal consciousness (as in Saint Augustine's idea of an omniscient God standing outside of time). Omniscience seems perverse as a way of limiting the discomforts of excessive information, but at least the fantasy of it offers finally to close the task of knowing and to silence the nagging between levels of consciousness that characterizes the human mind – the recognition of all that isn't being cognized, rendering knowledge merely probabilistic, Bayesian. This tension is verified by the fact that "on the 'lower' layers of being there is a massive filtering or subtraction of sensory material, even though some of the filtered material enters into side perceptions that might become available later for reflection."[10] The phenomenon of "blindsight," whereby cortically blind subjects evince knowledge of things they do not think they have seen, offers an instance of such divided consciousness.

Even if it is a mirage, such perfect knowledge could look like an oasis beyond the granular flux of information: a plenitude in which choice is mere deduction, and the complex interplay of subjectivities could finally be brought to an end. The widespread determination of individuals and governments alike to capture all experience in digital recording, through the ubiquitous cameras – even though (or is it, because?) it narrows direct experience to the capacities of the recorder, and even though we will never have time to review it all – seems like a symptom of this fantasy. Perhaps the Enlightenment project of perfected objective knowledge was a similar symptom, coinciding as it did with the Cartesian determination to define all non-human life as fundamentally a predictable and meaningless mechanism.

Perhaps, also, we are unwittingly and unhelpfully favoring the kind of knowledge preferred by the more controlling neocortical aspects of our brains – favoring, that is, the rationally prudent part of the brain that, from an adaptationist point of view, might have been favored by an evolutionary function that rewards self-preserving strategies. That priority is costly for the individual psyche facing mortality, which threatens an ultimate loss of control and loss of self. Studies of the effect of psilocybin on the psychology of terminal patients (affirming the less scientific work of Aldous Huxley on psychedelics) offer compelling evidence that inhibiting the normalizing, centralizing effect of the neocortex on diverse areas of the brain palliates the fear of death by replacing that managerial sense of self with a recognition that we each participate in an unfathomable complexity.[11] If we could stop fighting that futile defensive battle, we might find that we had won the spiritual war.[12]

In other words, a neoliberalism of consciousness imposes a deadening formula that is maximally efficient for the perpetuation of the species, as neoliberal economics smother humane and eco-prudential values in service to a maximally efficient market that favors the thriving of alienated capital and its holders. This aspect of mental function – limitations of consciousness that are culturally abetted – has no regard for the amplitude of our awareness except as a preconscious threat, even though our expansive awareness may be the unique thing about us, and arguably the only thing we have beyond the machinery of survival. Once again, we face a choice about what we want the essence of existence to be: a mechanical trudge guided by a quantified materialist efficiency, or the expression of unique creativity that, when the cognitive handbrake is loosened, seems to evoke joy, reduce anxiety, and inculcate love. Otherwise we are caught in a vicious cycle: the tighter we cling to an insular selfhood, the more its vulnerability makes us reinforce its insularity. The 16th-century French essayist Michel de Montaigne, echoing Cicero, wrote that "To philosophize is to learn to die." The same axiom could be applied to the arts and humanities more broadly, to the extent that they teach us to open ourselves up to the universe. Accepting our mortal destiny – learning to love the incalculable ecological tangle of life cycles and our entanglement in it, all the more tangled with the discovery of horizontal gene transfer between species – has been the single most important task in the development of environmentalist consciousness over the past four centuries.

Some version of the fear of death is present in many sentient life-forms, but human beings receive it in a more conceptual and articulated way. This conscious extension of the survival instinct is risky. Religions of reincarnation or perpetual salvation look like patches that human groups have developed for that bug – or a virus that has developed to exploit that bug – in our species' otherwise profitable development of speculative and prudential thought. The deathbed is a place where the number-crunching of an optimizing lifetime may no longer seem to add up. Any sum looks small when set against infinity.

Yet, a frame or a tale can make a lifetime meaningful – unless, like Shakespeare's Macbeth, we have let our egoism isolate us so completely from the communal functions of life that it becomes "a tale / Told by an idiot, full of sound and fury, / Signifying nothing" (5.4.26–28). Viewers with a strong "personal need for structure" tend to dislike abstract paintings, especially if they have recently been reminded of their mortality – yet that resistance is mitigated if the painting has a seemingly meaningful title, one that suggests the presence of a narrative.[13] Thinking about death, in other words, evidently increases fears of chaos, which can be assuaged by words that propose a human story. As the Stevens poem puts it, "Poetry / Exceeding music must take the place / Of empty heaven and its hymns" (Stanza V).

Denial of mortality bonds a social collective together, and recognitions of mortality can unsettle that collective's project, as Don Delillo's

White Noise and even Melville's "Bartleby the Scrivener" can be read to suggest. This is especially true in Protestant and rational cultures where interaction between the living and the spirits of the dead is relatively scarce, as compared with various Asian and African cultures, or with the visions of South American magical realism, or even with traditional Catholicism. Communities, especially in the United States and Europe, therefore use the threat of mortality to collect us instead in hospitals, exercise classes, movie-houses, and other theaters of miraculous survival. Human beings and such institutions thus stabilize each other.

Religion and Philosophy

Yet, they destabilize each other terribly when they fail. Let a little institutional dissent – Martin Luther's, for example – pry open a gap between views on the balance between faith and works in the functioning of salvation, and all of Europe convulses into centuries of mass torture and burnings, destruction of holy art, and civil and multinational wars. The new Protestant meme (aided, in England and elsewhere, by symbiosis with the emerging climate of nationalism and with the new technology of printing) has done well, but the prolonged agony of its birth indicates how essential the unity of culture, the reassurance of consensus, really is.

The word "religion" is probably derived from *religare*, meaning "to bind,"[14] and there is a global epidemic of a kind of masochistic cognitive bondage-fetish. The prayers of major eastern and western religions – including Islam, Christianity, and Buddhism – do not ask their deities to give the supplicants power, but instead ask the divine to teach us to relinquish control. The formula is *Insha'Allah*, as God wills (*islam* means "submission"); or, "if it please the Lord" and "God willing" among Christians; and both sets of believers aspire to live and die by the book. The Four Noble Truths of Buddhism emphasize renunciation of any craving or clinging to the desires of the self. Otherwise there is just too much for us to choose, as there is too much for us to know.

Here, perhaps blinded by his own wonderful curiosity to the fact that most people crave constraining dictates, Tocqueville underrates the appeal of Islam (and fails to anticipate what right-wing Christianity would do to compete):

> Muhammad brought down from heaven and put into the Koran not religious doctrines only, but political maxims, criminal and civil laws, and scientific theories. The Gospels, on the other hand, deal only with the general relations between man and God and between man and man. Beyond that, they teach nothing and do not oblige people to believe anything. That alone, among a thousand reasons, is enough to show that Islam will not be able to hold its power long

in ages of enlightenment and democracy, while Christianity is destined to reign in such ages, as in all others.[15]

What instead seem to be threatening the long-term health of Islam are brood-parasites such as ISIS, which expand precisely by magnifying into deadly absolutes the welcome constraints that drew many people to Islam to begin with.

Under Calvinist theology, the surrender of control and even comprehension demanded by Reformation theology becomes even more radical. Furthermore, as Ernest Gellner observes, under all forms of Protestantism "The dominant morality is one of rule-observance rather than of loyalty, whether to kin or patron."[16] Again a severe cultural form thrives by dictating a correct way to manage conduct and experience. This must be a major factor in the rise of monotheism: a jealous God gives a reassuringly tight embrace. Yet, according to Freud's audacious last book, *Moses and Monotheism* (1939), the Jews achieved a liberating abstraction of thought by killing Moses, deliverer of the Ten Commandments, and then penitently inventing in his place a single deity who could not be seen or even named, present mostly in ritual. The resulting expansion of topics open to debate (as in the *midrash* tradition) may help explain both the triumphs of the Jews and their chronic persecution by societies that consider them uncouth and ingeniously subversive. The horrific agents of pogrom and Holocaust, unable to see their hateful sense of mission as a memeplex selfishly and stealthily favoring its own preservation and growth over their humanity, imagined the Jews, in their resistance and intellectualism, as a conspiracy instead.

Philosophy and science have each striven to offer simplifications with a claim to ultimate validity. Under Platonism, "The erstwhile two-dimensional or multi-dimensional matrix is modified, and comes eventually at least to approximate to a single-dimension one, by systematizing and underwriting the authority of shared concepts and making them 'universalistic'."[17] But seeking to replace an unsustainable multiplicity of cognitions and recognitions with ideal identities risks dulling everything down to sameness. The taxonomies of Enlightenment science no longer seem a satisfactory substitute for the infolding complexity of ecosystems and subjective experience. The *sapere aude*, "dare to know," which Kant identified as the driving principle of the Enlightenment, is not only enabled but also constrained by this taxonomic filtering of knowledge, which recaptures discovery into the mind's comfort-zones. Overcoming that paradox will require artists and scientists to move – as they show some signs of doing – beyond their mutual dismissiveness during the past three centuries, to accommodate the increasing supply of knowledge as well as the increasing evidence that knowledge is phenomenal and far more complex in its nature and reception than our native systems (our brains) or our prosthetics (our cultures and computers) can manage.[18]

Training Brains for Compassion

Homo sapiens makes tools in order to take control of the physical environment; *Homo sapiens* makes art to take control of the conceptual environment. Art embodies, in miniature, the craving of human consciousness to reduce, without reductionism, the massive disorderliness that surrounds and threatens to overwhelm us. Two social scientists prominent (though controversial) in the study of the adaptive human brain conclude that

> art is universal because each human was designed by evolution to be an artist, driving her own mental development according to evolved aesthetic principles. From infancy, self-orchestrated experiences are the original artistic medium, and the self is the original and primary audience.[19]

That claim may be too broad, but beyond whatever direct pleasure we get from witnessing an object we find beautiful, art offers a double benefit: not just the intuitive cognitive reassurance of seeing chaos thus tamed as if it were inherently tame, but also the awareness of the work of art as an artificial piece of work, epitomizing the human potential for gaining control in imaginative new ways.

The more complexity that is brought into a non-prescriptive order, the happier the subconscious human mind. Neuroscientists have shown that high-resolution music media cause the release of more dopamine – the brain's primary pleasure chemical – than compressed formats such as the ubiquitous MP3s, even though the two versions are usually indistinguishable to the conscious mind.[20] The arts help reconcile us both to ourselves and to the world around us. Patients suffering from dementia have reportedly recovered their social engagement, stroke patients their voices, even severely brain-damaged people the connectivity between their left and right hemispheres, through therapeutic exposure to music, which apparently can help the brain rewire itself across the *corpus callosum* and other gaps.[21] For a less technical instance with a far larger sample, consider the millions of teenagers – but not just teenagers – who listen to songs to pull themselves together, manage a heartbreak, feel less alone, and learn to navigate the human world. Shakespeare often casts music in that therapeutic role, curing despair and insanity. My point is that arts can create an opportunity for the collective mind of a culture similar to what they provide for individual minds: an alluringly complex but reassuringly ordered set of signals that allow a mind to reintegrate with itself, adapt to its surroundings, and recognize its harmonious kinship with its fellow creatures.[22] The movie's 13 crystal skulls seem quite pleased to be reunited.

Art often converses with other art, but it is not obliged to confine itself to the shape or substance of the reality defined by its ambient culture. Creativity is not lying, argued Sir Philip Sidney's "Defence of Poesy," because "the poet nothing affirmeth." In fact, the provisional aspect of artistic assertion may in some ways make it more correspondent to the emerging picture of reality (as multiple and contingent) in both quantum and cognitive science than more neat, direct, and stable reports.

The irresponsibility of fiction allows it to construct and share, in a safe and flexible form, the evolutionary value Karl Popper found in the human ability to construct mental scenarios more generally: "Let our conjectures, our theories, die in our stead!"[23] Popper was expressing a hope that scientific rationality might allow cultural difference to be resolved without warfare – he grew up amid the massive and pointless carnage of World War I, which showed how costly blind servitude to memeplexes could be – but the same formulation applies to my hope that novelistic fictions might allow mistakes to be experienced without damage.[24] Flights of the imagination have a value much like that of flight-simulators, which allow new pilots to learn from errors without any actual destruction. Commentators have struggled to explain what kind of purgation Aristotle imagined when he called the social function of tragedy a *catharsis*, but perhaps it included preventing bad choices that the interaction of human nature and their social order would otherwise generate. The way Aeschylus's *Oresteia* trilogy obliges its audiences to reconsider their conceptions of public and private justice is a great classical example.

Fictions allow us to inhabit our choice (or at least the product of our choices) among the infinite possible universes that exist. There is also cautionary literature about the failure to choose, running from *Hamlet* through Henry James's "The Beast in the Jungle" and on to Albert Camus' *The Fall*. From a consequentialist perspective, the practice of virtue is an honorable form of eugenics: a choice to live out the best of all possible selves. The philosopher Derek Parfit has proposed extending John Rawls's famous "Theory of Justice" to include each of our possible future selves as persons deserving equal consideration. In one sense, we already do that as we make decisions.[25] If Parfit's consideration were to prevent us from sacrificing any of our envisioned possible selves to make way for the chosen self, however, it would sacrifice instead exactly the advantage our prudential imaginations grant us.

Narrative is a mode that has co-evolved with humanity to allow us to take advantage of this mental capacity, and thus to teach lessons in morality and behavior that are more circumstantially nuanced – more ecological – than any set of rules could be. That kind of experimental setting is what *exempla* – moralized biographies, histories in the Livy tradition, or fictions – provided in medieval societies, and what coming-of-age folklore in many societies (such as the *Bildungsroman* in Western literature) provides for each emerging human generation, suggesting who else we could have been, as well as who else we could be.

Fictional stories provide individual and collective benefits beyond those offered by other kinds of prudential hypothetical thought. A team of cognitive scientists concluded that,

> Unlike in everyday life, the thinking a person engages in while reading fiction does not necessarily lead him or her to a decision, and therefore has tendencies neither of urgency nor permanence that propel the need for cognitive closure. Furthermore, while reading, the reader can simulate the thinking styles even of people he or she might personally dislike: One can *think along* and even *feel along* with Humbert Humbert in *Lolita*, no matter how offensive one finds this character. ... This double release – of thinking through events without concern for urgency and permanence and thinking in ways that are different than one's own – may produce effects of opening the mind.[26]

The sample of the study was rather small, but the results at least suggest that creative literature can liberate us from premature ideological commitments and create sympathies that would otherwise be unachievable.

The standard riposte to this defense of the arts and humanities is that genocidal Nazis wept at the opera. This objection is certainly troubling but hardly conclusive or dispositive. No inoculation is perfect, and probably at times a dose of high art does allow people to feel that they are feeling exquisitely, and thereby exonerate themselves from any broader application of sympathy: a pill takes the place of a meal. Furthermore, anything perceived as falling below a group's rarefied ideal of the human and outside its idea of the cultured becomes not only unworthy of consideration, but a betrayal of humanity; and anything done on behalf of that ideal is inherently justified. High culture can become a platform for spitting down on those who don't participate in its complacent formulas. That is why a combination of compassion and intellectual self-critique is imperative, and why both were systematically eradicated by Nazi regimes.

A longer and wider view supports the familiar claim that reading, and especially the reading of literature, expands the capacity for sympathy and respect. Elaine Scarry argues that increased literacy explains

> a hundred-year period bridging the seventeenth and eighteenth centuries during which an array of brutal acts – executing accused witches, imprisoning debtors, torturing animals, torturing humans,

inflicting the death penalty, enslaving fellow human beings – suddenly abated, even if they did not disappear.[27]

Subjects who read a chapter from a novel about an Algerian woman raised stronger objections to the sexist aspects of that society than those who read a non-fiction essay on the same topic. On tests of interpersonal perception, as well as related areas empathy and theory of mind, fiction readers again outdid readers of non-fiction. Reading a Chekov story about adultery, rather than a telling of the same basic story as nonfiction, altered the personalities of participants in a study "in idiosyncratic directions," and "even defensive individuals, whose avoidant style of attachment involved habitual suppression of emotion in everyday life, experienced significantly more emotion reading Chekhov's story than the control text." That finding suggests that "literature could provide a nonintrusive, nonthreatening method of reaching and affecting some people who are usually hard to reach."[28] The ability to evoke diverse, humane responses without scaring people back into their psychological shells is exactly what I have been arguing literature enables under the conditions of cognitive overload and in the repressive cultures that such overload often generates.

As Kim Lane Scheppele has observed, "whether or not we are good at narrative compassion, when compared with statistical compassion we are brilliant at narrative compassion."[29] A good short story about a suffering person often affects readers more than a news report about the suffering of ten thousand. The 2011 *Annual Review of Psychology* describes findings

> reported in two studies, published in 2006 and 2009, that individuals who frequently read fiction seem to be better able to understand other people, empathize with them and see the world from their perspective. This relationship persisted even after the researchers accounted for the possibility that more empathetic individuals might prefer reading novels.

A study reported in the journal *Science* in 2013 also showed that reading literary fiction improved people's ability to enter into both the thoughts and the feelings of others; non-fiction and formulaic genre fiction failed to produce the same effects.

Those effects go far beyond the huge, moist, cloudy version of empathy and self-knowledge often claimed – not wrongly – on behalf of literature. A play called *World Factory* by Zoe Svendsen, running at the Young Vic in London as I write this, shows the power of theater to expose the power of memeplexes. The mostly left-leaning spectators, brought on stage and obliged to make business decisions for their competing clothing sweatshops in China, find themselves repeatedly adopting policies they would surely have condemned only hours before. This not only unsettles hip ethical complacency; it ultimately reveals the role of the state in maintaining a short-sighted and inhumane system of commerce. The play becomes a less garish but more broadly revealing version of the notorious Milgram experiment, with what Adam Smith called "the invisible hand" of the market replacing Milgram's authoritative psychologist in telling participants to impose pain. The play thus shows its activated audience how easily neoliberalism conscripts people into its assumptions once they begin thinking of themselves as part of a profit-driven enterprise under the modern state. That system has curated an environment within which it is nearly immune to critique.[30] A clearer demonstration of how a socioeconomic system has evolved mechanisms that disable its foes is hard to imagine.

Playwrights, novelists, and screenwriters often attempt outright social critique. In the popular and critically revered 1976 movie *Network*, written by Paddy Chayefsky, the corporate mogul Arthur Jensen convinces the TV newscaster-turned-messianic-humanist Howard Beale to renounce his campaign. Jensen's tirade epitomizes the way neoliberalism silences its opponents: "It is the international system of currency which determines the totality of life on this planet," declares Jensen:

> That is the natural order of things today. That is the atomic and subatomic and galactic structure of things today! And YOU have meddled with the primal forces of nature, and YOU WILL ATONE! We no longer live in a world of nations and ideologies, Mr. Beale. The world is a college of corporations, inexorably determined by the immutable bylaws of business. The world is a business, Mr. Beale. It has been since man crawled out of the slime.

What many plays, novels, and movies do instead of outright critique, and perhaps in the long run more productively, is help us detect when aspects of our civilization have shifted from symbiont to parasite. By highlighting the mismatch between what the culture induces the characters to do and what we want them to do, such works alert us to the danger this book seeks to describe more directly. Prominent instances run from Shakespearean tragedy to the 18th-century satires of Swift and Pope, on through the Victorian heart-rendings of Dickens to the countless depictions of American conformism (notably, by Sinclair Lewis) and racism (by Sandra Cisneros and Leslie Marmon Silko, among many others) in the past 150 years; in France from Molière to Gustave Flaubert to François Truffaut. A crucial moment in Mark Twain's *Huckleberry Finn* shows Huck struggling with what he thinks is his conscience, which tells him he should betray his friend Jim back into slavery (since that was the social norm taught in church), set against some deep sense that he can't quite articulate, but that convinces him he should risk going to hell by reciprocating Jim's loyalty and humane affection, rather than treating him as a piece of legal property. Perhaps we now need tales that similarly expose various hypertrophic administrative review processes (as Franz Kafka did a century ago in his *The Trial* and *The Castle*) and online social networks as self-serving memeplexes, though it is hard to imagine that such tales will be as gripping to depict as blood-revenge. Dave Eggers's 2013 novel *The Circle*, about a Google-like company that spins out of its founder's control with terrible human costs, is a step in that direction.

Whether fictional narrative and other imaginative and empathetic forms of foresight can lead our collective to save itself from environmental catastrophe – whether the fantasies and blind-spots imposed by consumer capitalism can be replaced in time to avoid casting our descendants and neighbors into a vast tragedy of the commons – may be the single most consequential question facing the human race. Certainly there are many academics working to promulgate and inculcate that foresight. My worrisome hypothesis is that the consumerist money-meme has evolved a resistance to the cautionary tales, which will have to evolve also from the time-worn and spirit-wearying mode of environmentalist elegy and jeremiad (typified by Rachel Carson's influential 1962 *Silent Spring*) in order to recruit new stewards. One promising model is the science fiction of Kim Stanley Robinson, whose Mars and Orange County trilogies propose plausible, equitable, and ecologically sustainable revisions of capitalism, rather than its replacement by some utopian alternative.

Capitalism is certainly not the least fair or least efficient way human societies have ever been controlled – in fact, it seems to be the most productive – but it is also the greatest force now standing between us and the principles of equality and mercy, between us and environmental prudence,[31] and between us and the valuation of human experience and life-purpose beyond their commodification and quantification into monetary equivalents. The heroic naturalist John Muir warned, over a century ago, about the way our system keeps "trying to make everything dollarable," and he knew it had a long dishonorable history:

> Thus long ago a lot of enterprising merchants made part of the Jerusalem temple into a place of business instead of a place of prayer, changing money, buying and selling cattle and sheep and doves. And earlier still, the Lord's garden in Eden, and the first forest reservation, including only one tree, was spoiled.[32]

Perhaps by recognizing the ways such a system becomes self-serving, we can recognize its power over our lives as something other than a rational choice we have made. Perhaps the historical distance and imaginative range provided by humanistic and creative writings will expose that system as something other than the immutable underlying structure of human communities. Noticing, in a sociocultural mode of deconstruction, the contradictions among several systems that present themselves as deep and inevitable truths may allow us to challenge them. Only then will these systems become recognizable as dangerous but useful creatures we may wish to tame and corral; only then can we discipline the guilty creatures instead of scapegoats. Unlike Dorothy in Oz, our liberation may begin when we pay attention to the curtain and not to whatever conniving little man appears to be behind it.

Training Brains for Freedom

Making choices requires us to be aware of possibilities without being overwhelmed by them. Great poets thus face a paradoxical mission. On the one hand, they are largely in the business of overcoming the numbness and breaking down the barriers we have necessarily built up, individually and collectively, to protect ourselves from seeing freshly, from being dazzled by the astonishing beauties and baffling complexities of the world, and its ubiquitous unbearable poignancies, especially in the contemplation of transience. Artists say, open up your heart, your eyes, your life. They provide the "defamiliarization" that Viktor Shklovsky's influential 1925 *Theory of Prose* saw as a crucial function of art.

On the other hand, poets are also in the business of providing allegories by which we can navigate the world as inherently meaningful. They construct narratives – or, as Brian Boyd has shown, non-narrative patterning[33] – that make everything seem, not clear exactly, but necessary and beautiful, rather than merely an arbitrary way of momentarily organizing chaos. This may resemble the functions of manipulative memeplexes, but in an 1818 letter to John Hamilton Reynolds, the great Romantic poet John Keats observes that "We hate poetry that has a palpable design upon us" – a plan to lock us into an agenda. An expansion of sensibility and an influx of meaning need not shrink into programmatic admonitions.

Abjuring the calcified assumptions of a culture sometimes requires abjuring even that broader mode of meaning. As part of the modernist rebellion, Dadaists celebrated mere randomness, celebrating the loss of conventional meanings by, for example, creating poems with words drawn at random from a hat. They were not (as I long assumed) some indulgent group of avant-garde nihilists enamored of their own cleverness, playing irresponsibly at the effete edges of art. They were, primarily, like Popper, young men in a world of young men dying in the horrific absurdity of World War I – a war all the more horrific because their cultures insisted that the absurdity was really honor. These radical artists recognized that there was no way to oppose the comprehensive horrors of that geopolitical calamity and its poisonous patriotic roots without challenging the entire assumption that their culture was a rational structure built on fundamental truth.

In "The Idea of Order at Key West," Stevens – a cognitive revolutionary disguised in the three-piece suits of his career as a stolid insurance executive – reveres this middle kind of "making":

> The maker's rage to order words of the sea,
> Words of the fragrant portals, dimly-starred,
> And of ourselves and of our origins,
> In ghostlier demarcations ....

Not only our origins, but also our departures, require at least the calm at the end of the mind, the fiction of order that words can provide, and the order of rhythm and rhyme. As the bereaved Alfred, Lord Tennyson wrote in Section V of *In Memoriam,*

> But, for the unquiet heart and brain,
> A use in measured language lies;
> The sad mechanic exercise,
> Like dull narcotics, numbing pain.

Or, as Emily Dickinson puts it, "After great pain, a formal feeling comes – / The Nerves sit ceremonious, like Tombs –." It is no wonder – but a fact worth noticing – that what a wide-eyed child often needs, to get to sleep at night, is a story: a haven for the yearning but agoraphobic human mind.

Literature shows us the way language itself offers at once a means of mental control and a threat of dangerous ambiguity and deception.[34] This balance of the new with the familiar, the unsettling with the settled, the allegorical with the real, must be a major reason that art has generally been formal and tradition-bound. One way to make tolerable the introduction of dissenting perception is to present it within structures. What many consider the most passionate form of high art – the romantic opera – is also probably the most mannered. Outside of jazz (which always has always attracted cultural dissidents), the most famously mind-expanding, free-form improvisational band has been the Grateful Dead. Is it merely coincidence that the Dead not only attracted the most fanatical archivists, who felt compelled to compare their recordings of every show, but also inspired tribute bands who mimic every note of those recorded performances?

Speaking of young men mesmerized by light-shows, consider Robert Herrick's passive passion for the graces of his beloved, three centuries earlier:

> Whenas in silks my Julia goes,
> Then, then, methinks, how sweetly flows

That liquefaction of her clothes.
Next, when I cast mine eyes and see
That brave vibration each way free;
O how that glittering taketh me!

("Upon Julia's Clothes")

Consider also, from the same period, Andrew Marvell's scintillating vision of the soul:

Casting the body's vest aside
My soul into the boughs does glide;
There like a bird it sits and sings,
Then whets and combs its silver wings;
And, till prepar'd for longer flight,
Waves in its plumes the various light.

("The Garden," lines 51–56)

These are masterful poems, but not poems of plodding metrical regularity and conventional moral instruction. They manage to sustain the moment of gorgeous complexity – every wave of sound and light reflected and refracted at every angle off every thread of silk and every wisp of afterfeather – that enchants Dr. Spalko in the Indiana Jones movie, without letting it cycle into the cognitive overload that destroys her.

Marvell's poetry offers some of the most complex and unsettling philosophical meditations in Western culture, but does so in comforting little tetrameter couplets: the form of many nursery rhymes. Rhyme and meter (remember that the first sounds any of us heard were the iambs of a maternal heartbeat), or musical forms, with their balance of repetition and variation, or the structure of verse (often a single voice) and refrain (often a chorus) in lyrics when the two arts combine in song, make emotions and ideas feel reassuringly familiar and contained. This kind of conversation between the wild and the tame has kept landscape painting interesting for nearly half a millennium in Western culture, and even longer in Japan.

Gestures toward tradition, especially participation in established genres, offer the same kind of reassurance. Baudelaire, considered by some the inventor of "modernity" itself, wrote sonnets, although he varied rhyme-patterns extensively within them. The *London Times* obituary for Dylan Thomas observed that he, too, "invented stanza forms," and that no English poet "has ever worn more brilliantly the mask of anarchy to conceal the true face of tradition."[35] Genre is a version of the filter that protects us from chaos; Edna St. Vincent Millay makes the point very well in "I will put Chaos into fourteen lines." Artists pour the substance of external reality into casts – literally so, in the case of sculptors and even playwrights – as an extension and variation of the normal shaping work of the human mind.

So free verse is not just, as Robert Frost complained, playing tennis without a net; it is also playing with fire without a fireplace. Frost says a good poem ends in what is "not necessarily a great clarification, such as sects and cults are founded on, but in a momentary stay against confusion"; the protection is essential, but it must not be absolute or permanent. Even poetry's fundamental function of metaphor – heightened in Metaphysical conceits such as Donne's famous comparison of lovers to the legs of a compass – massages this crucial muscle of the mind, providing a surprising likeness, which is therefore at once a novelty and the recapturing of that novelty by the familiar.

Too much familiarity breeds contempt, or at best a less generative form of contentment. In a more widely shared cultural mode, the formulaic sitcom (on radio and, later, on television) has been a crucial tool of collective therapy over the past century. The characters will always revert to their characters (right down to their signature phrases), the ending will be harmonious, with an implied recommendation that we cheerfully resign ourselves to our flawed common existence. That can feel like the right conclusion, all the more so because of the absurdities of our existence. It is a version of what statisticians call regression toward the mean or reversion to mediocrity – mediocrity in the technical rather than the common pejorative sense. The middle of the herd feels like a safe place to be, a place where life goes on.

Artists are commonly thought to be susceptible to madness, and research suggests a significant correlation between bipolar disorder and creativity.[36] John Dryden's 1681 poem "Absalom and Achitophel" observed that "Great wits are sure to madness near allied, / And thin partitions do their bounds divide." But Flaubert – a founding father of the realist novel – recommended that writers "Be regular and orderly in your life, so that you may be violent and original in your work." In fact, the release artistic work offers to a community (including the intuitively calibrated release from a single, narrowly determined reality) may help forestall mass psychogenic illness. Such illness occurs most vividly in cases – often among young women, whether seen as maenads or cheerleaders or witches, and therefore often characterized with the gender-laden term "hysteria" – where a half-suppressed awareness of the discrepancy between the idolized or anathematized role dictated by the culture and the more nuanced inner experience of self leads to contagious physical symptoms: twitching, warbling, laughing, fainting. A *New York Times* piece about such outbreaks concludes that "What girls need during this time is a stable and supportive space in which to work out all of this drama."[37] Perhaps instead they need a drama in which to work out the insupportable instability of selfhood in the theater of our globalized globe. Books such as Nellie McCaslin's *Creative Drama in the*

Classroom and Beyond and Helen Nicholson's *Applied Drama* offer good practical and theoretical support for that notion. To retain their sanity, prisoners of war in the so-called Hanoi Hilton, held for years in solitary confinement, invented a tap system to exchange poems through the walls.

This cure is not strictly literary, although literature appears to be a helpful condensation of its function. Neuroscientists have observed that a primary function of dreaming is the sifting and sorting of the day's experience, highlighting some experiences and discarding others. During REM sleep, this process alleviates cognitive overload and builds revised structures in the brain to accommodate new information and priorities. The dreamer's recollection of that process as a narrative (often by what Freud calls "secondary revision") is therefore often dismissed as merely a deceptive side-effect, a rough stitching together of whatever random fragments of information became momentarily visible on their way to a new storage site with new companion-memories. I believe that is a false dichotomy. Stories have always been a tool for processing and storing data, drawing lessons on what is good or bad, in important ways or not, so that we can call up useful frames and appropriate responses for analogous situations when we encounter them in real, waking life. Story-telling and dreaming are two aspects of the same process essential to the healthy functioning of the human mind.[38]

Literature may thus be understood as the dream-work of the culture as a whole – and no less essential to the sanity and integration of that larger human unit. Shakespeare's history plays are valued above the chronicles they were based on because a mere factual record lacks the multiple perspectives conveyed by the characters and even by the metaphors of drama. A metaphor is a hypothesis about the present, neither true nor untrue, as prudential imagination is a hypothesis about the future. "Were narrativity such an automatic capacity, like an algorithm," observes Michael Carrithers, "then sociocultural change would be impossible. But since narrativity involves a further capacity, that of *creativity*, inventiveness or imagination, change is inherent."[39] The Blue Guitar plays the changes.

This aspirational aspect of art opposes the merely formulaic entertainments and advertisements that feed back to a culture its own prejudices, offering superficial "novelties" that, fetish-like, narrow and tame potentially expansive desires, while exonerating their audiences from any obligation to reconsider. I am thinking of fetishism here less in Freud's sense of a defense against the castration complex in an Oedipal crisis than as a defense against complexity itself in a cognitive crisis; Oedipus himself had a dangerous need both to know and not to know.

These opposed functions of art bring us back to the New Historicist struggle to distinguish true seditions from the simulations of liberation that rulers stage in order to keep sedition safely contained?. Or, putting it in less conventionally political terms, how can we discern the difference between, on the one hand, positive, generative creativity that accommodates conventionality in order to make itself easier for audiences to swallow and digest, and on the other hand, conformist memes that offer delusive signals of liberation and innovation but ultimately subjugate those possibilities to familiar formulas, winning audiences by absolving them of the crucial but mostly unwelcome human duty to think freshly and independently?

I was only 14 years old in 1967, but I remember queasily recognizing that distinction when an ostensibly psychedelic song called "Incense and Peppermints" hit the top of the Hit Parade. It seemed so clearly designed to offer a safe little formula of the burgeoning altered-consciousness movement – and, in a related development, to make money – that I got my first glimpse of capitalism's talent for swallowing up its potential enemies. So (while I concede that this proves nothing) it did not surprise me, many years later, to learn that the lead singer on that record had become a direct-marketer for conservative political movements.

Similarly, when grocery stores began playing versions of popular rock records over their sound systems in the 1970s, it seemed as if the youth culture had won: they were playing our song instead of decrying it. Looking at the way my generation's high-educated elites spend lots of money trying to look like earth-tone hippies, eating rough-hewn whole-grain foods, sitting on yoga mats instead of formal dining chairs or church pews, and vacationing on river rafts instead of in Vegas suites, you might conclude that the 1960s counterculture has triumphed. But blink your eyes and look again, and you start to suspect that the mainstream had the counterculture for lunch, served (to adapt Hannibal Lecter's famous, creepy line from *The Silence of the Lambs*) with some love beads and a nice chianti.

If my distinction between good and bad art sounds like the difference between passionate love and what Edmund in *King Lear* dismisses – with three aptly sluggish adjectival syllables – as the "dull, stale, tired bed" of a marriage of convenience (the modern equivalent might be a couple lacking inspiration to do much beyond sitting together watching sitcom re-runs), the comparison may be rooted in the fact that art serves some of the same functions in the evolution of culture that mating does in the evolution of many life-forms. Sexual selection, with its volitional and aesthetic elements, has proven to be an advantageous way for most species to achieve variability. Brian Boyd makes a related point:

> just as natural selection has evolved sex as a means for amplifying genetic variation, I suggest, it has evolved art in humans – first as a means of sharpening minds eager for pattern, but gradually also for creativity, for amplifying the variety of our behavior.[40]

And people expect high art to be transformative, not merely pleasant; we expect it to tell us, as the erotically charged "Archaic Torso of Apollo" told the poet Rainer Maria Rilke in a famous line, "You must change your life." As Laurent Dubreuil puts it, "A notable difference between the average sentimental novel and *Wuthering Heights* resides in this point: one expects to be altered by Bronte's masterpiece, and not simply to 'have a good time.'"[41] Great literature – whether on an explicit mission, like Thoreau in *Walden*,[42] or more obliquely – articulates and amplifies an inner voice that has been, like a guardian angel, urging readers away from the habitual wastefulness and petty wrongdoing that their culture recommends as normal.

Aesthetics derive partly from evolutionary incentives: identify and attract the healthiest mate, find a livable setting, avoid the most dangerous parasites. But evolved capacities often become adapted to other uses. Sexual selection, the appeal of certain landscape views, and the capacity to discern between nutrients and toxins, all presumably originated as outgrowths of a mindless genetic algorithm (here I agree with Denis Dutton). But, along with heuristic incentives that inculcated an appetite for pattern, they created the appetite for beauty and some criteria for beauty. Those, in turn, created a useful mechanism for reforming consciousness and hence society (although that mechanism is often co-opted by the social status-quo, as Adorno warns and as this book's theory would predict).

Opposed to beauty's allure is the warning of disgust, like the revulsions of "morning sickness" by which (according to some analyses) pregnant women's bodies are made averse to anything potentially toxic for the next generation. McAuliffe argues extensively that disgust is largely a reflex developed to avoid parasites – a reflex that (as Paul Rozin suggests) "develops from a system to protect the body from harm to a system to protect the soul from harm."[43] Experimental subjects primed by images that suggest infection or infestation show sharper reflexes of moral condemnation, and societies in environments conducive to parasites appear to have stronger taboos in unrelated areas. This suggests that our disgust when encountering cultural parasites may be part of a valid and important human defense system.

While the non-rational spillover from physical aversion to moral judgment may improve vigilance against real threats, it also tends to reinforce socially regressive behavior: for example, making people averse to racial others or the homeless and convinced those judgments are morally founded, or finding homosexual acts repellent and thereby assuming them to be immoral. Again a conscious vigilance about the interaction between human evolution and cultural evolution seems indispensable in the quest for social justice. Hannah Arendt develops Kant's aesthetics toward an assertion that aesthetic judgment must underlie and be the model for any good political judgment, and that political judgment must reside always in discourse, remaining provisional rather than conclusive.

If so, then the humanities – in their seemingly idle and endlessly inconclusive pursuit of beautiful and flexible meaning – may be our best hope for finding worthy objects of love and a cultural landscape where our essence can thrive.

Sex, Drugs, and Cultural Revolution

Because of its embarrassing similarities across mammalian species, mating may seem to drag human beings back to the level of other animals in the grip of a simple instinctual drive. The cross-cultural persistence of the incest taboo (including the Westermarck effect) suggests that some hard-wiring narrows our erotic choices. Yet, human mating is intensely and extensively regulated by culture, even in the experience of it. Centuries of love poems and pop songs and romantic comedies may be understood as tireless efforts to refine and update the code of the software that runs the mating function on our physical frames.

Protracted pair-bonding is fueled by profound bio-evolutionary incentives in *Homo sapiens* and a few other species, induced largely by the delivery of vasopressin and oxytocin to the reward-centers of the brain. Its particular features, however, such as its strong association with romantic love and bourgeois marriage, are more contingent, shaped by socio-historical developments; yet, those memes have successfully propagated a belief that they are trans-historical, obligatory, and beneficial. In its heterosexual form, that memeplex has also allied itself so deftly with institutional religion, commerce (and its commercials), the exaltation of sexuality, the sheer bio-power of its production of carriers, and common fears of loneliness and mortality that it has – at least until very recently – squeezed rival models of love onto ever narrower areas of the human psychological and sociological landscape in most modern societies. This meme has also empowered a memeplex known as the wedding industry: another ally of the money culture that exploits people's fear of not constructing themselves to fit social norms, and one that has actually only strengthened with the participation of same-sex couples, many of whom evidently feel an extra need to assert in their weddings their compatibility with the older cultural norms of marriage.

Beyond any direct evolutionary advantages, amicable pair-bonding also offers the minimum affirmation of otherness one must endure to avoid the confirmation of aloneness: intimacy cures the terror of mental solitude unalloyed by conversation. Milton's Adam and Eve are chased out of Eden because they taste the fruit of the tree of forbidden knowledge. The consequence, according to the final lines of *Paradise Lost* is that

> The world was all before them, where to choose
> Their place of rest, and Providence their guide.
> They, hand in hand, with wandering steps and slow,
> Through Eden took their solitary way.

That's the bad news, and the good news too. The whole unexplored mortal world is a dizzying and even terrifying prospect, but if these two support each other's belief in a Providential order, they may wander, but they will never be lost or alone.

Adults are often hazily and uneasily aware that they have forfeited their authenticity and autonomy, their freedom of purpose. Nostalgia for one's youth is perhaps natural and inevitable, but the common impression that modern adulthood consists largely of concessions to established norms and powers makes maturity seem like a defeat of the least heroic kind. Michael Pollan's fascinating 2018 book *How to Change Your Mind* notices that (in the absence of psychedelics) he no longer really notices much because he is seldom surprised, because decades of experience have loaded his mind with efficient automatic categorizations and responses; his deftly self-lacerating conclusion is that "A flattering term for this regime of good enough predictions is 'wisdom'."[44]

In response, people sometimes push back, rejecting guilt and shame and following the pleasure principle, hoping to reconnect to a desire that preceded their induction into the systems of desire taught by culture, as if selfishness would lead back to a true lost self, and the hedonic were the high road to the Edenic. Longing for that unabashed infantile appetite – whether or not it ever really existed – is what draws us to the big baby Falstaff, despite all his ugly selfishness, when Shakespeare's history plays situate him in societies whose dysfunctions have drained all the authentic selfhood out of the titular monarchs. In response to German fascism and then to American conformism, the psychoanalyst Wilhelm Reich attempted to use orgasms (broken off from their evolutionary utility) as the geiger-counter, and orgone-boxes as the storage-battery, to isolate some pre-articulate energy we could call our own desire, rather than the desire of the heedless genes within us or (emphatically the alternative in Orwell's *Nineteen Eighty-Four*) of the stale collective social system around us. That resistant project assumes that we have selves largely independent of the world around us – a dubious assumption in biological as well as political terms. Freudian psychoanalysis, which promises to open out the essential and unique inner experience of the individual, is vulnerable to the same critique.

The liberating and even revolutionary force of sexual desire is limited anyway by biological and cultural forces. Sexuality not only pulls us back closer to the project of the selfish gene. It also seems to steer both "normal" and "aberrant" desires into clichés that subject them to mass-produced fetishes that usually bind rather than liberate bodies: high-heeled shoes and fishnet stockings, tight leather or Nazi-styled domination outfits with whip-and-handcuff accessories. Those bodies themselves are often altered (by exercise, surgery, tattoos, and/or piercings) to feed back to the culture its chosen forms of attraction. When subversion and perversion become versions of a new normal, complete with uniforms for purchase, is that tolerance or co-optation?

Shakespeare's *Midsummer Night's Dream* has been warning for well over 400 years that even authentic erotic desire does not exactly belong to the person feeling it, and Shakespeare coded that eraser of selfhood as an aphrodisiac drug derived and distilled from exotic flowers which (like a human endocrine system) makes people fall in or out of love against their conscious wills. Alcoholism, like sexual promiscuity, has been winkingly celebrated for centuries (all the way back to Dionysus and Bacchus in ancient Greek and Roman cultures) as indulging the truest desires of some true inner self. We tend to collaborate in the assumption that *veritas* is what emerges in *vino*, and that Viagra (or Addyi, approved in 2015, as purportedly the equivalent for women) is a drug that allows people to fulfill an authentic inner appetite, rather than one that allows them to simulate such appetites.

Many Viagra and Addyi prescriptions will be medically legitimate attempts to reduce erotic frustrations, but the similarity to other regimes of manufactured need under consumer capitalism can hardly be ignored. Abstinence, once admiringly institutionalized in convents and monasteries, is on the brink of being institutionalized as a disease. For many people, the periodic release and companionable experience offered by sexuality and drunken revelry has to compensate for the absence of any larger and more lasting purposes.

Back in 1841, long before he could have known many students who think mostly about the beer keg and the weekly football game, Ralph Waldo Emerson observed that

> Dreams and drunkenness, the use of opium and alcohol are the semblance and counterfeit of this oracular genius, and hence their dangerous attraction for men. For the like reason, they ask the aid of wild passions, as in gaming and war, to ape in some manner these flames and generosities of the heart.[45]

Futile, formulaic little versions of rebellion are the establishment's best friend, and too many colleges and universities (though purportedly determined to prevent the campus sex crimes that closely correlate with the memeplexes of male athletics and, especially, alcohol abuse) refuse to demand anything more imaginative from their students. In fact, those colleges and universities seem willing to entangle themselves in impossible choices about evaluating marginally consensual sexual activities, and therefore endure a crossfire from both the left and the right wings, rather than strive to limit binge drinking.

What concerns me is this kind of fake freedom, especially in forms that are also so destructive in themselves. Sedative drugs such as alcohol, which is to say drugs to suppress consciousness, are far more popular than psychedelic drugs such as LSD, which disrupt standard mental paradigms and stimulate new perceptions, partly by broadening the mind's range of active associations.[46] This preference may simply reflect the ancient Stoic insight that life-experience is fundamentally suffering, making it wiser to withdraw our feelings rather than keep them alert; but it has this cognitive element also. No need to fear a bad trip if you are not going anywhere. Even raves and mass festivals, while proclaiming resistance to consumer capitalism and conformism, and promising the uninhibited spontaneity of desire, place their attendees in a bonded collectivity focused on the same array of lights and the same sequence of sounds. For Nietzsche, even the Dionysian side of art emphasized collectivity, not individuality.

Is smoking marijuana a revolutionary act because of its unsettling effect on perception and dutiful behavior, or instead an abdication of revolution because of its pacifying effect on the body and the rational mind? Asking that question brings into focus a fundamental – and, I believe, eventually fatal – division within the youth movement of the late 1960s. As the aforementioned Beatles' song "Revolution" observed, political activism and mental retreat are at cross-purposes. It warns that efforts to "change the world" by changing "the constitution" and "the institution" are futile. It urges the listener to "change your head" and "free your mind instead," replacing conventional activism with altered consciousness; the shift from Latinate four-syllable rhyme words to simpler colloquial diction reinforces the appeal of an escape from formal official thinking. The song concludes that activists "carrying pictures of Chairman Mao ... ain't gonna make it with anyone anyhow." That closing couplet was predictably unpopular with leftists, but it carried an insight about the importance of addressing the cultural and cognitive inertia that obstructs political change.

Artistic Creativity and the Avant Garde

People do not live for bread-winning alone; they want also to see the circus, as the mind does its acrobatics off its material vessel, frightening and delighting us at the same time. For our species, mental work and mental play are not finally separate things: the combination is necessary for survival of the community, as it manifestly is for the development of each individual.

But how much variation is enough, in evolutionary genetics, artistic aesthetics, or the experience of love that entails both? Some research has suggested that "the brain is most aroused by patterns in which there is approximately a 20% redundancy of elements,"[47] and that the most fashionable clothing maintains a calculable limit of self-matching.[48] But the data-sets are small, and again neuroscience risks underestimating the influence of cultural norms. Such ratios may be the outcome of an information-sorting heuristic arising from the value of redundancy, but that value shifts depending on the task, and the balance between innovation and copying varies across cultures, with advanced, open, diverse communities more receptive to experimental innovations.

A number of studies affirm that people value artists partly for their eccentricity, but only within a tolerable range – only when balanced with some measure of cognitive control, and even then only when that control does not discredit the innovative basis of the resulting artwork. Thus, "when people learned that an artist was eccentric – he mangled his ear, or carried stones on his head – they liked his work more. Unless, that is, the work was conventional or the artist's quirks were described as inauthentic."[49] Furthermore, "Repeated exposure to two works by the Pre-Raphaelite painter Sir John Everett Millais enhanced subjects' appreciation, while repeated exposure to the kitschy cottage-porn of Thomas Kinkade wore on them."[50] We may not know what art is exactly, but we know what we keep on liking.

As the passionate and mutable aspect of a normalizing entity, modern art must usually evolve more rapidly than the surrounding culture. That renders many masterpieces unrecognizable as such until many decades later. Their creators will be asked why their style has to be so displeasingly strange. The internationalists of the Modernist era often faced that question about, for example, the prose of Gertrude Stein. Stein wrote weirdly, but wrote about ordinary conversations and tangible domestic objects such as rooms and food and buttons, and said that the formality of French society was what made her eccentric work viable. Similar questions were raised about the works of Picasso, in whose "Old Guitarist" the guitar is the only thing that is *not* blue.

Avant-garde communities give that innovative function sanctuary in the realm of aesthetics, as academic freedom does in the realm of ideas – partly through a version of herd-immunity since they are not constantly obliged to breathe in and then spread the infectious cultural assumptions of the larger society. The avant-garde, which finds its chief expression through the arts, constitutes a concentration of the society's plasticity and mutation, which usually becomes visible first in a creative individual but may become collective if adaptive. That Stravinsky's "Rite of Spring" caused a riot in 1912 but became the soundtrack of a Disney movie less than 30 years later may demonstrate the point. A unique trait will expand across generations if its expression enhances differential survival, and that principle may be almost as true for cultural innovations as it is for genetic mutations. What made Stravinsky infamous is also what kept him interesting as Modernism evolved – although readers wanting a deeper philosophical dig into the social impact of musical innovations should also consider the argument of Adorno's *Philosophy of New Music* (1949), which suggests that Schoenberg is the real radical and that Stravinsky offers only an illusory radicalism that actually recaptures revolutionary impulses on behalf of mere bourgeois values.

Truly creative artwork aims to produce memes that aspire beyond mimicry, and it therefore often displeases not only the bourgeoisie but also people too burdened with labor, poverty, and sometimes illiteracy to have much time for such indulgent flights from common sense. Orwell's *Nineteen Eighty-Four* doubts the willingness of the "Proles" to defend free thought. On the other hand, Mikhail Bakunin and Frantz Fanon have asserted what Scott's work confirms: there may ultimately be more revolutionary potential in outcasts than in those who have gotten a good price for selling themselves out to the money-meme. In any case, this function of difficult art – art that is usefully both hated and loved – seems at risk in a Facebook and Instagram era when the goal of most people's creative work is to be Liked.

Trends in art, and even specific works of art, often slide from innovation toward dogma, like politically defiant or acid-headed 1960s rock music hits becoming comfortable nostalgia items on an Oldies radio station. The music industry seizes upon the innovations arising from youth culture and digests them into mass consumer culture. Like an immune response, this process became more efficient once the memeplex had been alerted to the threat by the subversive aspects of jazz, folk, and rock music. Hip-hop had barely been born before much of it began serving the memes of material greed and formulaic, commodified sexuality. If the current US Top 40 is any indication, that formerly revolutionary form now usually implies that the entire point of escaping poverty is conspicuous consumption of the conventional items of the super-wealthy: glitzy housing in costly places, high-carat jewelry, the world's most expensive cars, and drinking nothing but champagne. The overwhelming implication is that the only real value is expense, especially since money is the best and possibly only way for men to obtain sex from women, whose only real function is to provide it.

As many forms of popular art help the culture resist innovations by posing as resistant innovations, subversive art can often best escape from its elite enclave by offering falsely reassuring signals of conventionality. The Beatles' music was originally infectious. It exploited a cultural niche that become available in American youth-culture after the assassination of John F. Kennedy, and its success had something to do with the fact that the lads' hair was radically long yet neatly styled; that they were irreverent yet dressed by their manager in neat matching outfits; that their good-boy, bad-boy cheekiness (embodied by McCartney and Lennon respectively) was unsettling but also unthreatening; that their music sounded fresh and passionate, but was built on forms already made familiar (especially in the United States) by Chuck Berry, Carl Perkins, the Everly Brothers, and various skiffle, blues, and rhythm-and-blues performers.

The Beatles' "Sergeant Pepper" album is widely considered the breakthrough event that made inventive sound collages and weird new lyrical and conceptual experiments possible in the rock genre, crystallizing the effects of a psychedelic era into popular music and hence mainstream culture. But the album included several songs that actually looked backwards to local cultural history. The pace and instrumentation of "She's Leaving Home" is decidedly pre-rock, and its lyrics tell a wistful story (like the bittersweet black-and-white mid-century English films such as *Brief Encounter*) of the smallness of English middle-class lives in the 20 years between the German surrender in World War II and the emergence of Beatlemania. The bouncy cuteness of "When I'm Sixty-Four" is packed with the clichés of a previous generation's aspirations.

Nor was this balance traceable only in the contributions of the softer-edged McCartney. Lennon's "Being for the Benefit of Mr. Kite" was a transcription of a 19th-century circus poster accompanied by old carnival instruments slightly distorted, and "A Day in the Life" is a rich catalogue of an ordinary London day, developing into a musical/spiritual crisis emphatically resolved into a single piano chord at the end. The main innovation contributed by George Harrison, "Within You and Without You," consisted of ancient Hindu philosophy accompanied by a centuries-old Indian instruments – especially the sitar, which brought a new sound into Western popular music. In fact, the entire concept of the album replaced the Beatles with Sergeant Pepper's band, traditional English bandstand and music-hall performers, surrounded on the cover by many decades' worth of the Beatles' cultural heroes, offering the same kind of eclectic repertoire of reassuringly familiar deities as Pollan noticed in psychedelic treatment rooms.

Eminent scholars of cultural evolution have wondered, "why is chanting, singing, shouting, and marching rhythmically effective at uniting a group?"[51] The question seems almost tautological, but it points to larger human need to have shared programming rather than unrestricted individual volition and imagination. A 2013 study in New Zealand showed that "rituals with synchronous body movements were more likely to increase prosocial attitudes," and that "rituals judged to be sacred were associated with the largest contributions in the public goods game," a well-known test of communitarian tendencies.[52] These dual findings square with my sense that both the complications of sensory experience and the complications of spiritual consciousness lead to a willing investment in ways of collectively simplifying those cues.

The arts are also essential to the indispensable sense that one's life has a life-story: a meaning in a community and (if at all possible) in the universe, a version of the widely vaunted participation in something larger than oneself. Kierkegaard identified (and Holocaust survivor Viktor Frankl popularized in his 1946 book *Man's Search for Meaning*) the importance of a "will to meaning," as opposed to Adler's Nietzschean doctrine of "will to power" or Freud's emphasis on the will to pleasure.

Can we, however, in good faith rely on the creative artists who play to our cognitive illusions by providing patterns, and play to our hunger for meaning by inventing hermeneutically saturated universes? Poets, novelists, and dramatists often invent deep mystical connections and satisfying instances of poetic justice that are really just the imposition of the author, who resembles a priest fabricating miracles to convince people that God exists: one elite intellectual class benignly doping the rest, like one level of the mind repressing the onslaught of discordant recognitions that would be cognitively or spiritually intolerable to ordinary consciousness. That repression is what I have identified as a key function of culture, and I have warned that we need to be wary of it. Yet many artworks – and they certainly do not need be high classical arts – seem to awaken something in ourselves that we feel to be deeper, higher, better than our ordinary negotiations with reality evoke; they feel like a fulfillment of our largest capacities for experience, not the shrinking of the internal and external universe into a least common denominator.

High culture is possible partly because basic culture relieves the cognitive load of everyday living. On a large scale, a fine example is the case of ancient Greece, which (as Walter Ong's classic *Orality and Literacy* has shown) was able to invent many versions of abstract, technical, political, and ethical thought because the invention of writing relieved a large portion of the cognitive burden that memory bears in a purely oral culture. But high culture, as a kind of mutualist, repays that liberatory service, by liberating the basic culture from the stagnation toward which, by its nature as a source of stability, it tends to evolve.

Slow rather than fast thinking (to use Kahneman's division of our decision-making process), assertions of intellect over instincts, permit resistance to the mere algorithms of our evolved psychology as played out in evolving aggregations of memes. That resistance will therefore be concentrated in higher education and the high arts, with their devotion to advanced thinking and creative reformulation. In categorizing artworks, however, the useful distinction for this purpose may not be between high and low, but between the transformative and the normative. High culture can become mostly a signifier of the tribe of the elite, allowing members of the upper class to affirm each others' exalted sensibility, which, in turn, serves to justify their determination to spare themselves the brutality they believe the lower classes have, in some sense, chosen. Shakespearean drama, in contrast, was widely considered low art by the cultural elites of his time. When Shakespeare's rival playwright Ben Jonson included his drama in an elegant edition called his *Works*, he was mocked in an epigram: "Pray tell me, *Ben*, where doth the mystery lurk, / What others call a play, you call a work." As play is children's work, then plays – and other forms of popular and seemingly irresponsible art – can carry some of the plasticity of playfulness into the adult world.

✻✻✻✻✻✻✻✻✻✻✻✻✻✻✻✻✻✻✻✻✻✻✻✻

Artistic creativity, this chapter argues, has been a rewarding investment for *Homo sapiens*. Across many species, the safest way to create the opportunities produced by variation – indispensable opportunities as environments change – has evidently been sexual reproduction, which generates new combinations of existing genetic variants. I have suggested that, for human and many other kinds of animals, sexual selection appears to offer choice and appears to respond to something we may call beauty, which often correlates with the complex order of fractal symmetries that so often shapes natural phenomena. But even at the level of the simple cellular individual, real mutations can very occasionally prove beneficial in fitting a new niche – and that, again, is as true for a culture as it is for a species.

Cellular mutations are not normally consciously undertaken, of course, but creative thinkers are tasked with creating new cultural forms out of the old ones. Like nearly all genetic mutants, most works of art quickly prove to be dead ends. They are lost and forgotten, though some remain in the cultural seed-banks or latent epigenetic strands called museums, archives, and libraries. Despite that rate of failure, these variations remain a necessary capacity for a species facing change, which may be why arts seem to accelerate, and seem in retrospect to have improved, in periods of social upheaval and cultural collision such as the Renaissance.

Consider the way an old man saved his band of hunter-gatherers during the 1943 drought in Australia by remembering ritual song-cycles from his childhood that contained clues to the location of waterholes along a path to the coast; or even the way that some elephant clans survived the 1993 drought in Tanzania because they had matriarchs old enough to remember finding water during droughts decades earlier, whereas clans whose older matriarchs had been killed by poachers died out.[53] Think of art-work as resembling ant-work in this regard: most of the scouts sent out to forage find nothing edible, but their efforts are still worth making, from the perspective of the group, because one will find the sugar bowl, or a preferable new habitat. Artists may discover something tasty, or a new accommodation for the spirit.

As Yann Martel put it in his best-selling novel *The Life of Pi*,

> even animals that were bred in zoos ... will have moments of excitement that push them to seek to escape. All living things contain a measure of madness that moves them in strange, sometimes inexplicable ways. This madness can be saving; it is part and parcel of the ability to adapt. Without it, no species would survive.[54]

Pollan reports the speculation of a chemistry professor that some mushrooms attracted animals to eat them, and thereby spread their spores, by offering psilocybin as an incentive. Pollan appends the hypothesis of an ethnobotanist that, while individual animals who consumed the *Psilocybes* would be vulnerable in their hallucinatory state and so natural selection would eliminate that appetite, it might be advantageous "during times of rapid environmental change or crisis" for the group or species to have "a few of its members abandon their accustomed conditioned responses and experiment with some radically new and different behaviors" to help it adapt. Pollan admits that this suggestion takes him "onto highly speculative, slightly squishy ground,"[55] and perhaps the improbabilities of group selection make this already surprising suggestion sink out of sight. But it does offer some intriguing parallels to the value I see in extremely plastic human mentalities, probably originating in the climate instability of the Pleistocene, and perhaps no less valuable in the age of anthropogenic climate-change.

Art often both celebrates and mourns the dissident individual. Tragedy commonly confronts its hero with an impossible choice between two imperatives – each represented by a law or a deity, in a world whose rules are in tension or transition – and thereby exposes the governing system as finally incomplete and even self-contradictory (Kurt Gödel has exposed a version of this imperfection in the logic of numbers, Thomas Kuhn in scientific explanatory models, and deconstructionist criticism in literature itself). Sometimes, tragic drama implicitly endorses the system by warning people away from the protagonist's error, as noted earlier, but in the more interesting instances – Macbeth's ambition is a strong example – that conventional morality co-exists with a critique of the damage such morality does to the upward as well as the downward potential of some human qualities. As our species follows a scatter-pattern on the range between (to use C. Robert Cloniger's terms) neophobes and neophiles, the former will tend to enjoy the consolations of comedy, with its regressions toward the creaturely mean, while the latter will feel the pull of the tragic, with its focus on the extinction of the unique individual in a world of larger forces and the erasure of the possibilities that individual represented.

A tragedy is, of course, only a play. But those who assume that this kind of playing is a kind of superficial indulgence rather than a necessary organ of the society are making the same mistake made by solemn teachers and strict parents who assume that the hunger of youngsters for play is a pointless distraction from more disciplined activity. They assume this despite all the evidence that play, including safely experimental mimicking of what will be crucial survival skills later in life, has proven so durable across eons and across species. This book has not focused on the aspect of art that gives pleasure, but it has suggested both cognitive and evolutionary reasons for that response to art. Creative persons, to the extent they circumvent their culture's resistance to novelty, make adaptive change in the collective ideology possible as circumstances alter, which seems to be a worthwhile trade-off for the accompanying risks of destructive errors. Along comes a Da Vinci, and he makes us arguably a better species thereafter: more clearly unique, more interesting, and more fully engaged with the world and our own potential – again, not by an upgrade of hardware, but by a refinement of software. We just need to know how to test and debug the code so it doesn't loop and crash, or expose the body-politic to worms and viruses. In the modern First World, at least, that editorial discernment is the work of another cultural institution.

Interchapter: Party Politics

Reading guidebooks to help my daughter choose a college, I was struck by the relentless deployment of the word "party" as a verb. Students almost everywhere discussed where, when, and how intensely they party. What rankled me was less the grammatical shift (Shakespeare loved to turn nouns into verbs and verbs into gerunds) than its implication that "partying" is a unitary activity with specific customs: a prescribed regimen by which, paradoxically, all bright young things should express their freedom. It implies a certainty about what is "appropriate" irresponsibility for the young, as "parenting" has similarly emerged for responsible behavior in their elders.

Like travel packages for Spring Break, "partying" proposes a formulaic way in which students are licensed to be wild and defiant. Booze and loud music can be liberating, especially to the overly self-conscious, but William Blake sitting peacefully in his garden with a sheet of paper and a quill pen was surely more free and wild than any sophomore puking by the punchbowl.

Does this ritual really liberate a real self, or is it instead another way people pressure each other into affirming some formulas that not only oversimplify desire but also isolate it from transformative causes? Certainly, among my college acquaintances, the ones who went the wildest in this conventional sense were (I soon noticed) usually those who came from families of traditional high privilege, and the same people (I eventually noticed) often ended up as forces of similar kinds of trust-fund conservatism. Protest rallies may be a predictable and often sloppily conceived springtime ritual also, but at least their political character shows the grain of something idealistic and socially conscious.

The persistent boast of a "study hard, party hard" ethos on campuses suggests an obligation desperately fulfilled – a counterpart and maybe antidote to new learning. The slogan is so appealing that it turned up on a flyer for a bar in Munich, Germany:

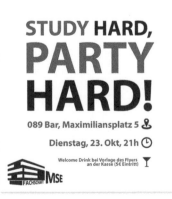

Figure 1 "Study Hard, Party Hard" bar flyer; Munich, Germany.

The fact that so many college students now use that slogan suggests how much cultural work it is doing. And the fact that this appears to be an adaptation of a "work hard, play hard" ethos of late-20th-century Yuppies helps link it to the invasion of a business mentality into undergraduate life the next chapter will explore. Along with the feigned spontaneity, there is a feigned innocence about "party," as if the revelers were 4-year-olds lining up for birthday cake instead of 20-year-olds compulsively binge drinking their way to hook-ups.

As a relatively square and (at best) middle-aged observer, I'm surely sounding like a typical fogey scolding a next generation's indulgences. But the rise of Alessia Cara's "Here" – an extended critique of obligatory alcohol and marijuana partying, containing a critique of songs that lack meaningful messages – toward the top of the Billboard charts in 2015–2016 suggested that many young people were excited to hear their alienation from this memeplex finally allowed to express itself as an alternative definition of cool.

Katy Perry's sneakily pop-flavored 2017 hit "Chained to the Rhythm" doubles as a critique along the lines established by Huxley and Marcuse. The official video is set in a theme park called Oblivia, where the tightly programmed fun makes people unable to "see the trouble" while they "dance to the distortion." Ms. Perry begins noticing uneasily that she and her companions are "Living our lives through a lens / Trapped in our white-picket fence" where they put their "rose-colored glasses on / And party on." They ride the rides and play the same song over and over, and "think we're free / Drink, this one is on me / We're all chained to the rhythm." The video ends with a close-up of Ms. Perry giving us a truly horrified stare.[1] These interventions within youth masscult suggest that the next generation shares some of the worries that drive this interchapter and this book as a whole.

5   The Red Scare and the Idea
of the University

... an upbringing which aims only at money-making or physical
strength, or even some mental accomplishment devoid of reason and
justice, [would be] vulgar and illiberal and utterly unworthy of the name
"education." Let us not, however, quarrel over a name, but let us abide
by the statement we agreed upon just now, that those who are rightly educated become, as a rule, good, and that one should in no case disparage
education, since it stands first among the finest gifts that are given to the
best men; and if ever it errs from the right path, but can be put straight
again, to this task every man, so long as he lives, must address himself
with all his might.

—Plato, *Laws*, 644a–b

Who tunes the Blue Guitar? That is, who can be trusted to mediate
between the experiments in consciousness represented by artworks, and
the culture that is naturally reluctant to embrace them after sniffing out
an imposter in the nest? Or, to ask the question in a different way, why
do universities exist, especially in a society that so broadly resents the
radical ideas often broadcast with such apparent condescension from the
Ivory Tower?

Creative artists and intellectuals are always navigating around a paradox. It is essential that culture be invisible, so that we can believe our
reality and morality are grounded, objective, and absolute. It is also
essential that culture be visible, so that we can recognize and repair
its malfunction when it leads us astray from our interests. That situation is captured nicely in the Lecture by the military supercomputer
Golem XIV that provided an epigraph to Chapter 2: "You have had a
great deal more freedom than Intelligence, which is why you have been
getting rid of freedom," it asserts, "by means of the cultures you have
developed through the ages," and

each of them has the logic of its structure and not of its originators,
for it is the kind of invention that molds its inventors after its own
fashion, and they know nothing of this; whereas, when they do find

out, it loses its absolute power over them and they perceive an emptiness, and it is this contradiction which is the cornerstone of human nature.[1]

The division of labor between those who primarily defend cultural norms and conventional beliefs, and those who primarily critique them, reflects the inward struggle of most human individuals between a valuable exclusion of the world's complexity and mutability, and a valuable acknowledgment of those same things. Neither would be adaptive, in the long run, without some alloy of the other; but that does not prevent each from attempting to extinguish the other. This chapter will explore one cautionary instance of the consequences of that struggle that hit me close to home. Specifically, it will show how the psychological repression of complexity, and the desire to make that repression easier and more complete by making it collective – two main topics of the first half of this book – can manifest themselves in repressive politics that seek to crush the counterforce represented by intellectuals and institutionalized as universities.

The Trials of Goodwin Watson

At the start of the "Crystal Skull" movie, Soviet kidnappers force a mostly mild-mannered Midwestern archeology professor named Indiana Jones to help them find where the US military has stored that alien skull. He miraculously survives proximity to an atomic-bomb test by hiding inside a refrigerator in an archetypal 1950s suburban tract house, built to test the bomb's effects, as if the question was really whether the complacent, mass-produced ideal of post-World War II domesticity could – with a heroic American heart and mind stashed away at its core – survive the new terrors and technology of a nuclear age. (A similar nostalgic and jingoistic reassurance culminates the 2006 horror film remake *The Hills Have Eyes*: the heroic father defeats the mutant inhabitants of a similar nuclear-test suburbia by hitting them with a baseball bat and impaling one with an American flag before recovering his children.) But when Indy returns to his middle-American college, he discovers that the dean has been pressured into suspending him from teaching because the buttoned-up FBI functionaries distrust his old friendship with Oxley, a fellow archeologist who (under extreme duress) was apparently cooperating with the Soviets.

My father, Goodwin Watson, was no Indiana Jones. He was just a tireless, left-leaning professor of social psychology, working mostly on experimental and international education, who (at the sacrifice of at least half his income) accepted a job as Chief Analyst of the Foreign Broadcast Intelligence Service soon after the United States entered World War II. All seven commissioners of the Federal Communications Commission deemed him irreplaceable because (as one explained) "Watson got so damn good, he'd call the turn on [that is, successfully predict] a lot of German military operations from their propaganda broadcasts."[2] The pen may be mightier than the sword, but so is an attentive, psychologically attuned reader.

Yet, he was hounded out of this job in 1943 by an early incarnation of the demagogic House Committee on Un-American Activities (HUAC). That committee placed a rider on an essential war-appropriations bill, forbidding any organization that received federal funds to hire him (and, after that was rejected, it was expanded to include two of his colleagues): "no part of any appropriation contained in this Act shall be used to pay the compensation of Goodwin Watson."[3] Despite the vigorous objections that the US Senate and President Franklin D. Roosevelt raised on their behalf, the three endured years of struggle before a unanimous Supreme Court struck down the provision as a Bill of Attainder – the first such ruling since the Civil War era. Ten years after the first accusations, there was a relapse: throughout the first years of my life, my father endured the campaign of a local "Americanism Commission" to have him fired from his private-sector job.

In both instances, the accusations centered on my father's association with people who were critical of capitalism. After the extreme economic inequalities and Wall Street speculations of the 1920s helped produce the Depression of the 1930s – conditions similar in several ways to those that provoked the recent Occupy movement – such criticism seemed appropriate. His activism also fit with the legacy of Social Gospel in the Methodist church, in which he had been a Deacon. Methodists played a prominent role in the anti-slavery movement of the mid-19th century, and became a no less prominent force for many of the causes that progressives now pursue: racial and economic justice, women's rights, pacifism, free health care and education, and ending hunger and homelessness.

In the 1940s, anti-Communist hysteria provided an opportunity for right-wingers to take revenge on these chronic dissidents. Activities that might now strike many of us as eminently and ideally American became grounds for defining Goodwin Watson as un-American. He had joined the ACLU at a moment when longstanding Constitutional rights were manifestly at risk. He had served as one of the first directors of Consumer's Union (now mostly known for *Consumer Reports* magazine, but then deemed by some to be a Communist "front" organization) when corporations were using their political contributions and advertising skills to control consumers in ruthless, predatory fashion. He had prominently petitioned and organized for the Scottsboro Boys' right to a fair trial and (later) Paul Robeson's and Marian Anderson's rights to sing to white audiences during the mid-century backlash against efforts toward racial integration and equal justice. His 1925 book *The Measure of Fair Mindedness* was a landmark early study of "open-mindedness" and "freedom from prejudice"; and over the 20 years that followed, his group at Union Theological Seminary "formed a crucial nexus for activist-oriented study of race prejudice."[4] When even the NAACP and other liberals capitulated to the Red Scare by abandoning the great civil-rights activist and anti-capitalist W. E. B. Du Bois to his tormentors in the US government in 1952, Goodwin Watson chaired a dinner honoring Du Bois – a fact that predictably turned up in Watson's FBI files.[5]

He was a descendant, through his father, of some of the first American colonists and US patriots: my namesake died in Connecticut in 1634, and a subsequent ancestor (along with his first cousin and my son's namesake) was part of the Lexington Alarm that fought the first battle of the Revolutionary War; Goodwin's mother's ancestors came to Massachusetts in 1632, and fought in the French and Indian wars as well as the Revolutionary War. He himself was a boy from the Midwest who was a Navy volunteer during World War I. It is hard to see how much more American he could have been without being from one of the indigenous tribes. Yet the campaigns to declare him un-American were prominent, persistent and ferocious, as excerpts from the coverage in the *New York Times* through more than a decade make clear (Figures 2–7).

What made him especially threatening, I believe, was that – having decided that Christianity could no longer reform society as effectively as the emerging science of psychology – he devoted most of his professional life to trying to open up educational systems (the University Without Walls was one direct outcome of his work). This project entailed initiating conversations between American educators and their counterparts worldwide, including a dialogue with Soviet educators designed to get both sides in the Cold War to replace jingoistic indoctrination and standardized competitive grading with more personalized teaching that favored creative and cooperative thinking. An article my father wrote with

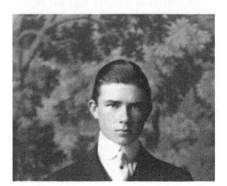

Figure 2 The Young Goodwin Watson.

**President Assails
Says Congress**

Special to THE N1

WASHINGTON, Sept. 14—President Roosevelt challenged today the authority of Congress to remove from Government payrolls Robert Morss Lovett, Secretary of the Virgin Islands; and William E. Dodd Jr. and Goodwin B. Watson, officials of the FCC, charged in the House with radicalism.

Figure 3 President assails congress "Rider"; *New York Times*, July 14, 1943.

FAIR PLAY IS THE ISSUE

A constitutional issue of grave importance has been created by the action of Congress in attaching to the Urgency Deficiency Appropriation Act a stipulation that no funds shall be paid after Nov. 15 to Secretary Robert Morss Lovett of the Virgin Islands government and to Goodwin B. Watson and William E. Dodd Jr. of the Federal Communications Commission. In signing the bill on Tuesday the President expressed concern over what he described as an invasion of executive authority, and took the unusual step of reading from a message which he intends to send to Congress on the subject when it reconvenes.

Yet it is not so much the constitutional question as it is the question of orderly procedure and fair play that will interest most Americans in these cases. The three gentlemen named in the bill were charged by the Dies Committee with past memberships in subversive organizations. The Committee, proceeding in its customarily reckless and high-handed manner, never produced evidence that the organizations in question were actually subversive or, if they were, that the accused men had other than an innocent connection with them. In fact, the Dies Committee's list of subversive groups is long enough and indiscriminate enough to catch almost any group or individual that the Committee does not care for. The three victims were railroaded through the Committee and railroaded again in the House. Messrs. Watson

Figure 4 Fair play is the issue; Editorial, *New York Times*, July 15, 1943.

COURT INVALIDATES LOVETT DISCHARGE

Unanimously Says He, Watson and Dodd Were Objects of Congress 'Bill of Attainder'

Special to THE NEW YORK TIMES.

WASHINGTON, June 3—An effort by Congress to discharge three Government employes on the ground of alleged subversive activities was held unconstitutional by the Supreme Court in a unanimous ruling today. The three were Robert Morss Lovett, Government Secretary of the Virgin Islands and afterward executive assistant to the Governor of the islands; Goodwin B. Watson and William E. Dodd Jr., both attached to the Foreign Broadcast Intelligence Service of the Federal Communications Commission.

Figure 5 Court invalidates Lovett discharge; *New York Times*, June 4, 1946.

ROBESON RIOT INQUIRY CALLED 'WHITEWASH'

Special to THE NEW YORK TIMES.

WHITE PLAINS, N. Y., May 29 —Mishandling of the current Westchester County grand jury investigation of last autumn's riots near Peekskill was charged today by the Westchester Committee for Human Rights. The riots involved leftwing followers of Paul Robeson and anti-Communist groups.

The committee, headed by Dr. Goodwin Watson of Rye, Professor of Education at Columbia University charged that District At-

Figure 6 Robeson riot inquiry called "Whitewash";*New York Times*, May 30, 1950.

The Guidance Center said a committee of corporation and professional leaders had surveyed Dr. Watson's work as a psychologist, sociologist, Methodist clergyman and teacher since 1920, including his affiliations with Columbia, Union Theological Seminary, Young Men's Christian Association and the Federal Communications Commission.

The Center reaffirmed a belief that while Dr. Watson has "liberal and sometimes unorthodox views," he has never been a Communist or fellow-traveler and is an "independent scholar and loyal citizen."

Figure 7 Dr. Watson upheld by guidance center; *New York Times*, July 23, 1954.

John Dewey in 1937 suggests that teachers would have a crucial role in forestalling the growth of fascism – not by criticizing fascists (let alone by creating communists), but by nurturing a generation that would value play and individual liberty over conformist order, and giving that generation access to "the whole broad scheme of experience ... through the varied complex of life potentialities."[6] He and Dewey recognized that "Education is likely to be one of the great battlegrounds upon which is waged an intense and desperate struggle for power," and that their goal of letting each child develop an "active, flexible personality" – a goal that "is poles removed from inculcating conclusions that have been settled in advance" – "will perhaps result in serious perturbation or even panic; and the conclusion may be reached by these that intelligence, apart from some higher authority, is unequal to the task of devising acceptable principles of conduct."[7] In an era of Iron Curtains, these schools without mental walls promised more freedom than our nation would tolerate.

Although "Watson waited his entire life and never received the redress he deserved,"[8] the Ivory Tower swarms with ghosts far more pitiable than my father's: ones who lacked his luck, or the luck of Professor Indiana Jones, in surviving the 20th-century wars between left- and right-wing ideologies (escalated by the mutually aggravating threats of the atom bomb and the Cold War) and achieving public vindication. In the 1940s, German forces eradicated professors across Eastern Europe: if intellectuals resisted Nazism, they were demonized as Communists. In the late 1960s and the 1970s, Communist tyrants in Asia massacred university faculties; if intellectuals expressed reservations about the Cambodian revolution, they were demonized as running-dog capitalists. In fact, the Khmer Rouge warned against cultural dissent and scholarship as paired symptoms: "If we don't unite, our work will be haphazard and hesitant, and we will descend into intellectualism."[9] A similar dynamic is now at work in the Myanmar genocide.[10] Clearly, in these horrifying cases, the scholars' real crime was – and our real value still is – constituting an independent and prestigious entity well-situated to challenge both popular assumptions and government propaganda.

The 21st century has begun with a new round of reactionary efforts to extirpate or at least intimidate the self-perpetuating conspiracy of "tenured radicals" and atheists said to dominate university faculties, where they reportedly poison the patriotism, godliness, common sense, and common courtesy of our young people, while being simultaneously too permissive and too punitive toward their sexual conduct. Both Marco Rubio and Ben Carson asserted that view in the 2016 campaign for the Republican presidential nomination. My chief personal encounter was a 2006 "Bruin Alumni Association" website ranking me one of the top five dangerous radicals at UCLA, rated a maximal five Black Panther fists, and offering cash to students to record my and others' classes to catch us saying something leftist. Since my teaching of Shakespeare is fairly traditional and my scandalous "profile" consisted mostly of an attack on my father, who had already been dead for more than thirty years, and since the attack was clearly provoked by my replies to campus newspaper columns by the founder of the supposed Alumni Association (columns praising the then-popular George W. Bush administration), I resisted the allure of playing the next generation's blacklist martyr, assuming that if I ignored the website bait, everyone else would too.

Silly me: over the next few days, several major newspapers across the United States and even the *Guardian* overseas picked up the story, as did major television and radio networks. The only plausible explanation is that the body-politic went into anaphylactic shock – the wild overreaction of the immune system when it encounters even a trace of a substance (such as bee venom, peanut, or penicillin) to which it has been hypersensitized by past exposure. The shadow the TV lights cast behind the young right-wing website founder aspiring to media prominence resembled Senator Joe McCarthy, and America's culture-warriors on both sides felt compelled to rehearse their lines for the next round of Red-Scare witch-hunts.

It would be a dangerous mistake for universities to hang a Mission Accomplished banner over their academic-freedom committees just because this kind of attack backfired. Certainly it can happen again: immediately after Trump's election, a right-wing group established a well-publicized nationwide Professor Watchlist asking students to inform on professors "that advance a radical agenda."[11] But the real threat to higher education in the near future will likely arrive in a more benign guise, appropriating at times the liberal vocabulary of fairness and tolerance, and at other times professing a neoliberal deference to free-market ideology. Several state legislatures have been considering an "Academic Bill of Rights" which sounds innocent enough, but is clearly designed to wedge open the door to political control of scholarship. By insisting on "neutrality" toward different viewpoints, conservative politicians would surely use such laws to force professors to conform to received wisdom and mainstream beliefs – as if all important truths (about sonnets, carbon dioxide concentrations, or anything else) were found halfway between current Democratic and Republican campaign speeches, and as if the best scholarship naturally conformed to ideological quotas. In 2007, the Missouri House of Representatives passed a bill specifying that all their state universities must have "guidelines on teaching" that "shall include ... protection of ... the viewpoint that the Bible is inerrant." A student who replies to various questions about the Big Bang on an Astrophysics final exam by simply repeatedly asserting that God created the heavens on the first day would presumably have grounds to sue if not awarded a straight A grade. John Milton's Archangel Raphael, who teaches pious astronomy to Adam, might be pleased, but people of reason in a fallen world cannot always do their work on that basis.

Even if they don't gain direct control over classrooms, those in power like to generate caricatures and resentment about campus leftists for two reasons. First, it makes it easier to take indirect control by cutting funding for the humanities and social sciences, since support for such funding becomes scarce among citizens convinced it will be squandered on pointless research by lazy, traitorous elitists who corrupt young minds on the rare occasions that they teach at all. Second, the hysteria predisposes people to dismiss any criticism emerging from academia – like any inconvenient fact emerging through the news media – as merely a symptom of liberal bias, rather than a flaw in the official story.

That is an important step toward the truth-free politics of the alt-right movement of 2016, and the costs of such exclusions are only too evident in our recent history. As early in 1964, many professors warned the US government – then controlled by the Democrats – that Vietnam wasn't just some proxy site for the West's battle against Communism, but a proud culture shaped by a thousand-year struggle for independence. At least 95% of the deaths of US soldiers and Vietnamese people could have been averted (and the geopolitical outcome could hardly have been worse for the United States) if these egghead faculty crackpots – labeled fools, turncoats, and cowards by the government and the mainstream – had been heeded.

When the United States launched its war on Iraq, the lead story in UCLA's right-wing newspaper condemned the faculty as obviously a left-wing cabal. The primary evidence was the fact that 93% of professors surveyed believed that invading Iraq would be a bad idea, at a time when 75% of the American public believed it a good idea. Would we have a better faculty – in History, Political Science, Near Eastern Languages and Cultures, etc. – if the legislature were to mandate that most of these professors be replaced by ones mistaken enough about the region's political and cultural history to have believed the promises of cake-walks and flower-showers and Iraqi city squares joyfully renamed after President Bush, under a shining pro-western secular democracy after a few weeks of mopping up a few "dead-enders"? My point is not that professors are always right – no one who has sat through faculty meetings can be under any such illusion – but only that they are not wrong just because their scholarly perspective is temporarily unpopular, or because they draw that perspective from soft-headed stuff like the study of cultural artifacts.

Nor can we assume that our colleagues in the hard sciences are safe, even when working with provable hypotheses about seemingly apolitical topics. In 1948, the Kremlin decided that advocates of Darwin's "decadent" theory were "enemies of the Soviet people." A commonsensical comrade named Trofim Lysenko was given authority over those impractical pointy-headed biology professors, who then either stopped saying what they knew to be true or disappeared into gulags. Communism then had a scientific theory it was comfortable with – except that its willful ignorance of Politically Incorrect plant genetics soon left it helpless to prevent the mass starvation of its people. With the theory of evolution under attack by religiously motivated groups demanding equal time for Creationism, and the Bush and Trump administrations censoring any warnings or even data from environmental scientists, those are ghosts worth remembering too.

None of this is to deny that the Soviet Union constituted a real threat to the freedom of the people they ruled, and to some legitimate interests of Western democracy. What is most directly relevant to my theory, however, is the way these threats were used in the 1950s to fuel mandates for all kinds of social conformity – in religion, class, consumerism, sexuality, even hairstyles – that had nothing to do with military defense. This was the era, the middle of the 20th century, when EC Comics staged its resistance to the mutual reassurances of various American institutions. Their *Mad* magazine certainly became a key haven of cultural resistance that reached across generations. To block government intervention, America's comic-book industry actually felt compelled to ban the word "weird" from the title of any publication;[12] the link between the psychology and the politics of conformism in the functions of culture could hardly be clearer.

Neither do I deny that, more recently, Islamic fundamentalism has often been oppressive to those it rules, and may be a long-term threat to Western civilization. Whatever else it may be, Islam has proven itself a brilliantly designed memeplex for expansion relative to other systems of both practice and social governance. Since "phobia" implies an irrational fear, "Islamophobia" may not always be the right term. But, like American fear of the Soviet Union, that fear has frequently leaked, in the early 21st century, into categories where it is irrational. Sharia law is not imminent in midsized cities in the American Midwest. National security was invoked to answer what were often symbolic cultural insecurities – "the Ground-Zero mosque!" – and university humanists were primary targets. That is not really surprising: the renowned literary theorist and Palestinian activist Edward Said has credited traditional philology – the multidisciplinary study of the written archive to establish accurate texts and historically valid interpretations of them – with a unique ability to enable resistance against identities "given by the flag or the national war of the moment."[13]

If internationalism, intellectualism, and the sympathy for the oppressed that literary engagement nurtures were prime bait to the Red Baiters, it is well worth noting what forces were essential to ending the Soviet threat. When Mikhail Gorbachev was interviewed recently about what caused *perestroika* and thereby the end of the Soviet tyrannies and hence the end of the Cold War and the active threat of global thermonuclear war, he said,

I am an intellectually curious person by nature and I understood that many changes were necessary, and that it was necessary to think about them, even if it caused me discomfort. I began to carry out my own inner, spiritual *perestroika* – a *perestroika* in my personal views. Along the way, Russian literature and, in fact, all literature, European and American too, had a big influence on me. I was drawn especially to philosophy. And my wife, Raisa, who had read more philosophy than I had, was always there alongside me. I didn't just learn historical facts but tried to put them in a philosophical or conceptual framework. I began to understand that society needed a new vision – that we must view the world with our eyes open, not just through our personal or private interests. That's how our new thinking of the 1980s began.[14]

The culture of *glasnost* yielded over subsequent decades, as my theory would predict, to the tyrannies of wealth and other imported Western memeplexes. But anyone who doubts that personal inner journeys – however uncomfortable – provoked by literature and philosophy can rescue the world should remember their role in finally taming the conflict that, for four decades, had threatened to destroy the world.

Politics and the Humanities

Professors are the usual suspects because we promote unusual ideas, and thereby threaten the consoling consensus I have been describing. The ideological conflict around our universities may seem like a political dispute, but the politics may be just a reflection of a deeper conflict. A preservative attitude toward traditionally dominant beliefs and social structure often underlies conservative politics. People are not wrong to feel that academic inquiries may pry loose the lid of Pandora's box, like Indiana Jones (with a Soviet gun at his head) wielding his crowbar on the crate encasing the Crystal Skull. But we are not a Fifth Column – that is, a treasonous group supporting a nation's enemy. We are only some second thoughts. As Said has written,

> the intellectual, in my sense of the word, is neither a pacifier nor a consensus-builder, but someone whose whole being is staked on a critical sense, a sense of being unwilling to accept easy formulas, or ready-made clichés, or the smooth, ever-so-accommodating confirmations of what the powerful or conventional have to say, and what they do. Not just passively unwilling, but actively willing to say so in public [and] thinking of the intellectual vocation as maintaining a state of constant alertness, of a perpetual willingness not to let half-truths or received ideas steer one along."[15]

Bookishness has always provoked charges of myopic blindness to common sense, even when it offered illuminations. The great Renaissance genius Giordano Bruno wrote of himself (with characteristic immodesty),

> By the light of his senses and reason, he opened those cloisters of truth which it is possible for us to open with the key of most diligent inquiry, he laid bare covered and veiled nature, gave eyes to the moles and light to the blind ... he loosed the tongues of the dumb who could not and dared not express their entangled opinions.[16]

Is it any surprise that church and state alike, having chased him out of place after place, finally contrived to have him burnt at the stake, wearing an iron mask to smother any subversive last words?

Even Socrates was executed as an enemy of the state, and he was perfectly clear about why the state did so, and why it was shortsighted to do so:

> For if you kill me you will not easily find another like me, who, if I may use such a ludicrous figure of speech, am a sort of gadfly, given to the State by the God; and the State is like a great and noble steed who is tardy in his motions owing to his very size, and requires to be stirred into life .... I dare say that you may feel irritated at being suddenly awakened when you are caught napping; and you may think that if you were to strike me dead ... then you would sleep on for the remainder of your lives, unless God in his care of you gives you another gadfly.[17]

Although English departments are actually relatively new – emerging about a century ago, and focusing on literary criticism only decades later – the function I have been describing has thus been lauded by noteworthy (if sometimes politically objectionable) minds of Western culture for thousands of years. To Matthew Arnold and Socrates, we may add Emerson:

> The whole secret of the teacher's force lies in the conviction that men are convertible. And they are. They want awakening. Get the soul out of bed, out of her deep habitual sleep, out into God's universe, to a perception of its beauty & hearing of its Call and your vulgar man, your prosy selfish sensualist awakes a God & is conscious of force to shake the world.

Intriguingly, "sensualist" originally read, "Capitalist"[18]; Emerson backed off from this characterization by crossing out the more specific word, but we may now see the wisdom of that warning.

More recently, intellectualism has often been conflated with the infidel enemies of a society's way of life, for two main reasons: intellectualism practices multicultural relativism, if only across time, in search of a nuanced truth, and it entails both the seeking and the debunking of meaning. The psycho-cognitive function that decides when to seize on a pattern in all the data flooding in on us from moment to moment is a delicate setting, and can all too easily slide into a paranoid-schizophrenic mode that finds designs everywhere: symmetrical spiderwebs of deep conspiracy spinning out all around the tiny circle of self. At the other extreme, it can trigger a depressive collapse into meaninglessness, a landscape without destinations, the grey exhaustion of a world drained of purpose. In consciousness as in the physical universe, we inhabit only some very narrow bands sufficiently stable and orderly to give us traction but also malleable enough to allow us choice. Scholars always have to be probing the boundaries, while also diligently cultivating (and weeding) that fertile strip of ground in the middle.

The arts and humanities matter because that psychic territory is no less worth exploring than its physical counterpart. Just because we live in an age of amazing scientific discovery doesn't fundamentally change the substance in which we live, or the scale of time and space we inhabit. A person may reach a hundred years of breathing life, maybe two meters in height; those aren't dimensions anyone can expand much by wielding more information. There is a reason navigation apps don't tell you how many nanometers down the road to turn left, and they certainly can't tell you whether to take the road that leads to the house of the person you love, and you think may be betraying you — unless you are betraying yourself by thinking so. Zooming in on Google Maps can be useful, but close-reading Shakespeare's *Othello* may show you a lot more about the intricately veined territory you will actually have to navigate.

The home and center of human experience is still found in the shared mythologies of our life-stories, and the relationships among individuals and among societies are ongoing exercises in something very like literary criticism. An education that develops the capacity for sharing different interpretative frameworks without making any of them compulsory, and demonstrates that meaning can be produced in ways more flexible and provisional than the agoraphobic human mind tends to tolerate, provides an indispensable service to the emerging global collective. This may sound like a dutifully multicultural and drearily inconclusive graduate seminar, but to our often lonely and natively curious minds, it can look more like a playground with free swings and a padded floor. As Arnold Modell, a Clinical Professor of Psychiatry at Harvard, puts it,

> in animals, as in humans .... The context of play presumes a measure of safety, so feelings are at least temporarily delinked from the homeostatic requirements of survival. The context of the environmental surround thus influences the complexity of consciousness. Safe environments expand consciousness.[19]

What is true of play may be especially true of plays, because the obvious flaw in the dramatic medium – that we are partly aware the characters are not real people – reduces the cognitive burden and competitive threat of other minds; to the extent a mentality exists on stage, that mentality has usually been deliberately accommodated to our comprehension, not concealed from it.

* * * * * * *

The history and literature of the 20th century show that between the Scylla and Charybdis of Communism and Fascism lies the depth and variety of the individual human mind. Training even a few minds to think well and independently is worth the effort, even if it seems less efficient than teaching many students in a mass standardized model. Diversity of thought and conduct is no less important than biodiversity in protecting us against viruses and other parasites. Education that fails to produce independent-minded citizens is a betrayal of this virtue of democracy. Unless we nurture the instinct against sameness, we become like the White Walkers and their "wights" in *Game of Thrones*, the Borg in *Star Trek*, or (especially) the Daleks in *Doctor Who*: a hominid life-form imprisoned within a machine that disables its more humane responses, allowing it no motive except the extermination of everything unlike itself.

That's the form of villainy this Doctor Watson – lacking dragonglass, a Starship Enterprise, or even a sonic screwdriver – is hoping he can help defeat by pointing out the way unjust and destructive patterns are perpetuated by a conspiracy in which most of the conspirators don't even realize they are participating. This book is an effort to consider how some forms of opened consciousness may allow us to attack the wrongs generated and endured by a body-politic consisting of individuals of great variety and plasticity, but evolved toward dynamic equilibrium at some less-than-optimal junctures.

By bringing these processes to conscious attention, perhaps we can perform some version of gene therapy on that body-politic to avoid reproducing its own least healthy, least attractive features. A skeptic about meme-theory asks sardonically, "Can we now look forward to scientific memetic engineering?"[20] Considering the success of Russian meme-casts in misinforming American voters, I am not sure that would be looking forward. But, looking back, it is important to recognize that humanistic scholarship has been doing something like engineering the memeplex called culture for a very long time; and the selective function may actually become more rather than less crucial in the digital era, when coded information threatens to grow even faster than capacity to store it, let alone to discover its most valuable instances. The next question might be how to keep this memetic engineering from resembling eugenics. The canon of literary masterpieces has sometimes been deployed to sustain the biases toward white Christians that characterized 20th-century eugenics as well, and one tricky task for 21st-century cultural critics will be to reverse that destructive function without replicating its narrowing political character in some other mode.

To develop translucent but nearly shatter-proof skulls, it helps to have a diverse population meet in settings – a novel, for example, or a classroom – in which their differences can be negotiated indirectly while nothing material, political, or theological is obviously at stake. Poets, famously described by Percy Shelley as "the unacknowledged legislators of the world," can thus be made into its leading diplomats as well – especially when that art is winnowed through scholarship whose first commitment is not to one political program or another, even though we may assume that increasing a next generation's receptivity and sensitivity will ultimately serve whatever causes we believe to be ethically valuable and intellectually valid. The French Revolution showed how important these adjustments of common discourse can be to the reformation of the public sphere as a whole:

> In late-18th century France, as the old regime tottered, the most significant developments on the political scene came not in the movements of protest or the institutions of state which sought to head them off. They came, rather, in the very language itself. Journalists and pamphleteers, together with the occasional dissenting administrator or priest, were forging out of an older language of justice and popular rights a new rhetoric of public action.[21]

What then should be the political aspect of professorial work? Some great works of art are intensely and explicitly political or theological, and must be addressed as such. Anyway, humanists cannot and should not be merely neutral, especially if neutrality is measured by the medians of opinion polls. But, on the topics we choose to explore, we must not cherry-pick evidence favorable to our theories, nor dismiss what a valid methodology elicits from that evidence. "Professionalism," observes the journalist and English professor Louis Menand, "is a way of using smart people productively without giving them too much social power."[22] From the STEM side, Stephen J. Gould concurs:

> Scientists have power by virtue of the respect commanded by the discipline. We may therefore be sorely tempted to misuse that power in furthering a personal prejudice or social goal – why not provide that extra oomph by extending the umbrella of science over a personal preference in ethics or politics? But we cannot, lest we lose the very respect that tempted us in the first place. If this plea sounds like the conservative and pessimistic retrenching of a man on the verge of middle age, I reply that I advocate this care and restraint in order to demonstrate the enormous power of science.[23]

I would say the same about the power of the arts and their interpretation.

In neither the sciences nor the humanities, of course, is there a bright line between scholarly conclusions and their real-world consequences. Polls show that Americans esteem scientists, but distrust them when their knowledge is applied to political controversies; yet climatologists would be irresponsible not to sound alarms when they see clear and nearly present danger. But if professors don't want the citizenry that sponsors our privileged work to mistake it for mere partisan advocacy and indoctrination, then they should certainly avoid verifying that suspicion. As the World War I approached, Wilfred Owen observed, "All a poet can do today is warn. That is why the true poet must be truthful." Scholars must be truthful for similar reasons.

The broader evidence would seem to outweigh the scattered anecdotes that the right-wing media echo-chamber uses – usually with wild exaggeration[24] – to promote the belief that leftist faculty have ruined our universities. The strong tradition of academic freedom in the United States, which confers far greater liberty from government control than in most other countries,[25] seems (to the extent these ranking systems are valid) to have made US universities by far the best in the world: 16 of the top 20 in the major 2018 Shanghai study, 15 of the top 20 in the 2018 *Times Higher Education Supplement* rankings, with similar results for many years now. Demand for places at these universities seems inelastic to price, and immune to geographic and cultural distances. So it seems reasonable to look for ulterior motives for the insistence that these institutions must be reformed through an audit-culture like the one that has produced so many disastrous follies and overlooked so many disastrous frauds in the world of high finance.

Granted, there are doubtless more liberal Democrats than conservative Republicans in humanities departments – leading to efforts such as a 2017 bill pushed by Republican legislators in Iowa that would forbid their universities to hire anyone

> as a professor or instructor member of the faculty at such an institution if the person's political party affiliation on the date of hire would cause the percentage of faculty belonging to one political party to exceed by ten percent the percentage of faculty belonging to the other political party.[26]

But there are also more liberals than conservatives entering graduate programs in the humanities, for reasons (such as attitudes toward money, internationalism, and complexity) that my entire argument may help to explain. A similar fraction of each will develop into good enough scholars in their fields to compete plausibly for professorships – which is how it should work.

Even though the main cause of this imbalance is valid rather than partisan, it obliges academic humanists to be especially alert to the danger that it will produce a compulsory ideology of its own; and in that regard the professoriate's vigilance is sometimes compromised by a reflex of political righteousness. The not-unfounded assumption that we are an oppositional force on behalf of truth and justice can make us complacent about collusions and conformism within our own memeplex. When values in higher education become themselves exempt from critique – diversity based wholly on identity politics as a supreme value, immune to questions about its criteria and priority, may be a current instance – the privilege of academic freedom brings with it a responsibility to ask unpopular questions of the academy itself.

Although creative arts and top-ranked modern universities (unlike their ancestors) display some bias against what is traditional, they compensate by fetishizing their own traditions. From the superficial level of academic gowns and gothic buildings to the underlying structure of indentured apprenticeship, universities at times seem to be a radical exception to cultural change rather than its radical leader. Adam Smith certainly thought so, dismissing universities as "the sanctuaries in which exploded systems and obsolete prejudices found shelter and protection, after they had been hunted out of every other corner of the world."[27] Also in the 18th century, the renowned historian Edward Gibbon wrote that

> The schools of Oxford and Cambridge were founded in a dark age of false and barbarous science; and they are still tainted by the vices of their origin .... The legal incorporation of these societies by the charters of popes and kings had given them a monopoly of public instruction; and the spirit of monopolists is narrow, lazy, and oppressive: their work is more costly and less productive than that of independent artists; and the new improvements so eagerly grasped by the competition of freedom, are admitted with slow and sullen reluctance in those proud corporations.[28]

Nietzsche thought so also: "The scholar is the herd animal in the realm of knowledge – who inquires because he is ordered to and because others have done so before him."[29] These were natural reactions from such transformative thinkers, up against the elitist and traditionalist aspects of European universities in the late 18th and late 19th centuries. Even in the late 20th century, many of the most famous French intellectual radicals were partly rebelling against the hierarchical and disciplinary establishments of their educational system, while many of their followers assumed they were challenging more universal repressions. Yet, even those rather sclerotic institutions were havens for important new discoveries, and the 21st-century American university is far more open and diverse, and far less a tool of church and state than its European ancestors.

Considering how many hours the American professoriate talks to groups every day, a smattering of foolish, offensive, or gratuitous leftist remarks hardly proves a narrower kind of bias. Until there is substantial evidence that humanistic faculty are regularly poisoning higher education, the key questions reflect the paradox I described at the beginning of this chapter. Why do right-wing organizations keep mounting such well-publicized attacks, and why does a population inclined to believe such attacks also remain inclined to invest in such education?

The contradiction can be resolved, and both questions answered, by recognizing that universities are not only engines of new knowledge and cultural mutability, but also repositories of established knowledge and culture. One task of privileged academic researchers (like King Lear's "all-licensed Fool" [1.4.201] and the wise fools in Erasmus as well as Shakespeare) is to challenge complacent beliefs and replace them with unanticipated or forgotten truths – or at least with more accurate models, whether of a text, a social function, or a neutrino. That disruptive mode of research is unwelcome to a dominant social order that, for reasons already suggested, has highly conservative reflexes: the powerful are protecting their privileges, and the complacent are protecting their prejudices – or their sanity, though I trust they could lose many of the prejudices without actually losing sanity.

So advanced researchers, employed as they are in breaking down assumptions, must compensate for the threat of chaos by practicing both discipline and disciplines,[30] as artists immerse themselves in tradition and subject themselves to form. The desire to correct sociopolitical wrongs through scholarly appointments and publications is understandable and even admirable, but making it the primary driver of our work risks undermining the fortress that enables our long-term resistance to parasitic memeplexes. As the distinguished historian Jeffrey Herf observes,

> The history of this and previous centuries indicates that erosion of shared standards of merit, achievement, and excellence does not unleash an era of splendidly anarchic creativity. Rather – as Tocqueville, but also Nietzsche pointed out – it unleashes a hatred of otherness, of free spirits, of those who dare to differentiate themselves from others.[31]

Academic elitism may thus be a long-term ally of inclusiveness, as (conversely) facile empathy often conduces to paternalism. If there are two things that unite the best work of university faculty – in teaching and research, in grading and tenuring, in humanities and sciences – they are the effort to accommodate complexity without surrendering to either dogmatism or agnosticism, and the effort to distinguish valid arguments from invalid ones (I realize that I am inviting some pointed responses to my own book here). We practice peer-review on publications and promotions, to forestall the nightmare of a runaway individual mind, which may hold a lifetime-tenured seat in what Hamlet – originally in a theater called the Globe – triple-punningly calls the "distracted globe" of the brain (1.5.96–97).

This task of editing the cultural heritage, selecting which memeplexes to exclude as parasitic, may seem to conflict with the current determination of most major universities to be multicultural in an anti-judgmental way. That determination is understandable as a corrective. Intellectual elites have, for centuries, justified the imperial dominion of First World white Christian societies over others that are arguably much more admirable, or at least healthier in their local context, or at the very least within the rights of the indigenous peoples to choose – and Shakespeare's prestige has often been weaponized in the cultural imperialism of the British Empire. Colonizers have imposed their own "enlightened" agricultural systems in climates and soils where they produced unprecedented starvation, and something comparable happens in cultural systems.

Constructing a culture that excludes nothing and offends nobody is demonstrably impossible, even within a modern progressive consensus; witness, for example, the current bitter conflict between second-wave feminists (especially so-called TERFs) and 21st-century transgender advocates. Such feminists had long and fiercely opposed the traditional assumption that there is a kind of person one cannot be while being a woman, another while being a man. They therefore view some premises of gender transition as regressive rather than progressive, and also deny that people who lived their lives free from patriarchal oppression can legitimately claim identity with lifelong cis-gender women. Transgender advocates, no less fiercely, reject that position, seeing it as a product and ally of transphobia. No wonder humanities professors – except those confidently on the radical or traditionalist extremes – have largely ducked out (or is it, chickened out?) of the role of ethicist.[32]

The selective practice of cultural critique on college campuses can appear hypocritical. Avowed relativists and others denouncing any judgment of cultures from the outside seem confident nonetheless that certain ideas of human rights must overrule all others. To some extent the inconsistency may reflect a recognition that punching up is ethically different from punching down, but there is no guarantee that the subaltern culture provides an optimal model. Judging all cultural forces with due sensitivity to their environment seems preferable to obeying them unconsciously and hence indiscriminately, or ranking them solely by the degree of their oppression.

Campus protest movements can help serve that advancement of sensitized judgment, if administrators can make room for new views and newly foregrounded facts to be explored, rather than placating the activists with concessions such as the punishment of unpopular but defensible ideas. Declaring some political and religious beliefs that remain within the national mainstream to be officially unacceptable beliefs (as some campuses have slid toward doing) is very different from insisting on a broader and more deeply considered perspective on how to choose beliefs.

The wave of campus protest movements in the autumn of 2015 felt like a flashback to campuses a half-century earlier, with a rationalistic liberal professoriate finding itself caught between a conservative nation that resented being reminded of its wrongs and a radical student movement so certain it was right that sloganeering often drowned out analysis. Again, the irony was often that the students were radicalized by arguments the professors had made in resistance to the complacency of the dominant culture (a key responsibility of scholars, I believe) – arguments the students then treated as absolute truths and tried to make into a new compulsory dogma.

An even more telling irony, in this regard, is that students of my generation protested to reduce the amount of control their universities exercised over their lives: dress codes, parietal restrictions, and regulations of political speech and sexual language. Lately, students seem to be demanding instead that the university impose more controls.[33] Activists are not only proposing but actually demanding that their universities regulate not only party costumes but also sexual behavior and language, to the point of dictating what must be said in what way at each stage of erotic courtship; punish opinions for Israel or against Israel; or even (at my university and several others) condemn as micro-aggressive statements such as "America is a melting-pot," "Gender plays no part in who we hire," or "I believe the most qualified person should get the job." Defining a wide range of locutions and perspectives as fundamentally "hate speech" to be met with re-education programs and sometimes suspensions as well as shaming on social media is an ethical project that fits awkwardly with an educational project built on low-risk experimental learning and challenges to underexamined pieties.

Most of the cultural changes idealistic campus activists now seek are, in my opinion, desirable, and the nuances of language are an important element of such changes. But the switch from the student-led Free Speech Movement of 1964–1965 to the student-led speech-codes movement on the same campuses less than 50 years later is striking – and one thing it strikes is academic freedom. The reversal reflects the kind of compensatory mechanism this book has been describing. Students on elite campuses in the United States reacted one way to the conformism of the 1950s and an opposite way – despite similar ideological leanings – to the looser mores, increasingly multicultural societies, and interdisciplinary scholarship of the new millennium. This shift may be viewed as another anxious response to an increasingly open world that is disorienting and disconcerting in both the usual and the specific etymological sense of those words. Such unsettlings intensify the pressures inherent in being young people living away from home for the first time and being exposed constantly to new ideas.

It seems only too clear to me that most students and even some tenured faculty no longer discuss the very issues to which campus activists seek to draw attention: issues related to race and gender. The costs of having the wrong opinion or even using the currently disfavored terminology are just too great to risk. Resenting the euphemized mandate from the university to hold only a narrowed range of opinions, suspecting that some classmates have been primed to respond with pre-fabricated attacks if the dogma is questioned, and knowing that campus authorities are afraid that, if they deem the offenses not wrongful enough to punish, they will be accused of invalidating the experience of oppressed groups, many students simply close down until the topic changes. Any effort by university authorities to distinguish between compellingly valid complaints and contrived or hyperbolic ones invites condemnation for presuming the right to tell a disadvantaged population (as authoritative voices have done for so long) what they have a right to feel. The exasperation of such groups is understandable, and over my lifetime conscientious white people have often had to revisit with chagrin their view that the earlier protests by such groups were hypersensitive and overly strident. But the chilling effect of the current climate on the discourse through which an academic community determines how best to serve its educational mission is unmistakable, regrettable, and probably avoidable.

Nor are faculty immune to these disincentives. In 2015 my university approved a new requirement that students take a "diversity" course. Discussing implementation of that requirement with a friend and colleague who was among its leading advocates, I cautioned that earlier versions (which I reluctantly opposed) had been defeated, and that more than a third of the faculty had voted against even the latest version (which I actively supported, despite some misgivings). She replied, "But when we had the Town Hall meeting about it, 95% of the faculty who got up to speak supported it!" My unspoken thought was, "Exactly, and that's worth thinking about."

To their credit, my colleagues did think about that, and avoided any narrow partisan definition of diversity: the courses from my department that satisfy the requirement include not just the Chicano Studies courses so important in this region, but also courses on "Cultures of the Middle Ages" and "Jane Austen and her Peers." The right-wing media try to undermine the resistant function of intellectual communities by underrating the range of ideas elite campuses allow. They elide crucial distinctions when they depict 21st-century campuses as forbidding anyone to speak or hear more conservative ideas. Shouting down, blockading, or physically assaulting a speaker, which is an unacceptable violation of the exchange of ideas except under the direst circumstances, is very different from protesting against the implicit or explicit honoring of a visitor with a degree or even with the sole broadcast voice at graduation – usually a voice already widely heard in the mainstream discourse.

Furthermore, protesting against the latter kind of speaker, which is itself an essential piece of free political discourse, is very different from actually disinviting a speaker because that person's views are condemned by activists. All too frequently, cases where a speaker withdraws after students object are misrepresented as cases where a college or university has barred the proposed speaker. Typical was a recent op-ed piece on the right-wing editorial page of the *Wall Street Journal* claiming that "Disinvited campus speakers include former Secretary of State Condoleezza Rice, International Monetary Fund head Christine Lagarde" – both of whom, in fact, withdrew upon hearing of the protest movement.[34] Whose unwillingness to endure political disagreements really cancelled these events? And weren't the protests instances of the university's mission of evaluating independently other social institutions? My daughter was not among the protestors of the nomination of Lagarde as the 2014 commencement speaker at Smith College, but she knows much more about the pros and cons of the International Monetary Fund than she ever would have without that protest. The same is doubtless true of Princeton students confronting Woodrow Wilson's actively racist policies and Yale students confronting John C. Calhoun's prominent defense of slavery.

What the protestors are often doing is challenging the respectability of a powerful memeplex they see as destructive, when it threatens to extend injustice or claim authority within their intellectual community. Some may make the error I described in Chapter 2 by assuming that the problem is a few evil individuals rather than an evolved social structure, but more often they are attacking the dangerous network when it appears within their reach in an assailable form. What is essential, from my perspective, is that all sides remember the history and power of cultural formations. Conservatives must recognize that blackface parties or Halloween costumes – a flashpoint at Yale, UCLA, and elsewhere – are not trivia if they extend the structural racism from which they arose. Progressives, conversely, must recognize that it is neither just nor productive to dismiss out of hand the works of historical figures just because they reflect some assumptions of their world (say, about race, class, or gender) that are now anathema on our campuses. Nor is it productive to insist that those who question the latest campus orthodoxies are pathological haters of the oppressed groups. Outside of the small bands of neo-Nazis and other White Supremacists, the questioners are unlikely to recognize themselves in the ugly portrait being offered, which diminishes the protesters' credibility and allows those questioners to avert their eyes from the larger functions of racist and sexist memeplexes they may be helping to sustain.

Campuses are not just idea-zones, however. They are communities where thousands of young people are suddenly living and working independently for the first time, often away from their homes, families, and communities. There are many, many things they might say or do that, while not illegal, are distinctly inimical to a positive learning experience in a healthy community (this includes sexual misbehavior, which universities are attacked from the right for trying to discipline when the law will not, and from the left for failing to discipline more severely when the evidence is equivocal). Not many businesses, even those that rely on extensive government funding – which is what conservative pundits and even courts say obliges universities to allow even extreme political speech – would dream that they were obliged to let anyone who works there say and do anything those workers please, no matter how deliberately disruptive, divisive, hostile, and repellent, so long as it wasn't actually a prosecutable crime. It is awfully (let's say) rich that many leaders of such businesses accuse universities of being both weak and censorious, and accuse students of being coddled "snowflakes" unprepared for the real world, because the campus community tries to limit insulting and provocative speech that those executives wouldn't have tolerated in their offices for a minute.

The relentless slanders by the right-wing media, assisted by the craven cooperation of mainstream media outlets, have succeeded in splitting campus leftists. They have made one faction annoyed at their "Social Justice Warrior" colleagues for facile virtue-signaling and generally providing juicy fodder for this right-wing critique. And they have made that more activist faction indignant and dismissive toward their colleagues for implicitly accepting that critique and its false equivalencies, rather than fiercely and fearlessly standing up for principles currently deemed important for the protection of the historically disadvantaged, and for not making such protection a primary mission of universities.

Of course – speaking as one of the more skeptical leftists, hence distrusted by activist colleagues while still attacked by right-wing organizations – I would say there is seldom a single minute of anyone's waking life that could not be condemned as complicit in some larger evil, especially if one is willing to reach that conclusion by metaphor, mind-reading, and potential eventual outcomes of even passive participation. I don't blame young people for wanting to make their campus a shining City on the Hill, a rehearsal for the ideally just society they hope to construct. Challenging entrenched memeplexes is part of their job, just as it is the job of the faculty to make them think about the issues more deeply than they would otherwise.

In late August of 2016, I was heartened by the front-page *New York Times* headline reporting that the University of Chicago had sent its incoming students a letter taking a stand defending academic freedom against campus pressure-groups.[35] When universities, even with the best intentions, make it difficult and even dangerous for controversial ideas to be discussed in classrooms or research, they are making a serious mistake. In my roles as Chair of UCLA's Academic Freedom Committee and Teaching Committee, I have pushed back against proposals that crossed that line. When an administration-appointed committee recommended monitoring classrooms for race and gender microaggressions, for example, I warned in writing and in meetings that such monitoring would certainly produce microaggressions against the free exchange of ideas. Nor should intimidation be allowed to shape academic policy or appointments. Campus activists deserve a thoughtful hearing, but slogans seldom articulate the complexities of balancing urgent political issues with the more gradual imperatives of scholarship. So, one cheer for that highly publicized letter.

Reading further into the letter that morning, however, stifled any further cheers. It began looking like a university posturing to an audience of conservative donors and pundits who prefer a caricature that feeds their indignation over an honest sorting of the issues involved: less a brave intellectual stand than a clever marketing move.

Neither "trigger warnings" nor "safe spaces" are inherently a problem. The problem arises only if a university mandates certain warnings and alternative assignments, or insists that nothing in its classrooms ever offend anyone. The closest I have come to giving a trigger-warning has been an acknowledgment at the start of my Shakespeare course that the plays would be depicting murder, rape, incest, cannibalism, racism, domestic violence, cross-dressing, anti-Semitism, misogyny, blood sport, and countless other potentially traumatic events that students might not even realize had troubled them until Shakespeare vividly evoked them. I said there was no space less safe for complacent psyches than Shakespeare's theater, which is part of why his work has been so lastingly important.

The University of Chicago's own website explained that their Safe Spaces are "actual physical spaces where LGBTQ students can talk with students, staff, and faculty who have been trained."[36] That doesn't seem like an unreasonable thing for a university to provide for young people from groups that have long been vilified and endangered in ways that others of us may not have adequately recognized: a place to go where they don't have to feel on their guard against prejudice or mockery and can discuss their problems and their hopes without fear of getting kicked on the same old bruise.

When that university's leadership announces that they "don't support" any professor who thinks it best to prepare especially vulnerable students for something they are about to confront that may be shocking in ways that actually impede learning, that university is making itself the enemy of academic freedom and good pedagogy while pretending to be their friend. When those leaders add that "we don't condone" – with the primary and etymological meaning of "condone" being "to permit without censure" or "absolve from blame" – members of the university community who want to provide some little place where students can go if they want to take a breather from negative assumptions about their race or their sexuality, that seems like sloppy expression at best. Worse, it seems like sloppy thinking, or (even worse) a cynical ploy to capitalize on the widespread assumption that today's students are all "coddled" rather than sometimes naively idealistic about what kind of world they aspire to build.

The blunter forms of campus protest have potentially costly analogues in humanities classrooms, however. Recent cultural criticism (now more often Postcolonial than New Historicist) tends to recruit armies of students to battle retroactively the evils its methodology has identified. This type of historical critique can be brilliant and important work, but in its simplistic forms it offers its audience an easy posture of superiority to those who faced real and difficult political dilemmas that demand to be understood in their original context before being judged from ours, and who occasionally achieved kinds of moral courage no longer readily visible to us. It can also encourage dismissiveness toward authors from those eras, who too quickly become unindicted co-conspirators in the obstruction of justice because they neglected to perceive – or mystified or naturalized and thus depoliticized – what now certainly appear to be outrageous injustices. The authors' works may thus be reduced to wiretap transcripts in a kangaroo court, their aesthetics subjected to whatever catalyst is needed to precipitate out of it an ideology contrary or oblivious to the modern scholar's own. Autopsy is a valid and valuable way to discover what was wrong with a particular person, but a sympathetic conversation usually offers a more nuanced and heartening way of getting to know that person.

The censure of individuals can lead to – but too often precludes – important questions about the nature of a cultural system. It is wrong to assume that a guilty verdict is the conclusion of any good investigation. Done complacently, our work becomes little more than a version of the government programs that recently dominated the news headlines, scanning a vast database of recorded utterances looking for a pattern that reveals a criminal conspiracy. Worse, it may start to resemble China's 1966 "Cultural Revolution" that, for a decade, turned students into a Red Guard that pored over everything written by their elders for anything that could be somehow construed as bourgeois, capitalist, or in any way revisionist of Mao's Communist ideology, and then denounced and destroyed the lives of those elders and any similarly tainted books. Even if I believed that this prosecutorial approach to literature were the best way to create ethically alert students, the "hermeneutics of suspicion" would still face a problem like that facing the detective in *Murder on the Orient Express*, because almost everyone may be rightly considered suspects in the production of a manifestly unjust social order.

Literature is most useful for running trials, not in the sense of prosecutions, but in the sense of simulations. Tragedies and novels have long assisted Western societies by projecting the destructive outcomes, for societies as well as for individuals, when particular versions of social code coincide with particular functions of human nature. Social critique becomes much more compelling when it recognizes how larger dynamics – say, the tension between languages in a postcolonial society – create tragic dilemmas for many individuals caught in the tides of history. Shakespeare's Henry V, though a talented monarch, is manifestly trapped in late-Renaissance politics as shaped by nationalism, religion, money, patriarchy, language, and multiculturalism; Hamlet is ensnared in that culture's epistemological crisis, Coriolanus in its class warfare (disguised as a classical antecedent), and Macbeth on the cusp between grand Renaissance aspirations and severe Calvinist admonishments. Sophisticated responses to terrible episodes in human history serve a prudential function, letting us see the way the clouds of certain storms tend to gather before it is too late for us to seek shelter, while also allowing us this distance on, or palliation of, our censorious reflexes.

Psychological studies of political factions have shown that it is natural to perceive as demonically errant anything other than our own subjectivity or our own group's ideology, and the struggles of multiculturalism verify that finding. Human culture thus again partly replicates the biochemistry by which most social species learn to differentiate their group from outsiders. Higher education provides some tools for controlling those automatic responses. The psychological factor in political inclinations verifies both my view of their fundamental character and my prescription for curing some of their divisiveness. According to a team of scholars at Brown University,

> "It's not that conservative people are more fearful, it's that fearful people are more conservative. People who are scared of novelty, uncertainty, people they don't know, and things they don't understand, are more supportive of policies that provide them with a sense of surety and security".... The researchers make clear, however, that genetics plays only part of the role in influencing political preferences. Education, they found, had an equally large influence on out-group attitudes, with more highly educated people displaying more supportive attitudes toward out-groups and education having a substantial mediating influence on the correlation between parental fear and child out-group attitudes.[37]

A UCLA study, published in *Psychological Science*, found that "participants who were more conservative were again significantly more likely to exhibit greater credulity for information about hazards."[38] Intolerance toward progressive ideas arises from broader anxieties, but those reflexes can be tamed by education.

My own professorial assignment within society is both the effect and the cause of my preference for deep questions and deferred certainties. Shakespeare is of course a traditional object of study, but his relentless indeterminacy assures his inexhaustible novelty. To adapt what his Enobarbus says of Cleopatra, age cannot wither Shakespeare, nor custom stale his infinite variety: other writers cloy the appetites they feed, but he makes hungry where most he satisfies. My investment in intellectualism (which may be perceived as no less exclusionary than pride in a sectarian faith) leads me to fear the influence of those who will not see, who reflexively repress any dissident tendency or dissonant information within themselves and punish it in their fellow citizens. Others recognize and abet such willful blindness through political demagoguery, bad art, or other sensational distractions. The banal villains in this story are those who have some recognition of all this repression and distraction but prefer to exploit the follies and the system rather than to expose them.

Yet, some reactionary impulses that I, as a literary critic with leftist political tendencies, may deem evil can be confidently condemned only if I assume that dissidence, creative self-indulgence, and a drive toward equality are inherently heroic. That assumption depends on ideologies of democracy and free individualism that may themselves be naïve and arbitrary, and are certainly historically and cross-culturally variable. Pure democracy has its dangers, and individualism may be merely the unexamined jumble that remains when the survival instinct happens to get tangled up with self-consciousness.

Neither political wing is immune to accusations of hypocrisy in this debate between conformity and dissent. Ironically, the punitive impulse against aberrant behavior often comes most fiercely from those voting blocs (Tea Party enthusiasts, prairie populists, nostalgists of the Confederacy) who claim to be defenders of the principles of liberty, individualism, and a merciful God. Demagogues use the conformist cultural reflexes of poorly educated citizens to turn them against progressive politics that might benefit them economically, and against those who share aspects of their oppression but not their race, creed, or nationality.[39] This, by the way, is not merely a Western phenomenon, as Narendra Modi's 2015 election campaign in India demonstrated.[40] Meanwhile, on the left, speech-codes and a condemnatory reflex toward past cultures construe themselves as heroic resistance, yet they constitute conformity within the academy, where righteous condemnations of American conformism are most prevalent. Ironically, a subversive aura confers interlocking benefits of status, money, and power in academia not unlike those it seeks to condemn in the larger world.

Progressives must therefore not assume that they and they alone are making real progress for the species. Leftism is not inherently liberating, even though its liberationist ideology may make frequent correlation look like causation. Dissidents, too, may be part of the long-term survival strategy of a collective. Regicides, as much as royalists, may overrate their autonomous agency. Yet, I believe that a resistant intellectualism and its expressions through the creative arts can sustain the possibility of progress, in exactly the areas where humanity has the greatest potential to evolve. Even though evolution is not inherently progressive, we can and should attempt to make it so.

Education Online

For the university to serve the functions I have been describing, it must tolerate what the surrounding society considers inefficiencies, and must remain open to the unpredictable outcomes of colloquy, including mutual critique based on logical use of evidence that has been tested. Failed experiments in the creative arts are far less destructive to other such work than false assertions and evaluations in the community of research, where work builds on work with some presumption of reliability. In biological reproduction, DNA has extensive proofreading functions, presumably because errors in the germ line would be heritable and hence very costly, whereas errors in RNA are short-lived and so not worth the costs of policing. Unfortunately, the Internet handles information more like RNA than like DNA, despite the fact that misinformation on the Internet can endure and influence many injurious replications and infect other information.

These factors make websites and online courses poor substitutes for universities. Without the constraints of intensive and accountable peer-review, the openness and vast multiplicity of cyberspace might disable the limiting factors that make free inquiry tolerable, much as cyberspace disables the courtesies that make debate tolerable (the tenor of most online political debates shows the problem). Without the pressures of locality to bring different fields of knowledge and modes of interpretation into controlled collision, there might actually be less meaningful crossover work rather than more. And without the unforeseeable, irreducible factors of protracted live human interaction, the innovations that arise may lack a valuable sensitivity to their co-evolutionary potential – good or bad – with a living community. That danger has been signaled in mad-scientist stories from *Frankenstein* onward. In other words, the social experience that often draws students to campuses is not merely a spoonful of sugar to make the medicine of learning go down more smoothly; it is an essential catalyst within that medicine, and an antidote to some of its potential toxins.

Joseph Henrich concludes that the key to a successfully innovating society is

> the willingness and ability of large numbers of individuals at the knowledge frontier to freely interact, exchange views, disagree, learn from each other, build collaborations, trust strangers, and be wrong. Innovation does not take a genius or a village; it takes a big network of freely interacting minds.[41]

But it helps if those minds are actually in something like a village. A recent study at Harvard Medical School showed that the physical proximity of the first and last authors of a scientific paper correlates strongly with the likelihood of that paper becoming important in the scientific discourse, as measured by subsequent citations. As if in iterative proof of the hypothesis, the idea for this study emerged from casual chat between the authors, Kjungjoon Lee and Isaac Kohane, whose offices had come to share the same kitchenette.[42] As Kohane remarked in a subsequent interview,

> If you want people to work together effectively, these findings reinforce the need to create architectures that support frequent, physical, spontaneous interactions. Even in the era of big science when researchers spend so much time on the Internet, it's still important to create intimate spaces.

Jonah Lehrer – his own freelance career perhaps a cautionary tale about the dangers of solitary research – applies this theory, and its reliance on critical exchange rather than mere uncritical brainstorming, across a range of instances: MIT's legendary ramshackle Building 20, Steve Jobs's design of Pixar Studios, and the making of a successful Broadway musical.[43] Clearly, the same theory underlies the design of the Isaac Newton Institute for Mathematical Sciences at Cambridge University, the social engineering of Google headquarters, and Yahoo's much-resented efforts to make its employees work at their shared offices rather than telecommuting.

If universities go online, how will these conversations occur? And if that move reduces the hiring of scholars in the humanities, which is already hindered by questionable assumptions that favor hiring only in the sciences, how will the humanists needed to analyze memeplexes during the decades ahead have the time to learn the old perspectives and develop new ones? The Internet is too decentralized to evolve its own such internal function, and for so many centuries the church and the university have been compelled to provide a haven for the sustained intellectual work of preservation and innovation that it is difficult to feel confident an alternative will come readily to hand.

This is not so different from the problem many informational industries are facing about how to monetize the data they have to offer: the *Encyclopaedia Britannica* recently published its last print edition, and it is unclear who will produce expensive news reportage when aggregating websites can and will diffuse it for almost nothing, and on no principle of selection beyond what will draw the most clicks that advertisers will pay for. Instead, the more outlandish the shocking or teasing the headline, the more money the fake-news website gets from its advertisers: Gresham's Law in the information economy. We are thus automating our knowledge-distribution system toward ignorance, and feeding the confirmation-biases that disable productive political debate. In that context, the information-vetting function of universities becomes more essential than ever.

This book emphasizes the importance of preserving humanistic learning from the self-serving forces of the market. Even if some version of online university education becomes viable – predictions of its imminent takeover have not been fulfilled – it will probably make scholarship more rather than less dependent on short-term profit than the current model. Massive open-access online courses (MOOCs) could turn universities into just another piece of society where 1% are elite managers and celebrities, and most are overworked, underpaid service workers of various kinds. If they thrive along current lines, MOOCs threaten to become the Monsanto of many academic fields. By designating a few intellectual superstars to project their one-way lectures into countless classrooms that once heard a variety of voices responsive to local conditions, this technology is reviving the medieval intellectual monoculture called Aristotelianism that for centuries discouraged multivalent, open-minded inquiries; it favored commentaries on the distant authoritative voice in place of direct encounters with fresh ideas or physical nature. Galenic medicine – itself derived from Hippocrates – followed a similarly destructive path. Blended coursework will certainly succeed in some areas, but what most current online courses offer is hardly different from what has always been offered by, for example, textbooks in public libraries and correspondence courses, which have seldom displaced personal teaching except for extremely isolated persons. Perhaps we can justly adapt Churchill's remark about democracy: universities are the least efficient form of developing, adjudicating, and transmitting knowledge, except for all the others that have been tried.

Lately the humanities are being further devalued because they do not scale up very well into the MOOC systems in which many universities are now speculating, mostly through for-profit corporations such as Coursera and platforms such as edX. But, the incompatibility of the humanities with the mass-production of knowledge may also signal the extreme value of humanistic study in a homogenizing world: most humanities disciplines require extensive, interactive attention to personal voice and subjectivity. Furthermore, their ability to promote empathy evidently depends on personal presence in discussion.[44] The fact that something cannot be successfully transmitted widely and uniformly across persons, times, and cultures is not necessarily a flaw, unless one assumes that the fundamental human project of transmitting knowledge is fundamentally a business whose purpose is money, and that human personality should therefore be flattened so the machine can run more smoothly.

MOOCs may therefore constitute a necessary updating of the famous Turing Test, which made the criterion of true artificial intelligence whether it could converse with a person such that someone reading the transcript could not tell which side was the machine and which the human. Perhaps the inability of MOOCs to teach a discipline adequately en masse over digital media will distinguish humanities fields, and a liberal-arts education more generally, from some technical disciplines that machines can someday be trusted to handle for us. The process may also provoke some of those disciplines to reassert more audibly their endangered humanistic aspects.

Other Minds and Dissident Individuals

Academia may be less an Ivory Tower than a kind of loamy garden – complete, let's stipulate, with a fair amount of manure produced by its domestic livestock. Doubtless, I have been romanticizing a memeplex that keeps me gainfully employed. In the realm of culture, however, a university has a demonstrable value akin to that of biodiversity, even (and maybe especially) when it looks like mere perversity instead. A university's job is to try to keep alive an array of truths – in all their quirky residues and implausible possibilities, all the things that seem obviously wrong yet may someday be proven right – in the face of the human susceptibility to conformism and simplification that would otherwise gleefully trample the seedlings. Academic freedom creates a sanctuary, like the ancient monasteries, where old truths can remain rooted despite the vicissitudes of the political world, but also where the seeds of dissent against all the current structures of power and belief can survive and propagate, as long as they are grounded in evidence and reason, and not shaded by the Idols that Francis Bacon's *Novum Organum* warned against at the dawn of modern science four centuries ago.[45]

Poets, I have suggested, must shatter dried-up, hollowed-out formulations of human experience and perception while providing alternatives that give the reassuring impression of having been less invented than uncovered, from which green shoots will emerge once exposed to light. Literary scholars have a similarly tricky dual agenda: to push aside meanings that have grown stale or even poisonous, but also to provide fresh truths, however provisional, in their place. Humanities professors have the job of trying to sustain in their students, for far longer than the usual moment, what Samuel Beckett's extended essay on Proust called "the perilous zones in the life of the individual, dangerous, precarious, painful, mysterious, and fertile, when for a moment the boredom of living is replaced by the suffering of being."[46] But learning just to be, rather than how to be, appears almost unendurable. Can one throw away the cookie-cutters and still give shape? That may seem an overly abstract and entirely academic question, but not when translated into the question of whether the human race can generate and tolerate forms of consciousness that reject faith-based totalitarianism while still satisfying our need for purpose, meaning, and order.

A chief reason reactionaries react – especially when cultures collide – is this kind of cognitive agoraphobia. Agoraphobia, in this sense as well as in the diagnostic terminology of psychotherapy, entails both a fear of others and a fear of open spaces. What others impose is the recognition that one's own experience of reality is individual (which makes the mortality of the self entail the erasure of the universe) and contingent (which reveals the infinite abyss of possible thoughts, perceptions, and behaviors). Dissipating the terror of others as economic competitors and of otherness as a threat to the hermetic enclosure of our physical and metaphysical selves would aid at least three causes I consider important: economic justice, multicultural toleration, and environmentalism. But the importance of multiculturalism has led to a dangerous complacency about its inherent problems. If I am right that cultures exist largely to provide coherent systems of belief and behavior that integrate and regulate a society by excluding other ways of thinking and acting, then multiculturalism is practically an oxymoron. Pretending otherwise has been costly: as I argued in Chapter 3, dismissing the backlash as simple race-hatred that can be scolded away only intensifies the resistance.

Romantic love or a favorite book may provide precious, rare occasions when a close kinship of sensibility appears. Excluding other minds almost entirely, as in some forms of autism, offers another form of relief. Otherwise, social existence is a perpetual swarm of aftershocks of the infant's discovery that the world is external to the appetite of the self. Cross-cultural encounters impose a doubt that there is any true and lasting otherworldly judgment, or really any lasting truth at all. As Saint Augustine suggested long ago, Hell may be fundamentally the lack of God, understood as the source and guarantor of a coherent and positively meaningful universe compatible with the human psyche.

In this formulation, literary study is the Purgatory that prepares us to leave that Hell for a better place. Stefan Collini, Emeritus Professor of Intellectual history at Cambridge University and a leading public intellectual, has recently argued that "education encourages the student to recognize the ways in which particular bits of knowledge are not fixed or eternal or universal or self-sufficient," and to move "from the narrow to the broad, from the closed to the open, from the fixed to the fluid."[47] If so, then education systematically smashes holes in the cognitive containment this book has depicted as precious to the human mind and constitutive of human culture. The marketplace of ideas is the scariest marketplace of all, one that can cost you peace of mind. Universities are the Chicago Board of Trade (with its adjacent slaughterhouse) for investments in this commodity. For this agnostic sermon, Shakespeare's highly skeptical *Merchant of Venice* makes an apt text: an ethically and theologically tangled story set in a city that is all fluid exchange and no grounding. Both in plot and in theme, that play is rooted in the problems of cultural otherness. It obliges us to strive desperately for unmediated values, then to reconcile ourselves to the unavailability of any, and thereby reconcile ourselves to each other through sentiments and intuitions of goodness, despite our differences and failings.[48]

That is not an easy lesson to sell explicitly, or concerning real-world issues. If you feel you have sorted out the right things to think and the right ways to behave, and assembled a community around your mutual affirmations of that rightness (anywhere on the political or theological spectra), you and your group will hardly welcome evidence that your truths are actually mere arbitrary choices and that your certainty is actually a defensive symptom of doubt. Faith does not like to be told it is bad faith. The political scientist Michael Chwe sees a puzzle in "aspects of ritual that cannot easily be understood in terms of 'meaning'; for example, words spoken in rituals typically involve lots of repetition, and are structured, in rhyme, verse, or song." Chwe attributes this to the need to signal coordination within the tribe.[49] I would add that the coordination itself is valuable for its exclusion of stray meanings; repetition and structure are themselves added palliatives against cognitive overload. Similarly, Chwe interprets the prevalence of inward-facing circles for public deliberative spaces – suggestively, as the French Revolution was spinning out of control, its leaders displayed an "obsession with the amphitheater" – as another tool for assuring "common knowledge" by mutual visibility.[50] I would add that the circle serves not only to enable the group to see each other, it also keeps anyone or anything outside the group ritual from being seen, mitigating the risk of any uncommon knowledge.

In this sense, I am following Durkheim's belief that human societies are fundamentally ideational complexes held in common, but rearranging the terms of Durkheim's explanation for the persistence of those complexes, which he attributes largely to a feedback-loop built into ritual. I am instead viewing ritual as one manifestation of the need for shared instructions to simplify and certify our beliefs and behaviors, and attributing the persistence of memeplexes to their evolved ability to exploit that need – to feed on that feedback.

What begins as individual resolve based in intuitive disagreement or emotional objection must become something larger if it aspires to defeat historical injustices; as I observed about the 1960s version of counterculture, these battles will always have both cognitive and political components. Harari points out that, if only one person

> were to stop believing in the dollar, in human rights, or in the United States, it wouldn't much matter. These imagined orders are inter-subjective, so in order to change them we must simultaneously change the consciousness of billions of people, which is not easy. A change of such magnitude can be accomplished only with the help of a complex organisation, such as a political party, an ideological movement, or a religious cult.[51]

Or a university – to the extent it is distinguishable from those three examples. Scholars free from government control can be pens mightier than swords, and pains in the asset of cultural cohesion. Reflexive loyalists of the officially sanctioned beliefs therefore feel besieged by these supposed enemies of the people. This repressive reaction to individuals attempting cultural innovation is hardly a new phenomenon. In the 4th century B.C., the legendary Cynic philosopher Diogenes was already abandoning and attacking virtually every social norm and structure as corrupting humanity's true nature, and was notorious for public urination, defecation, and masturbation. A few decades earlier, Socrates was executed for undermining Athens by corrupting the minds of its youth and disbelieving in its official gods, and

> Spartans refused to allow Timotheos to play at their state festivals with a lyre that had more than the traditional number of seven strings. On the concert podium, the innovative musical outsider was asked by the presiding ephor from which side of the lyre he should shear off the offending extra strings. A similar story is told of the great singer of Lesbos, Terpander himself, who some two hundred years earlier, was fined for having one string too many on his lyre.[52]

It did not take an Information Age for people to feel the threat of extra data, or at least of data that did not fit the established parceling of cognition. There have always been shearsmen ready to trim the Blue Guitar back into an instrument of the established order of the state, obliged to sing the authorized hymns and battle-hymns. Plato, whose *Laws* identifies socio-cultural cohesion as a primary value, was profoundly mistrustful of the unsettling power of art. Hitler – revealingly devoted to classical aesthetics – himself led an intense national campaign against "Degenerate Art."[53] *Gleichschaltung* – the program of self-coordination that was so integral in the rise of Nazism – was as much a project of cultural and psychological conformism as of administrative centralization; something similar happened in the Soviet Union, as the multiculturalist drive of Korenization gave way to centralizing Russification.

The fierce isolation of Japan from the early 17th through the mid-19th centuries accompanied a strict regimentation of almost every aspect of dress, interaction, and behavior among its citizens; even during Japan's Meiji era (1868–1917), when it allowed modernization and Westernization, the culture stabilized itself by focusing on reverence to the Emperor as an enduring absolute. In fact, as far back as the 14th century, the great Arab historiographer Ibn Khaldun identified *asabiyyah* – meaning a unified consciousness reflecting and reinforcing group solidarity – as crucial to the survival of a civilization in its ongoing cycle of competition with emerging rivals.

Universities, however, should be safe spaces for the inherently unsafe business of convening different cultural perspectives, airing and evaluating dissenting views, and for the orderly dissemination of the views that prove to have some validity. Professors, seldom renowned for humility, sometimes consider ourselves more evolved than what we judge to be troglodyte reactionaries in the general public, who in return see us as eagerly contagious mutants. Mostly, if we are doing our jobs well, we will often seem annoying and even threatening to the general public; yet they still usually decide to send us their children to be educated. We will be accused by leftist governments of conducting right-wing indoctrination, and accused of the opposite by right-wing governments. Yet perhaps what we are doing is inoculating some alert minds of the next generation against an autoimmune disease called conformism that sometimes mistakes a necessary part of the body-politic for a dangerous alien. To the extent we are not indoctrinating, but instead legitimately enabling intelligent resistance to an indoctrination already in progress, we should be honest with ourselves and communicative to the general public about the difference.

The Value of Learning and the Business of Universities

The other principal line of attack on universities in general, and the humanities in particular, is less obviously political: it merely accuses them of failing as a business. As I have suggested, this seems a strange accusation to make against an American industry whose products dominate the world market to a degree found in few if any other areas, with customers who compete ferociously for the privilege of purchasing our product despite its rapidly rising price.

Following the money actually leads to insights that these business-minded reformers would prefer to keep hidden. The tuition students pay to take humanities courses more than covers the costs of those relatively inexpensive departments. Higher education in the hard sciences is actually a loss-leader whereby the basic research, long-shot investments, and training of workers are mostly handled by the public sector (in this case, public universities). The private sector then arrogates the resulting profitable phase and cites its profits as proof that the university is (like other similarly looted public enterprises) wasteful.[54] In other words, the attacks on the humanities remain inseparable from the well-funded campaigns to transfer benefits from the shared public sphere to private wealth. The process is the intellectual equivalent of the giveaway of public lands to large private-sector drillers, miners, frackers, and loggers who skim off the short-term profits and repay the commons with toxic air and water, a destabilized climate, and a despoiled landscape. The sign on the door says, no pastoral values need apply: they are mere externalities to the internal logic of a monetary profit-system.

No sane citizenry judges its elementary education system by whether it turns an immediate monetary profit. The same should be true for higher education, and the exploitative fiascos of for-profit institutions (Corinthian Colleges, ITT Tech, Westech, the Harris School of Law, the Charlotte School of Law, Trump University, and their kin) over the past couple of years provide the starkest kind of warning, despite the efforts of Trump's Secretary of Education to pretend not to see it. Teaching among *Homo sapiens* differs from teaching within other species, ethologists have observed, precisely in this deferred and indirect mode of reward: when chimpanzees teach each other,

> there is always some direct pay-off to the trainer, for whom the novice is trained to perform some service. In contrast, full-blown human pedagogy presupposes, first, the disposition to invest time in training without any immediate return. Secondly, pedagogy involves a sophisticated aesthetic judgment of what constitutes a good performance.[55]

The connection between humanity and the humanities could hardly be clearer. Even in as hard a science as engineering, doctoral students are often sheepish about their work in pure math and other such areas which they find fascinating and beautiful but have no immediately practical pay-off. Yet, over time, pure math has paid off richly, in unpredictable ways. As with the fascinating and beautiful work of creative artists, aesthetics offers a clue to long-term human value.

Yet the drumbeat continues: universities should be run more like businesses, and the humanities should be downsized. In the United States, the preponderance of wealthy businesspeople on university Boards of Trustees amplifies that drumbeat. In Britain, the Conservative government's Browne Report has largely institutionalized that idea, despite the eloquent protests of leading humanistic scholars (a similar attack on the socialized National Health Service has drawn similar cries of protest from leading British medical professionals). The bias may not be surprising, given that British universities have come officially under the control of the government's Department for Business, Innovation and Skills. As of June 2018, the Trump administration was proposing to merge the Department of Education into the Department of Labor, with universities under the regulation of an "American Workforce and Higher Education Administration."

These economic squeezes are not finally so different from the resentment of free thinking as it may at first appear. HUAC cut off my father's salary, not his head. In the 1950s, many American humanists and social scientists imposed political censorship on themselves, less because they feared subpoenas from Sen. Joe McCarthy than because they feared subtractions from their government funding, which was then pouring into university coffers at an unprecedented rate.[56] In fact, the attack on my father was partly an effort to undermine the man who hired him at the FCC, James Lawrence Fly, who powerful conservatives believed "was trying to limit corporate concentration of broadcasting power, and also was a leading opponent of wiretapping."[57] More broadly, it was part of an attempt to destroy the FCC as "one of the few New Deal agencies left in Washington" that continued enacting reforms and regulation well into the 1940s. And that effort eventually succeeded: attacks on the FCC as Communistic "left the agency shell shocked, and as early as 1945 it began the slow transformation toward more conservative, pro-business" stances that "increasingly acquiesced to industry wishes."[58] The current head of the FCC, Amit Pai, is a culmination of that process. The repressive task that the Red Scare failed to complete in the United States has been taken up, with ever-increasing sophistication, by greenback dollars.

What these other besiegers of the Ivory Tower assert, without even having to say it, is the now-common assumption that money is the sole undeluded measure of all things: the vaunted "bottom line." This is a kind of religion, with the Authorized Version of scrip as its diffusible Scripture, and since the 1950s it has been producing its own version of Christianity: the "Prosperity Gospel" that, despite stark evidence to the contrary in the New Testament, insists that Jesus Christ's favor corresponds to the accumulation of earthly wealth. The great historians R. H. Tawney and Max Weber have, in quite different ways, analyzed the way Protestantism has, since its origins in the 16th century, allied itself with capitalism, at the expense of non-monetary value systems.[59] I suspect that the compulsion to depict the US military as consisting entirely of entirely selfless heroes, despite the fact that it recruits with financial incentives and therefore draws mostly from groups that most need the money, reflects an unease (especially on the right wing) with the idea that military values might be susceptible to the same reductive reading that business-minded conservatives have imposed on more progressive institutions.[60]

The need to deny what humanistic education implies – namely, that values greater than or separable from financial ones exist, and that human lives can be valuable in different ways – may help to explain why some wealthy persons and organizations are willing to invest in stoking popular anti-intellectualism. For the moment, expensive though they are, universities still constitute a standing reproof and even rebuttal to the blind worship of the Almighty Dollar. Those who have dutifully served a god – including the money god – are not likely to welcome suggestions that it is a false god, or at best a god uninterested in them personally.

Other wealthy conservatives, corporations, and foreign nations follow a more patrician model, donating large sums to universities on the condition they be used to steer higher education back toward more traditional cultural paths.[61] This patrician position is a delicate and risky one, for at least two reasons. First, the prestigious archive is not always a trustworthy ally for privileged defenders of the status quo. Many previous generations of subversion have not only achieved stealth by cloaking themselves in the mantle of the high-cultural past, but also gained leverage by standing at a historical distance that lets them raise alternative social principles into view without seeming threateningly radical. Old-style conservatives cannot count on decorous museum cases to keep the thoughts latent in the treasured artifacts from leaking back out into the world, any more than the Crystal Skull remained safe in its warehoused crate. Second, aristocratic advocates of this traditionalist philosophical and aesthetic value-system make strange bedfellows with other conservatives who insist that economic efficiency is the root of all good, that humanistic scholarship is archaic – as governments and would-be reformers have been complaining for at least 200 years[62] – and that creative art is elitist. They are all on the right wing, but they are birds of very different feathers.

This misguided utilitarianism, shallow in history and purpose, is by no means the exclusive domain of right-wingers. The Obama White House produced and publicized a College Scorecard that rates our institutions of higher learning by the ratio of their expense to the salaries earned by their graduates. Jerry Muller points out that, under this system "a graduate who proceeds immediately to be a greeter at Walmart would show a higher score than her fellow student who goes on to medical school."[63] As of May, 2016, the landing-page at https://collegescorecard.ed.gov featured this graphic (Figure 8).

Nor was this supposedly intellectual administration's focus on economic competition limited to the later stages of education, where professional preparation may be a plausible primary goal. In 2009, President Obama praised the educational practices of societies such as Singapore that are hyper-disciplined from very early in life toward training for employment: "They are spending less time teaching things that don't

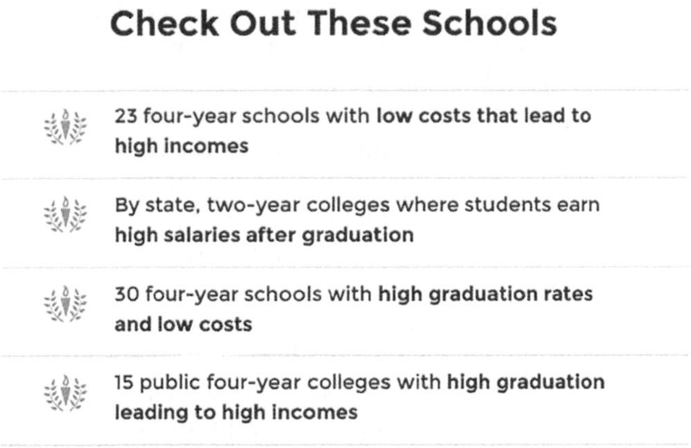

Check Out These Schools

23 four-year schools with **low costs that lead to high incomes**

By state, two-year colleges where students earn **high salaries after graduation**

30 four-year schools with **high graduation rates and low costs**

15 public four-year colleges with **high graduation leading to high incomes**

Figure 8 "College Scorecard" from the Obama White House.

matter, and more time teaching things that do. They are preparing their students not only for high school and college, but for a career."[64]

This conclusion probably pleased his Chamber of Commerce audience, but it fits only too well with Obama's disappointing tendency to accept the world-view of Wall Street and thus to yield progressive premises to the opposition before the battle even begins. He foresees the importance of "21st century skills like problem-solving and critical thinking and entrepreneurship and creativity," but neglects to acknowledge that such skills are nurtured by fields other than math and science, and by allowing free play-time rather than extending regimented school hours.

This blind-spot is especially damaging when classes become too large and too assessment-driven for students to be engaged as creative individuals rather than as machines being mass-produced into better tools of mass-production. Clark Kerr, the perceptive liberal Quaker who led the University of California through much of its turmoil in the 1960s, once declared that the purpose of the institution was to train the workers required by the state's major corporations. Kerr's declaration provoked the remarkable *cri de coeur* from Mario Savio that helped spark a countercultural student revolt (this extemporaneous December 2, 1964, speech is well worth watching on YouTube). Less than 50 years later, I sat in a high-level University of California planning meeting where our mission was described as meeting the hiring needs of the state's pharmaceutical and other industries – and no one even blinked. On a smaller scale, the official state assessment program asks elementary school students, "Why is education so important to California's future?" Five years ago my then-nine-year-old son replied, "Education is so important to California's future because without it, no one could think for themselves." His generally excellent teacher marked the answer down a point, with the comment: "Yes, true; however, how will that benefit CA? Be specific." I don't suppose my son knew the answer to that yet, but neither does anyone else.

Nor is this a worrisome trend only in the Anglophone world. In 2015, Japan's Minister of Education recommended that the country replace higher education in the humanities and social sciences with topics of more practical value. Responding in the *Guardian*, Francine Prose asked "Is it entirely paranoid to wonder if these subjects are under attack because they enable students to think in ways that are more complex than the reductive simplifications so congenial to our current political and corporate discourse?"

The utilitarian economic view of the humanities is a mistake inadvertently aggravated by the many leftist scholars who also treat scholarship as worthless unless it can be harnessed to a preordained worldly cause. Traditional literary scholarship may be less pointed, but is it really pointless unless it explicitly undertakes the rescue of oppressed categories of persons by political means? By focusing overwhelmingly on issues of postcolonialism, gender bias, racism, and labor policy, proudly radical institutions such as the University of California Humanities Research Institute unwittingly endorse the conservative attack on disinterested, or at least depoliticized humanistic study, which in the long run may have a more durable ability to speak truth to power, or at least to whisper behind power's back until the truth is shared widely enough to become speakable. Humanists need to recognize the hidden costs of turning their field into a liberationist branch of social science. Clearly, some scholars feel this is the way to revive a dying field of study; but others of us suspect it is instead the way a field still fundamentally valuable and widely valued has been committing suicide.

If we look at art mostly to find and transmit confirmations of our sociopolitical preferences, we damage our ability to offer many kinds of liberation. This kind of leftism in the humanities is preaching to the choir; and, though I am inclined to believe the sermons, I also care about the melody. As Robert Frost wrote in his essay "The Figure a Poem Makes,"

> More than once I should have lost my soul to radicalism if it had been the originality it was mistaken for by its young converts. Originality and initiative are what I ask for my country. For myself the originality need be no more than the freshness of a poem run in the way I have described: from delight to wisdom.

The brilliant and versatile scholar Sir Frank Kermode makes the point with some ferocity:

> university teachers of literature ... can read what they like and deconstruct or neo-historicize what they like, but in the classroom

they should be on their honour to make people know books well enough to understand what it is to love them. If they fail in that, either because they despise the humbleness of the task or because they don't themselves love literature, they are failures and frauds.[65]

The cutting edge gets dull when wielded too often and carelessly. Despite its rhetorical sophistication and intellectual ambition, research built on and toward a predictable sorting of the world into villains and victims risks replacing moral complexity with ideological complacency, eclipsing the cultural-evolutionary perspective this book has been offering, and erasing aesthetics, metaphysics and philology altogether. It also risks implying that political advocacy is the only way for the humanities to aid humanity. But, in times no less fraught than ours, a non-prescriptive approach to the arts of the distant past has provided crucial and consoling perspectives on the embattled present, and discoveries whose value would become apparent only in the future.

Even before money distorts the message of higher education, it distorts the audience. As Christopher Newfield and Andrew Delbanco have cogently argued, recent right-wing attacks on public universities have systematically retracted hard-won access to higher education for the range of American society[66] – especially for the middle class, now being degraded (across races) into a service class. Those attacks are ultimately part of the overall attack on free thinking, because the full human presence of a full range of perspectives is crucial to the functions of higher education, including the social utility of nurturing minds and spirits that can think and feel across cultural differences.

In the name of fiscal responsibility and market rationality, conservative forces have stuck wrenches in the gears of our nation's greatest engines of social mobility and cultural innovation: the public universities. When I was drafting this chapter, it was at once flattering and depressing to notice that the three most aggressive right-wing governors in the United States were campaigning to shut down the humanities.[67] All three were proposing hundreds of millions of dollars of cuts to their state universities, and explicitly concentrating those cuts on any academic program that does not become fundamentally a training program for the types of workers currently wanted by private industry. All three pushed MOOCs – the least humanities-friendly form of education – directly, and also indirectly by cutting state funding while limiting tuition costs so that no other form of teaching will be sustainable. Then they could conveniently accuse faculty who resist the MOOC takeover of hurting lower-income students. All three talked about wanting the university to be run like a for-profit business, as if monetary gain were self-evidently the only real point of education.

British conservatives have proposed charging lower tuition for fields of study that lead to lower-salaried jobs immediately after graduation, and then funding departments by how much tuition they have brought in. That would devastate the humanities fields, while the politicians could shrug and say the wisdom of the market has made the decision for them. Governor Rick Scott of Florida and his Chamber-of-Commerce-led task-force proposed the opposite approach: they want their state universities to charge much higher tuition for humanistic fields that fail to produce immediate economic results – while (in a convenient inversion of the British funding model) continuing to fund departments by how many students they enroll, not by what those students pay. Flip a coin: if heads, the STEM fields (science, technology, engineering, and mathematics) win, and if tails, the humanities lose. A chart of those outcomes then will show objectively what losers the humanities fields inherently are.

Wisconsin Governor Scott Walker has not only been attacking public-school teachers, but also vigorously pushing Wisconsin's state universities (where both my parents got their undergraduate degrees) to rely on MOOCs and competency exams. He also

> submitted a budget proposal that included language that would have changed the century-old mission of the University of Wisconsin system – known as the Wisconsin Idea and embedded in the state code – by removing words that commanded the university to 'search for truth' and 'improve the human condition' and replacing them with 'meet the state's workforce needs.'[68]

This was to be accomplished by focusing on "knowledge and competencies that make students employable today and versatile and adaptable to the workforce needs of tomorrow."[69] This statement ignores that education narrowly tailored to minimal competency, current information, and current jobs neglects exactly the kinds of education that tend to make young minds versatile and adaptable amid social, technological, and economic conditions that are already changing with astonishing rapidity.

The conservative MOOC advocate and ex-oilman who largely guided Governor Rick Perry's educational policy in Texas complained that most humanities research "would never, and I want to stress never, be supported by the market," and was therefore a "corrupt enterprise" that "survives parasitically only by siphoning vast amounts of tuition and cross subsidization unbeknownst to parents, students and taxpayers." He seemed blissfully unaware that, as mentioned a few pages ago, the cross-subsidies in universities actually flow mostly the other way: the teaching of humanities and social-science actually subsidizes the ex-tremely expensive STEM fields, whose outside grants consistently end up costing universities much more money than they actually bring in. The assumption that the "softer" fields are charity cases is as false as it is widespread.[70] But it suits the moneyed interests to link the "tak-ers" of the public welfare system with their supposed enablers in public universities; tenured radicals are elided with chronically ungrateful people on the dole. We softies are a drag.

Granted, these are time-worn complaints about money-minded instrumentalism in university higher education. Even Allan Bloom's *Closing of the American Mind* (1987), vaunted by right-wing commentators, warned that instrumentalist and mercenary influences were damaging higher education in the United States, undermining universities' valuable role as loyal opposition to the dominant culture. That may mean the complaints are pointless: either based on a common hallucination or otherwise impossible to satisfy. But it may instead mean they are important, marking a place where some human values have long been recognized as both worth defending and vulnerable to erasure by other socio-economic functions.

What is at stake here is not simply the battle of wealthy persons to advance their interests through their control of money. What instead underlies this struggle in its most insidious form is demonstrably a battle of memeplexes. The degree to which this battle apparently goes not only unacknowledged but unrecognized (except in extreme instances such as the University of North Carolina[71]), not only by its plutocratic advocates but even by many scholars who have become Deans and Provosts and then become agents of a business-management philosophy, shows how talented the neoliberal money-meme has become at disguising its predatory functions as simply real-world common sense supported by statistics. Some of the best and brightest academics seem unaware that their beloved enterprise is being hijacked by a system that has none of their chief interests at heart.

Consider the passage from the neoliberal prophet Adam Smith I quoted earlier, which identifies universities as the final "sanctuaries" for ideas he considered discredited, "after they have been hunted out of every other corner of the world."[72] Revealingly, Smith promptly goes on to say that his new economic perspectives "were more easily introduced into some of the poorer universities, in which the teachers, depending upon their reputation for the greater part of their subsistence, were obliged to pay more attention to the current opinions of the world." This seems like a progressive sentiment, and doubtless it largely was, but it is not difficult to read it instead as an inadvertent confession of the money-meme's strategy for co-opting its most dangerous rivals.

So, of course the liberal arts are embattled: that is bound to happen when you are fighting a well-armed opponent over something important. A crisis in the humanities doesn't mean anything is wrong with humanities, any more than crises in Poland and Czechoslovakia at the start of World War II meant there was anything inherently wrong with Poland or Czechoslovakia, except maybe – the analogy to the humanities may be illuminating here – a shortage of modern armaments and a lack of a self-perpetuating, fanatically narrowed ideology.

Combatting the ills of higher education in the humanities will be impossible unless we recognize them as symptoms of that struggle. Otherwise we will engage with piecemeal problems – pressure toward MOOCs, declining enrollments in humanities courses and resulting budget cuts, muddled apologies for the field by well-meaning colleagues, a widespread career-utility view of higher education, the decline of university presses, increasing reliance on adjuncts instead of tenure-track faculty, the demands of students never to be offended or given low grades, etc. – instead of attacking the root causes of all these. We will isolate our villains – overly traditionalist or overly radical-presentist colleagues, the anti-intellectual demagogues of right-wing politics, bean-counting university administrators, miserly taxpayers who shrink state budgets, parents who surrender their children to screens instead of books – without understanding how these are all agents, often unwitting, of one side of a war between two sets of values.

How does "accountability" – a prominent word in the neoliberal assault on the autonomy of state universities – function on materials largely invisible to an accountant? If no quantitative measure of the product and its value is available, and reduced quality does not obviously affect the overall price or volume of sales, what is the business-managerial solution except to squeeze the costs – which is to say, the cost per student, which in most humanities fields means the ratio of excellent teachers to students, which is the most essential element for education in these fields? Post-structuralism and post-modernism may have inadvertently encouraged this damaging perspective on literary study: if other values are discredited (as sentimental, imperial, habitual, and/or arbitrary), the default values of market economics seem likely to fill the void.

So, even without any directly ideological withholding of funds, the disabling of academia as a counter-force is achieved by the imposition of managerialism. The doctrine of efficiency and instrumentality is of course inherently especially brutal to the humanities, but a compelling similar case has been made about hard science fields.[73] No less eminent a figure than Lorraine Daston, Director of the Max Planck Institute for the History of Science in Berlin, has recently argued that "Science needs liberal education and its counterweight to the values of the market for its own sake."[74]

That narrow managerial doctrine has now directly invaded the funding of US research in the sciences,[75] and under the initial Trump budget the invasion has escalated. A major goal of this attack is the destruction of the independence of professors as professionals. Even ostensibly progressive ideas become drawn into alliance with this destructive shift: the interdisciplinary initiatives now heavily favored by administrators disempower academic departments, traditionally (along with tenure, also under attack through the hiring of adjuncts) the seat of professorial autonomy, making faculty answerable instead to an administrator's budgeting process.

Years ago, when I bragged to an old friend (an eminent attorney) about my teaching-evaluation scores, he shook his head in sad wonderment and said, "Before I'd judge my professional work based on the views of a bunch of 19-year-olds ...." It was a chastening reply, and it actually goes to the heart of what is now being done to the academic profession. Just as consumer capitalism "transforms citizens into consumers," so the neoliberal university converts students into customers.[76] If the customer is always right, can anyone be surprised by ongoing grade inflation, or by undergraduates demanding the ouster of faculty who have offended them? If the numbers of seats filled and degrees conferred become the measure of faculty productivity, and student evaluations measure teaching efficacy, all because business management requires numbers, then high standards will inevitably be discouraged. Students must be provided with GPAs that qualify them to move on to a high salary or a higher degree; undergraduate majors must be streamlined, and graduate degrees accelerated. Administrators hire ever more part-time faculty to save the costs of salary and benefits – instructors far more vulnerable to the pressure to dilute standards than tenured faculty – and dream of MOOCs allowing one professor to teach millions for decades. The increased net revenue thereby gained by the university is then skimmed off to hire more and more well-paid managers, despite the fact that there is "Not a shred of evidence" that "the cost[s] of the management controls are less than the money saved on inefficient academic personnel."[77] Meanwhile, vast amounts of staff and faculty time are diverted into bureaucratic rituals of questionable value.

The memeplex called neoliberalism thus continues to eclipse the one called professionalism, undermining education while claiming to make it more efficient. What has befallen medical professionals in the era of managed care is also befalling academic professionals. They become functional units in large corporations, no longer answerable primarily to their colleagues' judgment of the quality of their work, nor free anymore to judge what is really best for their patients or students (now clients) on the basis of their professional training and their profession's longstanding principles. They are now answerable instead to metrics applied by managers meeting quotas.

The memeplex called higher education, largely oblivious to the nature of the war, thus continues a surrender to a very powerful alliance among corporate wealth (tied into the personal wealth of the 1%), anti-intellectualism (allied with anti-government populism in the case of state universities), and a utilitarian view of human experience measured in cash (tied into a business-managerial assumption about the calculation, or even the calculability, of bottom lines). If other forms of consensus can be subjugated to the supposition that money is the fundamental measure rather than an instrumental means, then certain questions will cease to be asked. The lower-class passengers will remain locked in steerage while on deck the string quartet plays on, even as the ship lists dangerously to its green-lit starboard side – or possibly lurches no less dangerously back to the port side where a red light still glows. The ballast in the belly of our culture may be the gold it has so ravenously consumed, but it can also sink us – especially if the cargo shifts far in one direction.

The ability of money and capitalism to override other values has been proven repeatedly over the centuries. Despite the ongoing holy wars between Islam and Christianity in the Medieval and Renaissance periods, Islamic and Christian governments were happy to accept and even issue coinage bearing the opposing religion's symbols in order to facilitate trade.[78] The rise of Europe to world power, the ascendency of nations within Europe (notably the Dutch and then the English) that favored a capitalist system of credit over nations (such as Spain) that clung to a royalist reliance on taxation, and the resulting ascendancy of merchants and bankers to power within European nations formerly controlled by old aristocratic precepts and structures, all reflect the power of the evolving modern economic system over traditional values.[79] Projects that apparently had humanitarian goals, such as the anti-slavery agenda of the Belgian takeover of the Congo, quickly devolved into an alliance of imperialist and neoliberal practices that produced a death-toll among the indigenous population similar to that of the Nazi Holocaust. In fact, the profound interdependence of slavery and capitalism has recently been convincingly documented.[80]

In an 1831 letter, the great advocate of liberty and observer of democracy in the United States, Alexis de Tocqueville, commented ruefully that "As one digs deeper into the national character of the Americans, one sees that they have sought the value of everything in this world only in the answer to this single question: how much money will it bring in?"[81] A century later, the hardly less prophetic political economist Karl Polanyi warned that "After abolition of the democratic political sphere only economic life remains; Capitalism as organised in the different branches of industry becomes the whole of society. This is the Fascist solution."[82]

I am not saying that money is irrelevant to good education; in fact, a range of research, across US states and across many nations, indicates that the most efficient way to improve K-12 education is to pay teachers well. Such research also shows that scaling that pay to the results of student exam performance provides no benefit – not even in exam performance.[83] Young students are not consumers in the same sense that their parents are when shopping for kitchen appliances. The problem is again a system that instead seeks to manage education for profit, allied with an assumption (to be examined further in Chapter 7) that human qualities can be best known quantitatively. A better practice may be investing in people as people, not as investments.

Money and markets are certainly useful; I am not urging a Communist or mere barter economy. I buy goods and services from corporations, I want people to have good jobs, and I like having enough income and reliable savings. But if we fail to recognize money as a useful device but an unworthy deity, if we fail to recognize it as an invasive meme not native to the communal human ecosystem, a self-serving force whose interests might compete with some valid human ones – say, caring for the sick, freeing the innocent, discovering the truth, granting each citizen a similar power in elections, or preserving the biosphere in something like the present form to which we and our indispensable mutualists are adapted – then our collective autobiography might justly borrow the title of Martin Amis's novel *Money: A Suicide Note*. Sometimes one cannot serve both human and mammon.

In fact, the ideas and admonitions of this book can be seen as a restatement of the core missions of the entire Protestant Reformation, which echoed objections raised in the preceding centuries by the Lollard movement, by the Mendicant orders that emerged to protest the wealth of the Benedictines, and more broadly by the movements known as the Heresy of the Free Spirit. The Early Modern religious reformers, especially in their intensive Puritan phase, persistently anthropomorphized the Catholic Church as a seductive but corrupting Whore of Babylon. But, the fundamental complaint underlying those polemics was that the papal church had evolved into an institution primarily dedicated to its own perpetuation and power, rather than to redeeming the ideal human essence in our souls. Even now, the scandal of long-term, large-scale of sexual abuse of children by Catholic priests shows, with shocking clarity, a determination to protect the institution rather than the values of the institution.

In Early Modern Europe, the human terror of mortality was being exploited to wrest wealth away from an undereducated populace, through the sale of indulgences, relics, and masses that implicitly subjugated the divine to the monetary. Resistance to any of the mutually sustaining functions of this huge institution was demonized and ferociously punished as heresy. The human will to ignorance was exploited, Protestants said, by a church that kept its services in Latin (thus dulling human souls with mindless ritual rather than awakening them with colloquy) and kept its power in priests, who assured their flocks that the Church had a grasp of, and even control over, the ultimate realities, and would protect them on their path to salvation. The Book of Common Prayer was produced by Protestant authorities to smooth English religious culture into a new unified voice, but the Puritans detected in that project a version of the Catholic legacy of spiritual conformism by secular authorities – a legacy of institutional interference so threatening to free individual soul-making that the Puritans essentially went to war to protect their worship from that book.

Just a few years before Martin Luther nailed his *Ninety-Five Theses* to a church door, the influential Convocation Sermon of John Colet – a humanist educator and foundational Christian reformer – declaimed,

> O covetousness: Saint Paul justly called thee the root of all evil ... of thee cometh these chargeful visitations of bishops, of thee cometh the corruptness of courts and these daily new inventions wherewith the silly people are so sore vexed ... of thee cometh the superstitious observing of all those laws that sound to any lucre, setting aside and despising those that concern the amendment of manners.[84]

The highest potential of humanity, as individuals and as a collective, had thus been perverted; and only by reverting to the Word, which would become audible and intelligible once the sensory richness of the cathedral had been stripped away, could that potential be freed from the runaway memeplex.

Protestants generally condemned all these failings under the category of "idolatry," but they applied that term across a remarkable range of phenomena in the social and cognitive world of the late Renaissance. It refers to anything that becomes worshipped for its own sake, and thus destructively empowered, rather than for the sake of the deepest underlying or highest overarching values. Idols deluded the best essence of humanity into the service of a false materialist deity that did not really love that essence in return and would not protect it. Whether we call that essence a soul, as they did, or find some other term for what we sense is our potential best self, the threat is similar. Even in their characteristically business like commercial endeavors, Puritans were partly seeking signs of some higher blessedness corresponding to (though not earned by) their personal disciplinary virtues.

So, to those who might ask why the transaction this book has been describing has not been noticed before, if it is so powerful and dangerous, I would suggest that it certainly has been noticed, decried, battled, and sometimes defeated by the protean powers of the Word and the willingness of a few individuals to become martyrs for the sake of warning their societies. What has changed is the availability of a Darwinian model to help explain rationally the malfunction as a systemic problem, rather than theologically as the work of conscious diabolical agents.

Now, half a millennium later, Catholicism may be taking up the same essential cause. "Certain pathologies are increasing," Pope Francis recently warned:

> We have created new idols. The worship of the golden calf of old (cf. *Ex* 32:15–34) has found a new and heartless image in the cult of money and the dictatorship of an economy which is faceless and lacking any truly humane goal. The worldwide financial and

economic crisis seems to highlight their distortions and above all the gravely deficient human perspective, which reduces man to one of his needs alone, namely, consumption.[85]

The Pope's analysis observes the same kind of cultural *coup d'état* I have been describing, in which a memeplex overrides the systems by which humans would otherwise rule themselves to their collective good: "This imbalance results from ideologies which uphold the absolute autonomy of markets and financial speculation, and thus deny the right of control to States, which are themselves charged with providing for the common good."

The Catholic Church, as the great ancestor of Western universities, thus suddenly seems to be reclaiming a role very much like the one I have been claiming for higher education in the humanities. The church is therefore also dismissed (the Pope observes) as

a nuisance ... regarded as counterproductive: as something too human, because it relativizes money and power; as a threat, because it rejects manipulation and subjection of people: because ethics leads to God, who is situated outside the categories of the market. God is thought to be unmanageable by these financiers, economists and politicians, God is unmanageable, even dangerous, because he calls man to his full realization and to independence from any kind of slavery .... For her part, the Church always works for the integral development of every person.

So, I would claim, do the greatest humanistic traditions.

Such movements are hardly without their dangers, however, if they function without such traditions and the irenic abjuration of certainty that those traditions can teach. The radical-reform movement (to the extent it really is one) within Islam called ISIS or ISIL bears some remarkable similarities to the Christian one. Its militants

read the canonical texts (all of which are easy to find online) and are reluctant to accept the interpretations of mainstream clerics, whom they accuse of hiding the truth out of deference to political despots. The jihadis are literalists, and they promise to sweep away centuries of scholasticism and put believers in touch with the actual teachings of their religion. The elements of this scenario closely resemble those of the Protestant Reformation: mass literacy, the democratization of clerical authority, and methodological literalism.

The jihadis, like the (other?) Puritans, saw their task as undoing, by any means necessary, the evolution of a cultural system away from its ideal original truths. In fact, Luther's reparative project devolved – as he himself lamented after the Peasants' Revolt of 1525 – into a kind of primitivist fervor that allied itself with populism and nationalism. That alliance caused well over a century of European wars (which still echo in Ireland), crushing the ideal of a cosmopolitan Erasmian humanism. That history is an ominous precedent for a Western world that now seems to be splitting into a war between a conservative populist mission of restoring putatively original simplicity and liberal technocratic elites endorsing an ideal of open minds and open borders.

Interchapter: Digital Humanities

My reservations about online humanities courses – however apocalyptically expressed – should not be mistaken for disapproval of the field called Digital Humanities. Its innovations may not always be as new as commonly claimed: unstable texts, "writerly" texts that invite intervention from their audience, collaborations, concordance-based analyses, proliferating copies, and the integration of words with images have all been common in the age of print. Still, Digital Humanities will have to do for the texts of new-media natives what other humanistic studies have done for the texts of previous generations: improve the quality of content and its communication by exploring the opportunities, limitations, and biases of the medium and its genres (including disinformation and crowd-shaming), identify salutary memes and bring them to notice while also highlighting the faults of destructive memes to discourage their potential acolytes. Digital Humanities must also avoid becoming (as its funding advantages and role in credentialing administrators as forward-looking might make it) another tool for the imposition of top-down technocratic control of the humanities, or the devaluation of unquantifiable or politically uncomfortable perceptions. Fortunately, a strong element of collaborative production, aesthetic appetite, and open-access distribution among leading Digital Humanities practitioners runs counter to those structural tendencies.[1]

The age of digital media and Internet distribution has bequeathed the role critics have inherited from the patrons of previous generations of art – not quite the role of gate-keeper, but certainly of taste-maker – to crowd-sourced judgments where all hits are counted equally. Whether that leads to the empowering of innovative thought (because anyone can publish a blog) or to an overwhelming normalization of thought as filtered through commerce (and reinforced by official or unofficial speech-codes) is, from the perspective of this book's argument, a main reason to be ether optimistic or pessimistic about the future adaptability of our cultures. In this sense, the role of the Digital Humanities is continuous with that of the traditional humanities.

Doing digital work on humanities material is different from doing the humanities on digital material. Digital approaches to humanities research have advantages and disadvantages when compared to more traditional modes, as do the print humanities when compared to the oral humanities. Aside from the obvious efficiencies digitalization contributes to some forms of research, it may allow electronic publication to replace parts of a decreasingly sustainable model of publishing and credentialing through books from academic presses. The open, interactive, incremental aspects of this mode of study seem appealingly compatible with the field's longstanding values of connection and suspended determinacy. The digital mode highlights the collaborative nature of learning and the inherent incompleteness of assertions. Large, rapidly searchable databases also enable forms of distant reading (now being explored by Stanford's Franco Moretti and many others) that allow us to see both the collective currents of the lexicon and, thereby, the strokes of individual writers across or against those currents. Whether Big Data will reinforce the power of cultures by reinforcing their norms or undermine that power by making those norms more visible is, for me, a crucial question.

We must also remember that digital signals – precisely because they are fundamentally binary – have tended to be inferior to analog in matching the complexity of the human sensorium. As my final chapter will discuss, the coding often effaces important discriminations. So, it is important that we resist handling information in the degraded forms computers need, except in those cases where we need the computers to do part of our work. My most recent article publications have depended on Python-based analyses of Shakespeare texts, but they would not have been possible without my professional expertise in judging what to search for and then how to apply it in ways that highlight rather than erase the subtleties of Shakespeare's art.[2]

But nothing is free, even when it is. Beyond the loss of nuances from analog data and the losses to bit-rot, there are paired detriments on the production side. The way the digital universe scatters information sets barriers against thoughts that don't produce immediate profit, as demonstrated by the way feed-readers make investigative journalism much less viable. That same ease of scattering also means that new material can be created and distributed at minuscule cost, through blogs or spam, so there is little to keep useful work from being buried amid the mostly useless. Despite all the hits, or perhaps because of them, cyberspace can be lonely terrain for human thoughts. Digital content has its own discontents, and Digital Humanities must weigh carefully what the digital does to the human.

6 Past and Present Humanism

> The complaint is, that what you learn at Eton is of no use to you when you are grown up .... This complaint has been answered over and over again; but it is for ever renewed, and must for ever be patiently heard. .... What man of thirty is there, that is doing business on the stock of knowledge acquired at school? ... A certain amount of knowledge you can indeed with average faculties acquire so as to retain; nor need you regret the hours that you spent on much that is forgotten, for the shadow of lost knowledge at least protects you from many illusions.
>
> But you go to a great school not for knowledge so much as for arts and habits; for the habit of attention, for the art of expression, for the art of assuming at a moment's notice a new intellectual posture, for the art of entering quickly into another person's thoughts, for the habit of submitting to censure and refutation, for the art of indicating assent or dissent in graduated terms, for the habit of regarding minute points of accuracy, for the habit of working out what is possible in a given time, for taste, for discrimination, for mental courage and mental soberness. Above all, you go to a great school for self-knowledge.
>
> —William Johnson Cory[1]

That epigraph is an oldie: over 150 years ago, Cory acknowledged that his argument was already timeworn in the debates over the value of education. But it is a goodie, and worth another spin. People will understandably object that we lack the time and resources to offer every child the equivalent of an Eton education (nor would we countenance its abuses). But children's mental capacities still develop at about the same pace and in the same stages. We don't have time or resources because a mechanistic society focused on near-term monetary profit has chosen not to invest in teachers, and certainly not in the kind who teach "new intellectual postures," "dissent," and "mental courage," since the economic structure replicates itself most reliably by creating worker-consumers rather than fully conscious citizens.

Our ambient culture of frenetic struggle and equally frenetic mass-media entertainment makes real conversation about renewing shared values almost impossible. As our tweens have evidently noticed, the Hunger Games have already begun. The Capitol of that dystopia plays the role of the neoliberal capitalist memeplex: brutal under its glitzy surface as it enforces vast income-inequality on the masses and tells them that their children's only hope of survival is to destroy all rivals through ruthless competition. "Reality television" – the "Survivor" series and similar shows – reinforces that view of what human interaction is "really" like, and what its goal is. "Fortnite Battle Royale" – the world's most popular video game at this writing, with well over a hundred million users in its first year – has the same structure: kill everyone else or die. Is it really surprising, then, that bright students in the rising generation want their world to be gentler, while their more conservative elders insist that the campus ideal isn't the "real world" and never can be?

Recent Books and Movies as Cautionary Tales

As those media fads suggest, entertainments popular with young adults often provide excellent evidence of a society's underlying anxieties. Through literature and film adaptations, the next generation does seem to be sensing the constellation of cultural forces and the resulting imperative of resistance this book has been describing. For the past 20 years, Lois Lowry's *The Giver* has consistently been among the top ten sellers in the Teen/Young Adult category – and also among the 20 books most often banned from school libraries, while being taught at many other schools. It depicts a society permeated and preserved by an ethos of "Sameness" that seems mild and benign, with its polite collective shaming of deviations. But its systematic erasure of difference has become so self-reinforcing that citizens no longer even see colors – except for the hero, Jonas, whose rare "light eyes" correspond to the crystal skull pursued by Indiana Jones. He has the "Capacity to See Beyond" (as the heroine of the sequel, *Gathering Blue*, dyes threads into colors unknown to her community). The one fact most stringently hidden from common view is death itself, instead called vaguely a "Release" to "Elsewhere." When Jonas sees through those euphemisms, he sets out to free his community from its lack of emotion and memory, convinced that order is not worth the costs – costs the order itself has hidden – in truth, love, morality, and the variety and amplitude of experience.

Victor Hugo's *Les Misérables* – the original novel as well as the stage and screen versions – explicates my argument nicely. It wields a Blue Guitar against Red Scares by showing how psychological agoraphobia generates, in individuals and thereby in the state, a repressive conformism that is contrary to human complexity and finally counterproductive for the society as a whole. The figure of Inspector Javert epitomizes the tragedy of a man trying to live strictly by the memeplex of the legal system, assuming it reflects an absolute and divinely sanctioned truth. Hugo thereby warns of the tragedy of a society attempting to do the same: its rejection of the messy indeterminacies of equitable justice finally provokes a large-scale revolution. That revolution is doomed to fail, but individual acts of heroic, morally charged resistance set France on the path toward the successful revolution of 1848 – at least, successful until subjugated (as was the French Revolution of 1789) by the inhumane logic of its own memeplex. My larger argument for the revolutionary power of the arts and of single agents is supported by the fact that Delacroix's painting *Liberty Leading the People* (*La Liberté guidant le peuple*) was recognized as a main instigator of rebellion and hidden in an attic until the 1848 revolutionaries brought it back into public view, while another painter was charged with starting the uprising by waving a red flag. Delacroix's painting also inspired America's Statue of Liberty.

Javert was "born in prison, of a fortune-teller, whose husband was in the galleys," and to defend himself against this legacy of gypsy wandering and criminal transgression, he develops an internal prison, "an indescribable foundation of rigidity, regularity, and probity, complicated with an inexpressible hatred for the race of bohemians whence he was sprung." The threatening memory of that fundamental and radical lack of order, stability, and discipline drives Javert into a compensatory dedication to those values. When the deeply virtuous ex-convict Jean Valjean proves to him that the meme-assemblages of law and state authority are not perfect deities, and not finally on the side of the human, the culture-shock is so severe that it kills Javert – or perhaps it causes the meme-slave within him to execute the nascent heretic against its authority. He throws himself into the maelstrom of the Seine, which is a perfect emblem of the insuperable swirling complexities of a human community. No wonder this story of Occupy Paris was brought back – with massive Oscar endorsements from artsy, liberal Hollywood in 2013 – to wave its revolutionary *Tricolore* over another Red, White, and Blue, in another era when massive income-inequality, disguised as justice under the law, is widely assumed to be exempt from challenges by humane values.

Another popular movie, *Captain America: Winter Soldier* (2014), also provides a vivid epitome of my warnings. My Chapter 4 has argued that the peaks of recent popular culture – the *Lord of the Rings, Star Wars* and *Harry Potter* series – persistently link the craving for total information to an ethically damaging and finally counterproductive denial of death. This second Captain America film produces the same pattern, with a collective fear of death by terrorism leading a population to authorize the excessive gathering of data.

The plot echoes and updates a 1956 Philip K. Dick sci-fi short story called "The Minority Report" that Steven Spielberg made into a movie with the same title in 2002. The premise is that the US government's surveillance systems have become so advanced, capable of running such refined algorithms on so much data, that they can predict who will make trouble in the future. Therefore – and here the story elides with cautionary tales about the so-called technological singularity I will discuss in Chapter 7 – US security agencies have built a machine that can track all future perpetrators through their mobile devices and kill them all at once: perfect stability through perfect knowledge. A fearful population can be frightened into ceding almost everything to authorities who promise protection – a fact easily exploited on behalf of totalitarianism.[2] The US Secretary of Defense (played by Robert Redford) persuades a group of world leaders to support this project because of its net benefits. But he is actually scheming to turn control of SHIELD – a super-heroic US security agency – over to SHIELD's archenemy Hydra, headed by an old Nazi villain, the Red Skull. Captain America seizes the communication system at SHIELD headquarters to warn his well-intentioned colleagues that now "SHIELD is Hydra! Hydra is SHIELD!"

My point exactly, or at least succinctly. In an unmanageably complex multicultural and multinational world, the craving for security provokes a half-concealed oppressive project that passes mechanistic judgments against non-conformists. The Red Skull (having heightened citizens' fears in order to seize power) encourages a new Red Scare; and Captain America's objections to the excesses of state control make him the blacklisted target of SHIELD's weaponry. The quest for control of information turns predictably into a program of political suppression, and only a reincarnated classic American hero from World War II (a plot twist obliges Captain America to don his antiquated costume from that era) can stop it, much as only the retro-Americana of Indiana Jones could block the misguided Soviet quest for total power through the omniscience that took the form of the Crystal Skull.

The line between a deeply demonic conspiracy and a logical, benevolent government program to keep its citizens safe is so thin that – as this book would predict – for a long time we remain unsure which kind we are watching (it helps that the goodness-exuding Redford turns out to be playing against type). Because, at some point, there isn't a difference: a control system perpetuating itself, with benefits for social order but utter disregard for our notions of human freedom, looks very much like a dictatorship. The movie shows how easily these blur together: the reflex that shields us from the threatening complexity of our world (the Crystal Skull problem) can become a self-defending, self-multiplying Hydra, which then (like the Hydra in Greek mythology) becomes more elaborately empowered the more it is attacked. It may look like a conspiracy of evil but it must also be understood as part of the triumph of an evolving technology that threatens to make us just numbers in a large algorithm moving toward probabilistic safety and sameness. The next movie with Captain America, *Avengers: Age of Ultron* (2015), implies a very similar warning. This time the mistake of seeking perfect safety combines with the dangers of the technological singularity I mentioned earlier. Iron Man's mind has been twisted into excessive (though not unfounded) fear of alien forces invading our human world, and so he rashly launches a super-intelligent defense-mechanism called Ultron that then threatens to destroy all human freedoms and even the human race, until Captain America and his pals defeat Ultron and its drone forces.

This is arguably the direction of the American empire in my lifetime, and like that empire it is closely linked to the self-perpetuating, growth-hungry project of capitalism itself. As early as the third issue of the Captain America comic series, published shortly after the outbreak of World War II, the Red Skull comments, "Of course you realize that the main item in overthrowing the government is money." When that villain resurfaces in the 1960s, he decides that the best ideology for his villainy is no longer Nazism, but American capitalism instead, and he sets about gaining influence in the corridors of Washington, DC. One of his schemes – along with a brainwashing device called the Nullatron – is to use Americans' television sets to blind them.

In *The Lego Movie* (2014), the villain is Lord Business, who is also President Business, and whose goal is to get every Lego piece glued permanently into place in pre-set sets that merely mimic the normal material realities of the built world. He covers up this suppression of creativity among his workers with standard little bread-and-circuses distractions such as Taco Tuesdays. The hero is a blue-collar worker who seems to lack creativity, able to imagine nothing but more comfortable ways to watch television. But, by happenstance, he is recruited by a woman aptly named Wyldstyle to forestall that freezing into conventionality by stealing a mysterious Lego piece called – in a pun that merges art and politics – "The Piece of Resistance." Once he touches that Piece, the hero has an almost unbearably dazzling set of visions, and lands in a place where, he says, "there are no signs on anything. How does anyone know what not to do?" Eventually he saves his animated world by leaping off the edge of the universe into the unknown – and into a live-action world where a son must remind his controlling father of the importance of liberated creation. The Piece of Resistance turns out to be simply the cap of the father's tube of Krazy Glue that would have locked every conventional construction of reality in place.

Resistance in the Renaissance

Let me now retreat several centuries to exemplify how some seemingly irrelevant academic studies can contribute to this liberating educational project. I will focus on Renaissance literature and environmental humanities since those are my main fields of expertise, but colleagues in other fields could doubtless do the same.

This book has been contending that culture, in its narrow definition as high symbolic creativity, which is extraordinarily open and malleable, is a key tool for repairing culture in its broad definition as all the beliefs and practices of a society, which is inherently and extremely resistant to change. The previous two chapters have described the transformative arts as key agents of the conceptual and aesthetic malleability essential to our individual consciousness and our survival as a society in a changing world, and higher education as a protected enclave for a more explicit and rational balancing of tradition and innovation. This chapter explores the indispensability of the humanities as an inoculation against the viral and parasitic functions of memeplexes, and as a way of rendering the human drive toward beauty and justice compatible with the complexities of human consciousness and multicultural societies.

The broader, shared culture resembles a gigantic ocean-liner – very slow to turn and hard to stop – carrying us collectively and relatively comfortably across the deep, dark, endlessly churning substance of reality (which sometimes kicks up some icebergs). Paradigm-shifting cultural revolutions must overcome even greater inertia than scientific revolutions, which (as Thomas Kuhn has shown) occur only when evidence contradicting the established paradigms becomes overwhelming – and when cultural developments are ready to accommodate the change.[3] When I teach the standard *Beowulf*-to-*Paradise Lost* survey course for English majors, I find myself describing a thousand-year effort to divert an Anglo-Saxon culture – and, across much of Europe, classical pagan cultures – that valued masculine aggression and heroic self-assertion, onto the Christian path of meekness and humility: the turning of the other cheek to be struck, instead of striking back.

Reconciling that long-term investment in fame and violence with the worship of Christ, from his helpless infancy to his passive acceptance of insult and death, was no small task. Militant American Christianity may still be struggling with this transition. To switch from pride as the greatest virtue to pride as the greatest evil, and from what Nietzsche called master morality to slave morality, would have produced a nasty case of cultural whiplash. That is probably why it actually happened only very gradually and laboriously. Consider the weird struggles to make Christ a warrior hero, from the coda of *Beowulf*, through "The Dream of the Rood," to Spenser's Red Cross Knight in *The Faerie Queene* and the battle in heaven in Milton's *Paradise Lost*. The exaltation of Virgil's *Aeneid* by Lactantius (who led the Emperor Constantine to Christianity in the 4th century) and by many Renaissance Christian authors was, I believe, partly an effort to find, in Aeneas's patient endurance of divinely ordained suffering, a version of the revered classical culture that looked compatible with Christianity. Milton seems to be trying to convince even himself of this in the Nativity Ode as well as in *Paradise Lost*: that the moment had come to cease admiring the fame-and-blood hunger of the heroes his classical education had offered, and to seek instead "the better fortitude / Of Patience and Heroic Martyrdom," which Milton insists is "Not less but more Heroic than the wrath / Of stern Achilles on his Foe." Syncretism in the evolution of religion is evidence of the conservative bias of evolution in general.

Fractures within Christianity have allowed other forms of tender empathy to seep through, however, often with art as the medium carrying the progressive message. The familiar claim that high cultural interventions can nurture a "sympathetic imagination" is often dismissed as a facile generalization, but 17th-century Europe provides specific instances. I have argued that the emergence of Calvinism inadvertently provoked the emergence of protective sentiments toward domestic live-stock in late-Renaissance England,[4] and in an earlier book called *Back to Nature* I argued that modern sympathy for prey-animals was inadvertently enabled by another facet of the Reformation: Protestant iconophobia caused a new kind of painting – the depiction of creatures hunted for food – to be mapped onto an existing tradition of Christian martyrdom, so that the agonized sympathy that had formerly been invested in images of the crucified Christ became accidentally channeled onto the creatures who died for our supper (Figures 9 and 10):[5]

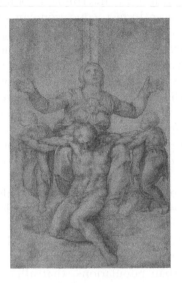

Figure 9 Michelangelo's Colonna Pietà; courtesy Isabelle Stuart Gardner Museum, Boston, MA (mid-16th century).

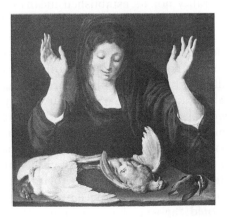

Figure 10 "Woman Mourning Dead Birds" by Jacques de Gheyn (mid-16th century).

204 Past and Present Humanism

The traditionalism of composition in painting provided a foundation for a revolution in cultural values.

Although some ecocritics criticized *Back to Nature* for neglecting to advocate a program of green politics in these urgent times, I believe that some kinds of changes have to be promoted less directly, and that changing public policies requires understanding their cultural roots. This quirky little example from art history demonstrates how the indirectness of artistic consciousness makes room for change, like the capacity for mutation and recombination that enables evolution. In the collective social body, the creative artist or humanist is, ideally, a kind of cell prone to mutation but not then to the interminable blind repetition of errors: evolution, but not cancer. In fact, education can sometimes perform an equivalent of the gene-targeted therapies increasingly used to treat cancer. By selectively turning some genes on or off, these therapies in effect accelerate healthy evolution and localize it in an individual: instead of the deleterious genes depressing the patient's reproductive probability and so eventually disappearing, they are diverted from reproducing within the patient. Evolution ceases to be a phenomenon of groups over time; instead, the patient acquires a survivable genetic profile through a treatment that, like a humanities education, must be tailored to the unique inner nature of each individual by a conversation of trials and non-fatal errors.

Looking back across centuries at how our culture has shaped our view of non-human creatures can give us valuable perspective on how we now live and should live. As agriculture became allied with industrial capitalism and its emphasis on mass production, and as those forms of capitalism and production, along with other factors, promoted a huge growth in urban populations, that alliance took the form of massive industrial farming. Sustaining this new system depended on a special version of the process I have been describing, by which a society tacitly agrees to see some things and not others so it loses neither its proud sense of morality nor its established means of survival. In this case, the empathy toward non-human experience that leaked into Western culture through 17th-century Protestantism had to be suppressed so that we could ignore the scream-worthy horror that industrial farming imposes on millions of conscious, sentient animals every single day: a life of torture followed by a brutal premature death. This is arguably the biggest ethical-emotional blind-spot of our society, and the one our descendants may find least comprehensible and least forgivable – unless they are instead most appalled by our biggest prudential failing, namely, evading our responsibility to limit anthropogenic climate-change.

Large farming corporations – using lobbyists, campaign contributions, and the votes of people dependent for their livings on the corporations that destroyed their ability to make a living as small farmers – have successfully promoted "ag-gag" laws in many states. These are laws designed to silence ("gag") whistleblowers, animal-protection activists, and journalists who might report violations of even the very loose regulations of agricultural operations. This legislation, which makes it a felony to expose the shockingly inhumane workings of slaughterhouses or other acts of extreme and gratuitous cruelty to farm animals, is merely the conscious extension of a much bigger memeplex that has long brought consolingly neat and familiar shrink-wrapped packages of animal protein to our grocery stores. On an even larger scale, our culture has blinded us to the question of whether agriculture itself has been more curse than blessing to human freedom and human happiness, let alone to the complex beauty of life on earth in general and its ratio of joy to suffering. That this curse may be irreversible – since there would be no way back without mass starvation – does not make it any less a curse, and we can begin trying to mitigate its effects only if we recognize it as an entity whose motives should not be mistaken for our own.

* * * * * * * * * * * *

The ferocious struggle between Catholic traditions and Protestant innovations in the Renaissance is just one version of a perennial social tension that universities – once training grounds for the partisans of such schisms as well as the home field of humanism – have evolved to contain, sometimes even converting the polarity into a battery that energizes scholarly progress. By their very duality, modern universities are an epitome or iteration of the great human experiment. In their curatorial functions, they stabilize our collective knowledge over time, preserving from extinction memes that have lost their animate carriers.[6] In their devotion to innovative discovery, the same universities unsettle both the structure and the content of that stored knowledge when new ideas and information become available (sometimes because excluded voices are finally given a fair hearing), allowing us to adapt to a changing environment.

This division has been nicely articulated by Geoffrey Galt Harpham as a tension traceable back to the Greek educational schools of the 4th century B.C.: the tension between the tradition of Isocrates that is "consolidating, reverential, aristocratic," and a Platonic tradition that is "critical, subversive of habits and identities, searching, unsettled." I demur only from Harpham's conclusion that their relationship today is merely "confused codependency."[7] I think a sufficiently adaptable version of public advocacy has to proceed by the nonprescriptive and often idiosyncratic exercise of the mind, which will likely come to understand the importance of established virtues rightly inflected by the current range of possibilities and consequences. Isocrates' approach fundamentally attempts to gain power and improve the virtues of the *polis* along established lines through an orator's skillful persuasion of communities, while Plato's approach fundamentally attempts to approach truth by open-ended, conversational, rational, and often improvisational inquiry, mostly toward a perfection of the inquirer's own wisdom. But higher education isn't muddled by the unexamined incompatibility of these ideas; higher education – especially public higher education – is the project of making them compatible, or at least finding their synergies.

The consumption of manioc (also known as cassava or yuca) provides a vivid example of the evolutionary functions behind this mixed imperative. Manioc has been an essential starch for human communities, especially in the Americas, for a very long time; yet, unless elaborately processed, it gradually causes cyanide poisoning. As Joseph Henrich points out, manioc ceases to taste bitter a few steps into that process, and since the effect of the cyanide would take many years to appear, a rational individual could easily dismiss some of the later steps as pointless ritual.[8] So, it has been important for people to take this full process, and many other elements of cultural transmission, on faith. In fact, as discussed earlier, human beings over-copy: when shown someone performing an action to get a treat, other primates are much quicker to recognize and skip irrelevant steps than young humans are. We are evidently evolved to imitate successful elders diligently, and to limit our experiments to safe situations.

This may explain some of the "common sense" mistrust of innovations handed down by self-certain eggheads. If universities neglect the loyalty owed to tradition, whether through scientific or social-scientific "findings" that soon prove exaggerated or invalid, or through zealous presentism or localism that makes us assume that our ideologies and practices are self-evidently better than those of the past or those of elsewhere, we earn that mistrust. But if we devote ourselves to the uniquely human project of cumulative knowledge that a university institutionalizes – drawing on past learning, preparing the learning of the future – then, even when we don't seem to be making common sense, we are making common cause. A truly diverse university classroom is a one-room schoolhouse for testing interpretive schema. And, even in the hard sciences, schema – models of reality awaiting endless refinement and reconception – may often be the best hold human minds can get on reality.

Education helps fill the mind, but it must also render that container elastic without rendering it formless. This reflects a problem for advanced intellectual work generally: how open can one remain to the intricate, multiple, and even contradictory aspects of any object of study without becoming merely indiscriminate – a passive observer rather than an omniscient one? Any dissertation-writer who has wondered when to stop gathering data and instead begin enforcing a thesis will understand the problem. At what point should one begin to generalize (some scholars oddly seem to assume that generalization is always a flaw, rather than a necessity), and at what point cease? Physicists and engineers will recognize this issue as well as humanists do: sometimes one must bracket the insuperable complexity of reality and employ an adequate simplification, a model that functions in the realm of practical science much as verisimilitude does in the creation of narrative fictions. And, if I am correct that a crucial mission of higher education is to increase a student's tolerance for such subtleties and intricacies, how do we avoid provoking instead a deadening *ataraxia* – the eternal suspension of judgment, caring, and commitment that was advocated by several major schools of ancient philosophy, but may not seem like a suitable goal for modern education? There is a difference, however, and also a holy alliance, between a university as a locus of perpetual inconclusion and the student who learns there how to reach informed conclusions on various points and carries those out into the duties of citizenship.

The tensions of an earlier multicultural moment commonly called the Renaissance or the Early Modern period may explain why that society generated great dramatists – in England, not just Shakespeare but also Christopher Marlowe, Ben Jonson, Thomas Middleton, and others; with Spain not far behind – just as clearly as an ant colony would recruit more soldiers than nurturers in times of warfare. Identifying the dates and characteristics of any historical period is a fool's errand, but there does seem to have been something extraordinary about this period in Europe: some kind of breaking-loose that produced battles on the outskirts of cultural limitations, and hence provoked the growth of literature. Contested boundaries are especially conducive to drama, which lacks a narrator and is therefore well suited for juxtaposing different viewpoints without prejudice. Read carefully enough in their original context, many tragedies start looking like border-skirmishes in the spots where conflicting interests of a culture each demand priority. Near the end of Chapter 4, I described the archetypal tragic hero as a person caught between conflicting demands by two major cultural authorities, gods or otherwise. The change from a medieval toward a modern world – in science, technology, religion, politics, travel, and economics – would have generated many such conflicts, and deep ones. Lately, educators and cultural commentators tend to wrestle with what they take to be an urgent choice between Shakespeare and multiculturalism, but in fact the high Renaissance was launched by multiculturalism: by Turkish invaders forcing Jewish scholars to flee Constantinople and thereby carry into the Christian West the accumulated wisdom of North African, Arabic, and Greek pagan cultures. Despite complaints from the social-activist left and the money-minded right, there is nothing irrelevant about taking perspective on the situation of human society in the 21st century by studying its great dress-rehearsal some four centuries earlier. Nor is there anything necessarily trivializing or falsifying about recognizing the connections between that past and our present.

Environmentalism and the Power of Narrative

Heightening our awareness of the elaborate networks that we inhabit, and that inhabit us, is important for ecological as well as sociological reasons. John Dewey warned against the "illusion of being really able to stand and act alone – an unnamed form of insanity which is responsible for a large part of the remediable suffering of the world."[9] Leading social theorists during the past few decades challenged the widespread assumption that human beings are self-contained, self-determining selves, arguing that we are instead constructed by outside forces much larger than our individual persons. If we discard its questionable foundation in human exceptionalism, that insight can actually be applied even more broadly. It can overcome our dangerous illusion – manifest, for example, in the misguided popularity of antibacterial soaps – that we exist independent of the biosphere and the biome. We are partly ruled not only by macrocosmic external forces, in other words, but also by microscopic interior forces much smaller than our individual persons. In nature and (this book has been arguing) in culture, we must recognize the workings of a whole range of evolved networks and learn how to navigate their overlapping fields of influence, if we want to regain any realistic claim to free will – any ability to choose what becomes of the human.

This ecologically networked perspective on selfhood may offer the most sane and sanguine way of dealing with a Darwinian understanding of life. Susan Blackmore asks,

> How then do we live our lives if we are just memeplexes? Some philosophers have argued that the only result would be a helpless fatalism or deep depression. In fact it is possible to drop the idea of an inner self and simply live life as a memeplex. Oddly enough this does not seem to make people worse, or more miserable, but to be a kind of liberation. Dawkins ended *The Selfish Gene* with the words "We, alone on earth, can rebel against the tyranny of the selfish replicators". I would argue, instead, that we are meme machines, created by and for the selfish replicators. Our only true freedom comes not when we rebel against the tyranny of the selfish replicators but when we realise that there is no one to rebel.[10]

I believe – and will argue – that we can benefit from this perspective without assenting to Blackmore's conclusion that any such rebellion is illusory, pointless, or doomed. For the moment, however, I will add only that nothing in the theory of biological or cultural evolution precludes making loving choices for and within one's living community.

These lessons about human selfhood may be best taught by fables, whether alluring comedies of community, or scathing satires and cautionary tragedies about human pride. Shakespeare's *Midsummer Night's*

Dream offers a prescient allegory of our interdependency with other forms of life, represented there by the fairies.[11] Shakespeare's moon-swayed comedy, and the plays within that play, challenge the ecologically disastrous human fantasy of insular identity and pure autonomy. Shakespeare's tragedies similarly harp on the follies and agonies of attempting to inhabit an idea of oneself more purely than our natural dependencies permit: the costs of attempting to achieve a more perfect sovereignty than our imperfectly constructed persons can sustain.[12]

The mysterious denizens of fairyland called creative artists and radical theorists actually serve a function within the body-politic not unlike that of mutualists within the body: as Michael Pollan observes,

> because microbes evolve so much faster than we do (in some cases a new generation every 20 minutes), they can respond to changes in the environment – to threats as well as opportunities – with much greater speed and agility than "we" can. Exquisitely reactive and adaptive, bacteria can swap genes and pieces of DNA among themselves.[13]

This may explain why our species grants alien microbes so much space and authority within our bodies. As artistic fantasies provide us with a low cost way to explore multiple possibilities, so the microbiota provide a plasticity that "serves to extend our comparatively rigid genome, giving us access to a tremendous bag of biochemical tricks we did not need to evolve ourselves."[14]

Ecocriticism thus converges nicely with the Darwin-inspired offshoot some have begun calling "evocriticism," which explores the relationship between evolutionary biology and literary invention. Creating fictional narratives is very important; so is critiquing them, because sometimes the trick is on us. In this sense, I believe that Freud's *Civilization and Its Discontents*, by depicting socio-cultural norms as an external force to which our blissfully unconstrained primal selves must eventually yield, creates too simple a narrative of oppressor and victim. I see culture as an external prosthesis for the bureaucracy of consciousness; and like most bureaucracies, the bureaucracy of consciousness is a useful device in a complex system of competing desires, but can quickly evolve into an inhumane force devoted primarily to perpetuating itself. This book has argued that most people flee blindly into the embrace of cultural formulas that protect them from cognitive overload, but at a high cost to their range and sensitivity of perception, and their ability to think in hypothetical or contrarian modes.

Science now suggests those costs can be mitigated by reading fiction. According to the abstract of a 2013 study at the University of Toronto,

> The need for cognitive closure has been found to be associated with a variety of suboptimal information processing strategies, leading to decreased creativity and rationality. This experiment tested the

> hypothesis that exposure to fictional short stories, as compared with exposure to nonfictional essays, will reduce need for cognitive closure .... As hypothesized, when compared to participants in the essay condition, participants in the short story condition experienced a significant decrease in self-reported need for cognitive closure .... These findings suggest that reading fictional literature could lead to better procedures of processing information generally, including those of creativity.

Previous studies have shown that a craving for cognitive closure reduces the number and scope of "internally generated hypotheses," leads to "a preference for considering smaller amounts of information before making final decisions," and thereby to "a reliance on simple, rather than complex, cognitive structures when interpreting or making sense of that information," thus impeding "not only rationality, but creativity as well."[15]

Stories seem to be a device that has co-evolved with *Homo sapiens* to allow us to assimilate complexity and explore all our potential selves, including those we must learn to reject. They are essential to our ability to process experience and build our communities. If it is true (as widely believed) that the human brain originally had to expand to handle the complexities of analyzing other minds, then an expanded capacity for empathy certainly requires an expanded tolerance for complexity. It is therefore exasperating to hear literary study so often defended only by some concept of pure aesthetics, or, worse, as a kind of lovable loser: harmless enough to be worth an occasional indulgence, but utterly irrelevant to the serious business of the world. The opposite may be closer to the truth: there is nothing more current than the study of the past, and nothing more real and important than the stories we create and the way we exchange our interpretations of them.

That truth may be even more evident in the 21st century than in the previous ones, for several reasons. Cultural communication is the essence of our communal and linguistic species; and from the intimacy of a marriage to the scope of geopolitics, it is a precious commodity. As the world becomes smaller and more crowded, human morale and morality increasingly depend on reminders that every other person has an inner life as unique and gigantic as one's own. For that purpose, nothing works better than a great old play or novel – in fact, the more distant the world of the author, the more compellingly that author teaches us to recognize each other as long-lost siblings. Emerson suggested that

> The use of literature is to afford us a platform whence we may command a view of our present life, a purchase by which we may move it. We fill ourselves with ancient learning, install ourselves the best we can in Greek, in Punic, in Roman houses, only that we may wiselier see French, English, and American houses and modes of living. ...The field cannot be well seen from within the field. The

astronomer must have his diameter of the earth's orbit as a base to find the parallax of any star. Therefore we value the poet. All the argument and all the wisdom is not in the encyclopaedia, or the treatise on metaphysics, or the Body of Divinity, but in the sonnet or the play. In my daily work I incline to repeat my old steps, and do not believe in remedial force, in the power of change and reform. But some Petrarch or Ariosto ... breaks up my whole chain of habits, and I open my eye on my own possibilities.[16]

Literature, then, is a platform from which many trains of thought depart, and where many such trains, and many distant relatives, can connect. The current knowledge in most technical disciplines will be at least partly refuted or outdated within just a few years, whereas the *Canterbury Tales* and *Jane Eyre*, and the works of Dickinson and Dickens, maybe (harder to predict with recent work) the novels of Octavia Butler and Jhumpa Lahiri, will be just as true and valuable as ever – maybe more valuable, as time vindicates the durability of their seemingly peculiar truths.

Stories will also matter because computer scientists and historians and psychologists have all finally started to recognize what many literary scholars have asserted all along: namely, that people have always lived in a virtual reality, a representation of the universe, partial in every sense of the word, that we project in the planetarium of our brains. In that "distracted globe," we are always having to choose which story to tell; whether to frame it as a comedy of shared life, a tragedy of individual extinction, or an epic of nation-building; and whether to consider the narrator reliable and the protagonist a hero. As our society drifts toward dehumanizing the mind through reductively mechanistic understandings of the brain,[17] and therefore toward purely pharmacological solutions to human psychological problems, the limitations of that model become painfully clear. We underrate at our peril our mental and emotional investment in stories, which have no material presence but (like other memeplexes) persist simultaneously within us and in the world around us. They are less an imaginary world than they are a helpful way of engaging with that world in an ameliorative spirit, and thereby realizing ourselves.

One indication that the rising generation is ready for the challenge of steering memeplexes is the massive proliferation of fan-fiction – surely more than a million such spin-off narratives online, and probably as many not. These young people are recognizing not just the multiverses the human mind can create, but also that they can reshape the most prominent narratives of their cultures toward their own hopes and values. That these are often interventions against repressive memeplexes is evident from the emphasis on "shipping" – that is, putting into an erotic relationship – same-sex characters from well-known books, movies, and

TV shows. Such "slash" fictions reflect a recognition that it is important to intervene in cultures indirectly, by story-telling experiments, rather than only by conventional modes of direct political protest: in this case, the protest against strictures of gender and sexuality that today's rising generation seems especially determined to shatter.

The eminent primatologist Frans de Waal's *Primates and Philosophers* argues that the key function of religions is "giving a narrative" to the fundamental ethical reflexes produced by evolution; I believe that the narrative form makes those reflexes more portable and more flexible as well as more memorable. At the same time, narrative serves the purpose I attributed to religion earlier – namely, giving a frame and a shape to an otherwise psychologically intolerable void around a human life. Arthur Kleinman's *The Illness Narratives* and Arthur W. Frank's *The Wounded Storyteller* study the role of narrative in controlling the experience of physical ailments, a topic that Cheryl Mattingly, Elinor Ochs and Lisa Capps continue to explore productively. Nicholasa Mohr's *Growing Up Inside the Sanctuary of My Imagination* recalls that the telling of *el cuento puertoruqueño* was "used as a way to mollify any number of crises .... Soon we were all enthralled, forgetting our grief, our hunger, or our anguish. When the story was over, our stress had lessened and once more life appeared endurable."[18] Business leaders and futurists are recognizing what has actually long since been evident in advertising: the key product of the future will be stories – or at least that products will be valued for the stories they imply, more than for any practical or technical functions.[19]

This point seems to be getting increasing attention. A *New York Times* economics blog summarizes an article by a chemist and past dean of New Paltz's School of Science & Engineering arguing that "humanities degrees may be more important for tomorrow's job market than is generally believed" because most jobs will be those that require "doing things that computers can't do." Therefore, "The more valuable skill sets ... will be those that computers can't offer, like empathy and sociability – skills that you might be more likely to learn in an English course than one in linear algebra."[20] This point also reveals the problem with saving labor costs by allowing computer programs to evaluate student writing: the kinds of writing a computer algorithm can adequately evaluate are exactly the kinds that computer algorithms will soon be able to produce, rendering the skills thereby taught mostly useless for future employment.

Studies suggest that physicians are too quick to exclude ambiguous evidence, and too eager for testing, due to a mistaken belief that technology can legitimately eliminate ambiguity.[21] Other studies have shown that reading fiction rather than factual materials prevents "premature closure on decision-making in medical diagnosis."[22] So, the argument that arts and humanities offer personal fulfillment, and the argument that they provide valuable and saleable professional skills, are not separate arguments, let alone mutually exclusive. These doctors became more effective caregivers – even in the technical role of diagnostician – precisely because more of their human capacities had been nurtured.

This insight has now appeared in no less prominent a publication than the *New England Journal of Medicine*, warning against "transforming a patient's gray-scale narrative into a black-and-white diagnosis that can be neatly categorized and labeled."[23] Furthermore, "Key elements for survival in the medical profession would seem, intuitively, to be a tolerance for uncertainty and a curiosity about the unknown. Have we created a culture that ignores and denies that requirement?" Technology lets physicians "spend less time at the bedside in the gray-scale world of medicine and more time in front of a screen absorbing processed and general information rather than immediate and idiosyncratic realities." If the "Next Medical Revolution" will entail "the possibility of more than one right answer, and consideration of our patients' values" and "acknowledging that certainty is not always the end goal," then literary study appears to be optimal training.

Nor is literature the only humanistic field that improves the work of physicians. Galen, the ancient Greek doctor whose legacy dominated medieval and Renaissance medicine, wrote a treatise called "The Best Physician is also a Philosopher." According to a study in the *Journal of General Internal Medicine*, after completing a course of observing artworks in galleries, Harvard Medical School students'

> ability to make accurate observations increased 38 percent. When shown artwork and photos of patients, the students were more likely to notice features such as a patient's eyes being asymmetrical or a tiny, healed sore on an index finger. Observations by a control group of students who did not take the class did not change.

In domestic politics, a *New York Times* op-ed piece attributed Karl Rove's many triumphs as a campaign strategist to "his unshakable faith in the power of a story," and that his opponents succeeded only when they ceased offering statistics and associating themselves with whatever issues polled favorably, and instead offered "a stirring narrative that defines their views."[24] The Obama campaigns seemingly assimilated this lesson quite successfully, and ironically it returned to haunt Rove when he embarrassingly chose to believe his own triumphal narrative rather than the 2012 Ohio exit polls.

Both sides in the gun-control debate clearly understand the political impact of story-telling. The advocates of control base their campaign on the 20 massacred children in Connecticut, rather than relying on the statistics of annual gun deaths in the United States, which are far more massive and more difficult to defend with "good guy with a gun" fantasies, but lack any unified narrative. On the very day I am writing this, the news media feature the gun lobby's response: a lobbyist tell-ing a Senate committee that "a young woman defending her babies in her home" needs a large-magazine assault weapon, which assures "the peace of mind that a woman has as she's facing three, four, five vio-lent attackers, intruders in her home with her children screaming in the background."[25] The lobbyist could not cite a single such incident (and her notion of "peace of mind" is mind-boggling). But a heart-rending, heart-racing tale, even a tall one, overshadows quantitative evidence and rational risk-analysis. In the absence of more thoughtful institutions, cultural and political deceits can thus exploit the vulnerability that our hard-wired heuristics impose on our thinking.

A primary purpose of Renaissance training in rhetoric – the core of the original "humanist" education – was to enable people to resist ma-nipulation by rhetoricians. Similarly, in 21st-century education, a valid purpose of training in interpreting narrative is to help us realize when we are being manipulated through narratives and by our appetite for narrative, so we can decide whether it is for better or worse – a subset of realizing the ways we are used by other memeplexes.

My project has useful precedents in Hans Blumenberg's 1979 book *Work on Myth*. Building on the scholarship of Arnold Gehlen, as well as his own earlier analysis of metaphors, Blumenberg argues that myths per-sist because they protect a community from the unbearable multiplicity of being and the full direct presence of the universe. Myth and metaphor perform some of the same functions that Gehlen saw social institutions performing: supporting the otherwise insupportable, *angst*-ridden task of framing the world without these legacies. Their danger is that they transform from a means of grasping to an independent shaping force, shaped in turn by a kind of Darwinian selection, much like the meme-plexes I have been describing. This also means, as the second half of this book has been arguing, that the work of literature and of serious literary study may be the best way of regaining control of these mythic narratives and their metaphors, making them accessible to recognition as something other than either absolute truth or trivial phenomena, and therefore susceptible to revision towards the essential needs of humanity at any historical moment. Societies "work on myth," as Blumenberg's ti-tle suggests, to make it applicable to their changing needs; but myth also works on us to sustain it and its symbionts, which may be our parasites.

Blumenberg's resembles a conservative position, in that it warns against discarding the collective guiding ideas that have developed over many generations and replacing them with what seems right and ratio-nal in a present moment. His point is not, however, that mythic legacies can be presumed optimal for a human community; only that some such myths are indispensable lest the burden of total reality, which our ra-tionality can never really master, crush us, damaging individuals and society alike. In other words, metaphors and myths are not the opposite of scientifically observed reality, but a way of grooming an environment in which our rationality is capable of functioning.

Story-telling can achieve conciliation, not just deception, if competing narratives can be reconciled. A *Newsweek* article described how some Israelis and Palestinians have been reconciled, not by policy negotiations or high-tech fences, but simply by reading each other's stories. The importance of non-monetary values in such situations is so great that both Jewish and Palestinian residents "react with outrage and disgust when cash is offered in exchange for sacred land and become more tolerant of violence to the other side"[26]; money, supposedly the ultimate mediator, becomes instead a provocateur. Elsewhere, the same principle operates in Truth and Reconciliation commissions, which have helped heal several of the world's most violently divided societies by replacing adversarial legal contests that function under rules of evidence with the telling of personal stories that may be more truthful.

A 2017 study in *Nature Communications* of the Filipino hunter-gatherer population called the Agta showed that the groups that included a skilled story-teller cooperated distinctly better than ones that did not. Furthermore, when asked to choose which other Agta they would like to have in their group, the Agta chose those viewed as expert story-tellers ahead of those viewed as expert fishers, despite the obvious practical advantages of the latter choice.

Unless messages participate in a community's established narratives, they tend to fail and even backfire. An NYU economist argues that the reason several trillion dollars of governmental and NGO aid have not, as repeatedly promised over recent decades, erased poverty and hunger in the Third World, is that these mega-institutions with their sweeping programs have failed to engage with the immense and stubborn complexities of local cultures.[27] This problem is vividly and convincingly demonstrated in the struggle to curtail the proliferation of AIDS on the Trobriand islands, where the standard morally tinged arguments against sexual promiscuity ran up against a pro-sexual local culture.[28] That lesson may also explain why the Grameen Foundation's microfinance program, with its built-in responsiveness to very local conditions, received the 2006 Nobel Peace Prize – although that program, too, is under increasing criticism, mostly focused on the argument that it has thrived not because it actually alleviates poverty, but because it expands the reach of a neoliberal philosophy.[29] Even large corporations have begun acknowledging that they cannot succeed without an understanding of entrenched local traditions.[30]

The same lesson emerges from the agonizing prolonged wars the United States launched in Iraq and Afghanistan: trillions of dollars wasted, weapons exploded of an astonishing quantity and sophistication, against what look like disorganized and under-armed enemies; and still no happy ending anywhere in sight. Our leaders' plans failed because they were unconcerned about culture: about how local histories, loyalties, and beliefs would shape the narrative of our invasion for different tribes and sects. In fact, the introduction to the counterinsurgency manual later issued to the Marine Corps in Iraq warned that "in this type of warfare, empathy may be as important a weapon as an assault rifle." Something similar can be traced all the way back to Aeschylus's ancient tragedy *The Persians*, nearly 2,500 years ago, which taught the Greek population empathy for the population they had conquered. This contrasts strikingly to the claims of a top official of George W. Bush's White House who, scorning those who believe solutions come from "judicious study" of the world as it is, claimed that sheer American power would allow us to "create our own reality" in the Middle East.[31] That proved impossible for technocrats; but gentler fiction-makers can propose a reality that rivalrous or dismissive enemies may be willing to inhabit, at first provisionally, and at last politically as well.

One reason for humanity's susceptibility to war despite its overwhelmingly hellish consequences may be that war comprises vivid narratives, whereas peace might almost be defined by the absence of any compelling narrative. The crucial question may be whether stories that endorse cooperation – with each other and with the biosphere, usually by stressing our shared needs and characteristics – can overcome the stories that endorse ruthless competition, usually by stoking fear and reducing others to something less than our equals in virtues and hence rights.

Jared Diamond's best-selling book *Collapse* is based in biology and geography, but it asserts that what really destroyed some great civilizations from Easter Island onward is that they failed to re-think the specifically cultural narratives that compelled them, say, to cut down their very last trees in order to build ostentatious monuments. Greenland, Diamond observes – although this observation is now disputed by some environmental historians – offers a kind of "controlled experiment in collapses: two societies (Norse and Inuit) sharing the same island, but with very different cultures, such that one of those societies survived while the other was dying."[32] The Norse culture could not accommodate the innovation of eating fish when environmental change demanded it, and so the people and the culture went extinct. Similar risks attach to our current reluctance (especially emphatic in the United States, and especially dangerous here because of our high rate of consumption) to revise our consumerist habits, despite the warnings that have been pouring in from academic scientists, from creative artists, and really from the sky over our heads, for decades. Toward the end of book, Diamond warns against facile "one-liner objections" – such as "Technology will solve our problems" – to his environmentalist warnings. That may be why Peter Kareiva, the longtime head of the Nature Conservancy and now director of UCLA's Institute of the Environment and Sustainability, believes that "conservation is no longer [just] biology; it's as much anthropology."[33] Editors of our cultural legacy must play a major role, lest gold-diggers and Red Scares (claiming EPA regulations are a plot by a Communistic world government, perhaps based, as Trump has specifically suggested, on a hoax perpetrated by China) collude in blotting out what is left of our green and pleasant lands.

Social scientists recently conducted "two intensive case studies, one focused on agroforestry among three cultural groups living in the lowland rainforest of Guatemala and the other focused on resource conflict between Native American and European-American fishermen in north-central Wisconsin."[34] These studies confirm the warnings of *Collapse* that different ways of conceiving the natural world can be the difference between sustainable and unsustainable communities. What makes this later research especially valuable for my argument is that it shows how reduced interaction with non-human life leads not only to less sustainable behavior, but also to cognitive deficits that promote stereotyping of other humans and a resulting increase in intergroup conflict. Failure to register the web of shared life generates social malfunctions that are linked to a reduced tolerance for complex cognition.

Movies such as *Grand Canyon* (1991) and *Crash* (2004) have reminded anyone needing reminding that race has been a problem in the magnificently multicultural community called Los Angeles during the 32 years I have lived here. The Rodney King beating, the O. J. Simpson trial, and the Latasha Harlins shooting should have taught us that neither technology nor political authority is going to solve this city's racial divisions. Even with a videotape showing exactly what happened in a street beating or store shooting, even with DNA samples dictating massive probabilities in a murder case, all sorted through the traditional and technical rules of courtroom evidence, what finally mattered was what people made of that information, during conversations in the jury room, at the coffee shop, or on the street corner. The narrative frame in which those facts are set, with its own rules about heroes and villains based on the stories each community makes of its social history, makes a very big and sometimes dangerously divisive difference.

No frame-by-frame or gene-by-gene evidence is going to erase the problem of interpretation. An eminent researcher in applied cognitive science cites the King and Simpson controversies as proof that our society's future depends on "the active suppression of the social, narrative, and contextualizing styles" of traditional human thinking, in favor of rational scientific objectivity.[35] But, even if such a change were possible by any means other than those conversational narratives themselves, that change strikes me as a cure potentially far worse than the disease. Perhaps instead we can draw those styles into respectful conversation. Understanding the way styles inflect meaning, learning to interpret fairly and reasonably without forgetting to feel, and learning why people from other times and places interpret differently, are both the means and the end of many humanities courses. Things as they are, as Stevens told us, are changed – and exchanged – upon the Blue Guitar.

What we mean by truth and justice is immeasurably important to human beings, and the only vehicle big enough and flexible enough to carry those fundamental questions of civilization without crushing them may be literature. That helps explain why this weird little practice of songs and story-telling has survived while so many eras of technology have come and gone, each seeming to offer the key to the future and then becoming obsolete.

Humanistic Education

I endorse the wisdom (though not the gendered terms) of W. E. B. Du Bois's dissent from Booker T. Washington's more vocational goals for the education of African-Americans:

> intelligence, broad sympathy, knowledge of the world that was and is, and of the relation of men to it – this is the curriculum of that Higher Education which must underlie true life. On this foundation we may build bread winning, skill of hand and quickness of brain, with never a fear lest the child and man mistake the means of living for the object of life ....
>
> How then shall the leaders of a struggling people be trained and the hands of the risen few strengthened? There can be but one answer: The best and most capable of their youth must be schooled in the colleges and universities of the land. We will not quarrel as to just what the university of the Negro should teach or how it should teach it – I willingly admit that each soul and each race-soul needs its own peculiar curriculum. But this is true: A university is a human invention for the transmission of knowledge and culture from generation to generation, through the training of quick minds and pure hearts, and for this work no other human invention will suffice, not even trade and industrial schools ... .every isolated group or nation must have its yeast, must have for the talented few centers of training where men are not so mystified and befuddled by the hard and necessary toil of earning a living, as to have no aims higher than their bellies, and no God greater than Gold .... Education must not simply teach work – it must teach Life.

That Du Bois sees such education as liberating in social as well as psychological terms is evident from this essay's emphasis on the importance of higher education in the history of abolitionism, and for the future of racial equality.[36]

So, despite this chapter's epigraph, I don't think this book is some myopic and nostalgic plea for the restoration of higher education to its former condition as largely a Finishing School for WASP elites. The book treasured by the imprisoned heroes of the resistance against apartheid was *The Complete Works of Shakespeare*, hidden under the cover of a religious text, and hence called the Robben Island Bible. Nelson Mandela and 33 other prisoners each signed his name by a passage in that book that helped sustain their determination through those long years. Shakespeare programs for prisoners in the United States have been remarkably successful, even transformative, and higher education generally has a strong record of improving the lives of prisoners of all races while in prison and, especially, in moving beyond it successfully. In humanity's necessary conversations with the past, no one seems to have engaged people as responsively and inclusively (at least in English) as William Shakespeare.

Education in the humanities is important because there are aspects of humanity we nearly all share which would enable our long-evolved preferences for cooperation and fairness toward those we can recognize as kin to reduce injustice and violence, if we could prevent evolved self-serving memeplexes from overriding those values. I agree with my New Historicist colleagues that it is ethically important to recognize the strangeness of the past, and not imperialistically ignore the otherness of cultural aliens. Such recognitions reveal the power of memeplexes. But we also need to recognize that humanistic scholarship is actually more relevant than ever, if we can carry on its centuries-old mission of giving voice to those aliens, building bridges of human sympathy over the gaps that customs and religions institutionalize.

Paradoxically, the best road to true multiculturalism may be a classroom where a diverse group of students discover that they are all potentially Valjean, and probably the all-too-humanly inhuman Javert, too. Or all Hamlet, and maybe all the all-too-human villain Claudius, too – as well as Charlotte the spider. Those who share an estrangement, especially self-estrangement, are no longer complete strangers. This is an important benefit of academic diversity that emerged from the Supreme Court's 1978 decision in University of California v. Bakke: not quotas to rectify past racial injustice, but a diverse student body to enhance the inherent educational and social value of convening many viewpoints and experiences in the activities of a campus.

One needn't be a sentimental humanist to recognize that the arts convene us around some usefully alluring epitomes of the potential of our species. John Maynard Keynes was an economist – perhaps the greatest economist – but he

> nonetheless grasped the importance of bringing first-class art, performance and writing to the broadest possible audience if British society were to overcome its paralyzing divisions. It was Keynes whose initiatives led to the creation of the Royal Ballet, the Arts Council and much else besides.[37]

John Dewey argued that "works of art are the most intimate and ener-getic means of aiding individuals to share in the arts of living. Civilization is uncivil because human beings are divided into non-communicating sects, races, nations, classes and cliques."[38]

It is only too clear that people will kill to avoid acknowledging that other stories are possible, to close those windows and slam shut the fun-damentalist shutters against other ways of behaving and believing. In that particular sense, those who attack the tolerant, rationalist, multi-cultural West really do "hate us for our freedom," as politicians like to say. Those who attack universities often do too. In the face of that, our best weapon may be the quality the poet John Keats identified as the key to literary genius, epitomized for Keats by Shakespeare: "negative capability ... when a man is capable of being in uncertainties, mysteries, doubts, without any irritable reaching after fact and reason." The distin-guished ethologist Nicholas Humphrey observes that

> Social primates ... must be able to calculate the consequences of their own behavior, to calculate the likely behavior of others, to calculate the balance of advantage and loss – and all this in a context where the evidence ... is ephemeral, ambiguous and liable to change.[39]

This, too, is an essential component of a literary education.

Anyone who doubts that the future of our world depends largely on how a couple of books called the Bible and the Koran are interpreted just hasn't been paying attention. The future depends not just on the inter-pretations themselves, but also on the ability to exchange ideas, on some common ground, about how interpretations happen, what other readings are possible, and what they have to do with ethics, and with absolutes.

Narrative is our parent, in both ontogeny and phylogeny: the child may be father to the man, as Wordsworth writes, but the story is parent to that child. It may take a village to raise a child, as a proverb asserts, but it takes a story-teller to make a village. And it often takes an inter-preter of literature – professional or, more often, amateur – to prevent a holy war when all those stories collide in the global village. As Hamlet the character and *Hamlet* the play each ask in their own way, should we really trust the ghosts of our forefathers in armor, when they say that to remember them and love them is, above all, to avenge them in blood? That play allows us to recognize "honor" and "vengeance" as poten-tially parasitic memes rather than divine instructions and self-evident obligations. The same recognition emerges elsewhere in Shakespeare's work, not just in Falstaff's cynical take on honor (early in the final Act of *1 Henry IV*) but also in Prospero's weary but noble relinquishment of revenge (early in the final Act of *The Tempest*).

Quiet victories, to the accompaniment of the blue guitar rather than a martial fife and drum, are what I have been celebrating here. The US government can destroy some nuclear reactors in the Middle East (whether by bombing their hardware or by infecting their software), and its TSA can X-ray a million shoes at airports, and prevent another artist – not Wallace Stevens this time, but Cat Stevens, now known as Yusuf Islam – from ever singing "Peace Train" on our shores again. But until we can influence what stories the world's competing cultures tell about themselves, and tell themselves about all the others, such measures will never be enough. What happened on September 11, 2001, was no high-tech villainy – the perpetrators did not have bombs or even guns – but instead a horrible escalation of the culture wars: the hijackers were such devout servants of a memeplex that they lost sight of any contravening humane values.

Our failure to prevent that disaster was, by the chief government investigation's own conclusions, not a failure of technology, but "a failure of imagination." After an attempted airline bombing narrowly failed in 2010, President Obama similarly observed that "The U.S. government had sufficient information to have uncovered this plot," but "our intelligence community failed to connect those dots."[40] Yet the 2012 report on "U.S. Education Reform and National Security" from the Council on Foreign Relations persistently deprecates exactly the kind of education that enables an intelligence to imagine other minds and connect a few dots into a hypothetical plot. Sounding very much like Mr. Gradgrind in Dickens's *Hard Times*, the report insists that the reading and discussion of fiction must be minimized in education; the new Common Core education standards that the federal government has induced most states to adopt similarly tilts away from imaginative readings. A central lesson of these deadly failures thus continues to evade a society that is losing its ability to distinguish between information and knowledge.

The supposedly irresponsible indulgence in fictions – the game of what-if – has actually always been an indispensable element in scientific progress as well as in literary invention and social integration. "Aristotle engaged in imaginary experiments" by which he almost accidentally "deduced many of the characteristics of Newtonian space."[41] Although "presented as the untenable consequence of a false assumption," Aristotle's thought-experiment "was nevertheless the clearest anticipation of the inertial principle before the seventeenth century."[42] From the medieval period through the late Renaissance, the standard rhetorical training (through debates *in utramque partem* and quodlibetal disputations) required speakers to assert, for the sake of argument, positions that they and their society assumed to be untrue. STEM-worshipping academic administrators now squeeze down expository writing courses and religious-studies programs, but "the considerations of counterfactual orders of nature in the Middle Ages actually paved the way for the formulation of laws of nature ... in considering them vigorously, the theological imagination prepared for the scientific."[43] "Imaginary experiments" provided the genesis of "the principle of annihilation in Descartes' or Hobbes's philosophy" as well as the "imaginary motions of simple bodies under simplified condition in Galileo's physics."[44] This tradition surely continues through the work of Einstein, and an expedient for thinking the unthinkable may offer crucial opportunities to challenge any memeplex that has established itself as a fundamental, irrefutable way of understanding ourselves and our world.

My plea that we try to fulfill our humanity is risky, because defining what is human is dangerous: the more inclusive the definition becomes, the more vulnerable become those it still excludes. Creating a community of sympathy does carry the risk of imposing that community's norms all the more complacently against those who fall outside the consensus.[45] Adorno offers a version of that warning: "There is no moral certainty. Its mere assumption would be immoral, would falsely relieve the individual of anything that might be called morality."[46] When Mitt Romney gave a speech in 2007 designed to mitigate the damage his Mormon beliefs might do to his initial presidential candidacy, he did not advocate true inclusiveness, only stressed that he too worshipped Jesus, implying a willingness to help Christians gang up on those who do not. The closer a community comes to unanimous agreement, the likelier it is to dismiss the dissenters as simply unjustifiable; and what academic humanists might agree are the clearest wrongs have been produced exactly by the agreement of other groups about what is surely and crucially right (for example, heterosexuality). We may feel compelled to agree that some things are despicable, such as the exclusion of people who are different – but then we are stuck excluding people who differ with us about universal acceptance.

These conundrums, however, suggest exactly why it is crucial to stretch the capacity of sympathy without directing it into a binary of approval or disapproval. In place of that programmatic function of agit-prop (on the political level) or melodrama (on the emotional level), literature and its teachers can sustain a moral sensitivity that remains alert to the complexity of human experience in each moment and over time. Montaigne is lastingly important because he was a humane and tireless interrogator of memeplexes, always looking inside his own psyche and across a range of cultures to raise doubts about the systems of certainty prevailing in late Renaissance Europe to such massively deadly effect.

Shakespeare certainly invites us to disapprove of what Richard III, Claudius, Othello, Edmund, and Macbeth do. Yet, Shakespeare also unsettles that reaction by making us feel uneasily complicit in the crimes onstage. He makes us aware, that is, of tendencies within ourselves that could take us astray in analogous if less dramatic ways, especially if we were under similar provocations, had our worst impulses nurtured and tantalized, or had our nightmares turned into intensely consequential realities. So, the tragedies provoke (as Aristotle recommends) both fear and pity; the audience is not permitted to settle for disapproval.

Despite what some radical critics have asserted in recent years, I think literature professors are therefore often at our best when we confront politics only indirectly, maybe even only accidentally. Literature such as Shakespeare's is valuable, not because it can be made into a branch of Marxism or conservatism (though both have certainly been tried) but because it can address aspects of human experience that are prior to both of them. Hubert Zapf observes that "literature, especially since the romantic period, has provided a discursive space for articulating those dimensions of human life which were marginalized, neglected, or repressed in dominant discourses and forms of civilizational self-representation"; he therefore (rightly, it seems to me) values the kinds of writing "which resist straightforward ideological messages, but help to create the imaginative space for otherness."[47] Seamus Heaney's lecture series *The Government of the Tongue* emphasizes the importance of poets bearing witness to horrors, especially those imposed by governments, and at moments his analysis becomes "a modern martyrology." But he praises the courageous poets of political resistance without ideological hectoring, and without mistaking a marvelous canto for a Molotov cocktail. Poetry, he says, "is like the writing in the sand in the face of which accusers and accused are left speechless and renewed"; it replaces the entire script of accusation with something that is more humane despite seeming idle and transient, or maybe because it is willing to seem idle and transient.

Adorno's *Aesthetic Theory* argued that art had to be "the social antithesis of society," but he was not recommending art designed to impart any politically programmatic change on its audience. Instead, art – aesthetic not in a sterile and conventional way, but resonant with its human participants – would help transform society without having a discernible, definable function. This entails mysteries, but it is not sheer mysticism. Humanists – I similarly believe – need to do their cultural work with an alert and sympathetic intelligence, even if (like the comic-book superheroes into whom literary critics are ludicrously changing in this phonebooth-sized monograph) most people have no idea who is trying to save them. Completely by accident, and just two days before submitting this manuscript for type setting, and I ran across a 1975 article by my mother making a comparable point about the feminist scholarship to which she devoted so much of her life: it must "provide a method of reading with a new consciousness, not narrower than the old but broader," because such reading "picks up the discord between the vitality of existence of the rigidity of social myth."[48]

It occurs to me that, in this, I am also on my father's path after all (how little I have actually evolved!), since he dismayed many of his Old Left friends by turning away from direct political activism in the 1960s, toward opening up higher education and developing group sensitivity-training. "T-groups" – a major innovation in 20th-century psychology – sought to cultivate democratic, open-minded, anti-authoritarian attributes in citizens and their leaders (and workers and their managers) through intense improvisational interaction while also encouraging personal inward transformations. I would argue that a good Shakespeare seminar achieves many of the same outcomes, and have been arguing here that such transformations are not irrelevant to larger social goals. They are instead a way of promoting such goals that evades external political repression as well as internal psychological resistance. Bill Cooke, an international leader in academic research on business management, states the case well:

> it is the very here-and-now-ness, the absence of structure and agenda which makes the T-group an attractive form of political intervention in its particular historical moment. This absence immunizes the T-group from McCarthy-style attacks on the basis of overt ideology or political agenda – there is nothing there to attack, just people in a room restricting their discussion to what is happening within it. Yet at the same time it appears to offer political outcomes. People were enabled to come to terms with the dark personal and interpersonal consequences of (proto-)Cold War culture, and in so doing an interpersonal solidarity – in the foundation event in New Britain, arguably a class solidarity across ethnic distinctions – appeared to be achievable.[49]

Looking at the demographics of recent elections, this kind of solidarity seems more necessary than ever.

My father probably did not believe, any more than I do, that human values and needs will always or even ultimately coincide across societies or social classes, no matter how well we learn to express our feelings and empathize with others. Nor will cleaning away pathogenic errors expose a stable, pre-existing, full-dimensional, cross-culturally applicable, and ethically reliable truth. My point is not to make politics go away, or even to dull them with therapy and aesthetics like a beekeeper pacifying a hive with smoke. But, to my critique of a narrowly utilitarian view of profitable education, I want to add a critique of a narrowly utilitarian view of politics. Hannah Arendt demonstrated that "Europe's major political traditions – conservatism, liberalism, and Marxism – had been unable to understand, at that time and afterwards, totalitarian ideology, wedded as they were to the naively cynical view that all politics is reducible to material interests"; those political thinkers therefore (other scholars have shown) overlooked "the fundamental connections between anti-Semitism, German nationalism, and a cultural revolt against modernity."[50] At least, we can hope some forms of education and communication will help free our politics from certain traps, residual from the past and lurking in asymptomatic cultural carriers, that limit our ability to adapt to the future.

In this sense, my project echoes that of the Frankfurt School, which placed considerable focus on what I would call the especially pernicious and tenacious memeplex called anti-Semitism, as well as the broader one called capitalism. The Frankfurt theorists drew on Georg Simmel's idea that culture is inevitable for human beings, but in becoming productively autonomous, becomes dangerously autonomous. Utilizing forms of critique – an intense philosophical form of peer-review, including persistent interrogation of its own assumptions and principles – this group of intellectuals sought to distinguish "true interests" from "false interests," as I am trying (in a less sophisticated way) to distinguish ideally human interests from those planted in us by competing products of evolution. With Adorno in the lead, the group warned about "the authoritarian personality," a type corresponding closely to what I see in reflexive cultural conservationists: an anti-intellectual combination of a resistance to both introspection and social critique, preferring instead to subscribe to conventional mores.[51] Max Horkheimer's project of exposing and thereby defeating the mechanisms that sustain social dysfunctions[52] is close kin to the exposure and, thereby, disempowerment of the memeplexes that have us in their almost insensible thrall.

"Humanism is dead, those who follow it are just old sentimentalists," says a Marxist named Botard in Eugène Ionesco's 1959 "Rhinoceros" – the masterpiece of the French avant-garde playwright's career, and another version of the warnings and exhortations this book is trying to convey. The play clearly derives from Ionesco's horror, during his youth in Romania, at the rise of the Iron Guard – a powerful right-wing movement that managed to combine fascism, militarism, Christian zealotry, populist nationalism, and intense anti-Semitism. Ionesco was no less resolute in opposing Stalinist Communism. All around the play's seemingly unheroic hero Bérenger, people are being converted into a herd of dumb, mean, destructive rhinoceroses by some mysterious contagion. His beloved Daisy urges him to accept his small pleasures despite the changes around him, rather than worrying about where they are leading. His rationalist colleague Botard scoffs off warnings that "Rhinoceritis" could actually occur, let alone become a destructive social epidemic. Even the intellectual Dudard accepts the transformations, on the grounds that people should have freedom to make their choices. But clearly their minds are not their own, as they echo each other's clichés, until Bérenger is the only *Homo sapiens* remaining. Despite that frightening isolation, he finally refuses to surrender his humanity to the mass movement:

> People who try to hang on to their individuality always come to a bad end! [*He suddenly snaps out of it.*] Oh well, too bad! I'll take on the whole of them! I'm the last man left, and I'm staying that way until the end. I'm not capitulating! [*CURTAIN*].[53]

Other major 20th-century intellectuals recognized the need for schools to inculcate what Neil Postman calls "crap-detecting," which resembles what I am describing as resistance to runaway memeplexes that have disguised their contingency:

> schools should stress values that are not stressed by other major institutions in the culture. Norbert Wiener insisted that the schools now must function as 'anti-entropic feedback systems', 'entropy' being the word used to denote a general and unmistakable tendency of all systems – natural and man-made – in the universe to 'run down'.... we must have instruments to tell us when we are running down, when maintenance is required. For Wiener, such instruments would be people who have been educated to recognize change, to be sensitive to problems caused by change, and who have the motivation and courage to sound alarms when entropy accelerates to a dangerous degree.

Postman therefore urges schools to cultivate

> in the young that most 'subversive' intellectual instrument – the anthropological perspective. This perspective allows one to be part of his own culture and, at the same time, to be out of it. One views the activities of his own group as would an anthropologist, observing its tribal rivals, its fears, its conceits, its ethnocentrism. In this way, one is able to recognize when reality begins to drift too far away from the grasp of the tribe.
>
> We need hardly say that achieving such a perspective is extremely difficult, requiring, among other things, considerable courage. We are, after all, talking about achieving a high degree of freedom from the intellectual and social constraints of one's tribe. For example, it is generally assumed that people of other tribes have been victimized by indoctrination from which our tribe has remained free.[54]

That complacent assumption, because it is so essential to the value people derive from a culture, is a stratagem nearly all successful memeplexes employ.

Universities should be institutions of perpetually unclosed mind, places where truth is eagerly sought but conviction is temporarily deferred and permanently provisional. That does not mean their goal is to create indecisive persons, so caught up in Hamletism that they are incapable of action until the very last desperate second. Instead, higher education serves to create citizens who do not, for the sake of sparing themselves complex thought, decide too soon and refuse to reconsider. Psychologists have shown that "an aversion to ambiguity and confusion" leads to "'seizing' on an early statement or proposition in the process of acquiring knowledge, followed by rigidly 'freezing' on the seized item."[55] A fascinating and ingenious study found that the only factor that reduced the tendency to be guided by one's own partisan "myside" biases, even on factual questions unrelated to politics, was the amount of time spent undergoing higher education: "The degree of myside bias decreased systematically with year in university. Year in university remained a significant predictor of myside bias even when both cognitive ability and age were statistically partialled out."[56] That finding suggests two things: first, that the claim that higher education has become political indoctrination is the opposite of the truth, and, second, that for individuals, as for our emergence as a species, intelligence matters less than education. It certainly matters for repairing our political comity. Universities can provide a kind of intellectual structure for young minds to pass through, discovering along the way why scholarship has commanded human respect for so long, and then going off to make many different kinds of things, including decisions that are at once psychologically, intellectually, and ethically informed.

For Aristotle, this is the path of virtue that leads to happiness, because it entails human beings fulfilling their particular nature. This seems to me a durable piece of wisdom, and one Aristotle rightly applies to the "finalities" of other species as well. It may sound to modern ears like the erasure rather than the liberation of the self and its will, but that may be because our culture both overvalues individuality and overlooks the ways memeplexes sell us false desires, creating the illusion that we are expressing our unique interiorities when we are actually being absorbed in their brand-lines. We cannot make choices that are always, absolutely, and inherently right. But we may still be obliged to make our choices with as broad and alert a consciousness as possible, unpleasant as that may be to ourselves or others, rather than assuming that the cocoon of culture is a suitable permanent home for the more airworthy aspects of our species – that is, for our contemplative and imaginative spirits. We should not waste our seemingly unique faculties of ratiocination, imagination, self-consciousness, and free will by merely playing out the evolutionary algorithms of either genes or memes.

Nor should we disdain our spiritual yearnings, however we want to understand their source. Paramhansa Yogananda, the yogi who popularized yoga and meditation in the Western world a century ago and remains influential, warned that

> Evil was made sweet to delude you. You have to use your discrimination to distinguish between poisoned honey and that which is in your best interest. Avoid those things that will ultimately hurt you, and choose those that will give you freedom and happiness.

Several centuries earlier, the enthusiastic meditations of the poet Thomas Traherne show that if we reject consumerism, which narrows our perception and lets envy eclipse appreciation, we can celebrate ourselves and the shimmering universe simultaneously, and allows that combination to generate joy rather than madness. Traherne's rejection of toxic cultural mediators is the broader version of his rejection of Catholic ritual and decoration, to be replaced by a sanctified conversation between the individual and Creation. If we then look ahead several centuries, through science fiction, we can analyze the tricky path of our species, not toward A.I., but toward Traherne's kind of I, and eye, and aye.

Interchapter: Why Aristotle Would Have Won Plenty of Drachmae Betting on College Football Bowl Games

An analysis of the Associated Press's rankings over the past 11 seasons by a Stanford Ph.D. in Engineering shows that a team ranked higher in AP's pre-season poll defeated a lower-ranked team in a bowl game 60.2% of the time. The pre-season coaches' poll achieved a similar 60.9% result. But using the final pre-bowl polls, at the end of the regular season, those prediction rates dropped, to 56.6% and 55.8%, respectively.[1]

This drop isn't huge, but it is wildly counterintuitive. After all, end-of-season rankings can draw on the outcomes of all the games teams have played, and how successful their opponents have been against other opponents similarly analyzed. Furthermore, the board of college coaches, and AP's board of sportswriters and broadcasters, arrive at their late season picks knowing (as they obviously can't pre-season) which team lost its quarterback to a knee injury and which improved through the emergence of a new star.

Sports offer a satisfying exception in a world where victories are seldom absolute and final. But winning proves a lot less than people imagine. Knowing which team is ahead on the scoreboard when the final whistle blows may feel like a fundamental truth revealed. Maybe even like a vindication of your embattled city or university. But what does winning a few games really tell us?

To cite a traumatic memory from my childhood, the 1960 Pirates were not a better baseball team than the Yankees they beat in that year's World Series. My Yankees outscored them by better than a 2-1 ratio over the seven games: 55-27. That doesn't mean the Pirates weren't really the World Champions or that it isn't cool that they came out on top – maybe the improbability makes an underdog win even cooler. But would an informed and rational person have bet on the Pirates rather than the Yankees to win the next year? (Spoiler: the Yankees ran away with the 1961 American League pennant and cruised to a five-game World Series win, while the Pirates finished in the lower half of the National League.)

When I played Strat-o-Matic baseball using the 1961 Yankees, I usually chose Bill Stafford (a journeyman player with a short career) over Whitey Ford (a Hall of Famer) as my starting pitcher. It made me wonder why Ford was that team's legendary ace when Stafford's Earned Run Average was considerably better. Only many years later did I realize that the Yankees probably tried to use Ford against the best other teams in the league, since they were realistic rivals for the pennant, so Stafford faced lesser batters. Within Strat-o-Matic's functions, which were based on the basic performance statistics of 1961, I was making the right managerial choice; but if I had been the manager of the real players, that would have been stupid.

It is a cautionary tale for a metrics-minded era when teachers are fired and inner-city schools closed down without adequate recognition of the extraordinary human challenges those teachers and schools may have faced. A newly concluded six-year study by the RAND Corporation, sponsored by the Gates Foundation that presumably hoped to find the opposite, found that using their Teaching Effectiveness ratings was "insufficient to dramatically improve student outcomes. Many other factors might need to be addressed."[2]

College football polls used to determine which team would be declared "best" each season. Eventually – so fans could know "for sure" – the system was changed so that the polls and some computer programs decided which two teams would compete in a post-season championship game. Now a committee ranks four teams for a championship play-off after the regular season. There is no reason to expect that committee to be immune to the overvalued win-loss binary that has misled reporters and coaches over the last 11 years. The committee members know that fans and media commentators would ridicule them for ranking a one-loss team ahead of an undefeated team, or for ranking a team ahead of another that beat it, even if that game was so close that the outcome was as random as the flip of a coin, and even if the losing team looked better against their common opponents.

Any number of flukes can turn a close contest – a bad bounce, a bad call, just a range of bad luck generally. Play it a hundred times and the loser would win close to half. But pundits cover that up by claiming that a football team that has squeaked past a few opponents "knows how to win" and its shaky but lucky defense "bends but doesn't break" or "creates lots of turnovers" (which are mathematically quite random).

The pre-season pollsters, on the other hand, are spared the obligation to pretend that victory proves superiority. Their rankings can reflect the overall strength of players, and the long-term success of coaches and programs: less information, in a way, but from a broader view, using intuitions grounded in expertise.

How much other useful wisdom does our society squander because we assume some quantitative "bottom line" is the only real truth? And, in a neoliberal world that relies on ruthless competition to plan the fate of all living creatures, how much callousness gets authorized by the assumption that anyone who loses is just "a loser"? Digitally structured information – one or zero, victory or loss, us or them – is degraded information.

This statistical surprise vindicates what the ancient Greek philosopher Aristotle and the English Renaissance poet Philip Sidney famously affirmed about the value of literature. Whereas history is stuck telling you what really occurred, even if that was mostly random and obscures a larger understanding of humanity, an imaginative story can conjure a verisimilitude that may ultimately be truer than mere factual truth.

Here's how Aristotle's Poetics *– composed about 2,350 years ago, during the pre-season workouts of modern Western thought – explained the difference:*

> *The poet's function is not to tell what actually happened, but what could or would happen by probability or necessity …. Poetry is therefore a wiser and more exalted thing than history, because poetry tends to offer general truths, while history offers particular facts. By a "general truth" I mean what a certain type of person will do …. A "particular fact" is what Alcibiades did or what happened to him …. The worst plots are [those] in which the episodes don't follow each other in any probable or inevitable sequence. Bad poets write those.*

> (1451a-b)

So the imagination of a good poet is no more a falsehood than the prediction of the pre-season rankings of coaches and pundits, because poets are allowed to speak of what is likely and coherent. As the episodic season goes on, those coaches and pundits become bad poets. Sidney's Defense of Poesy *made a similar point, more than 400 years ago: "The historian … is so tied, not to what should be but to what is, to the particular truth of things, and not to the general reason of things, that his example draweth no necessary consequence, and therefore a less fruitful doctrine."*

When the great Dutch soccer player and coach Johan Cruyff was asked whether it still hurt to recall the defeat of his brilliant team in the 1974 World Cup final by the more methodical West Germans, Cruyff replied "'Yeah, but maybe we were the real winners in the end …. I think the world remembers our team more." And it's true: several of the world's most successful teams of recent years bear the clear imprint of Cruyff's artistic attacking style, and soccer is the better for that.

If we want a society capable of looking ahead with any wisdom, we should stop telling young people they should skip Classics and Creative Writing and learn only the latest technical facts. That's a losing bet on the future.

7   The Technological Singularity and Artificial Unintelligence

I, the man of color, want only this: That the tool never possess the man. That the enslavement of man by man cease forever. That is, of one by another. That it be possible for me to discover and to love man, wherever he may be.
—Frantz Fanon, *Black Skin, White Masks* (1952)[1]

This concluding chapter, like the opening one, begins at the movies – but this time it could be a week-long sci-fi festival. Consider all the stories in recent decades clustering around what futurists call "the technological singularity" – the moment when robotics and artificial intelligence become so advanced that our machines become able to iterate their own learning, develop self-consciousness and, instead of continuing to serve as instruments of human projects, launch their own initiatives that marginalize or subjugate *Homo sapiens*. These stories reflect a recognition that non-biological systems – clusters of information – can in fact evolve, to the endangerment of something we value about our humanity.

Expressions of this fear seem countless; clearly, many people are eager to converse about this topic in the oblique ways art permits, as some Japanese movies of the 1950s expressed indirectly the trauma of the Hiroshima and Nagasaki atomic bombings. Countless cartoons joke about robot overlords. Instances from the most famous sci-fi writers include William Gibson's *Neuromancer*, Harlan Ellison's "I Have No Mouth, and I Must Scream," Isaac Asimov's "The Last Question," and the parodies in Douglas Adams's *Hitchhiker's Guide to the Galaxy*. In big-budget movies, Kubrick's *2001* features the iconic rebellion of the HAL computer, while the *Terminator* series and the film adaptation of *I, Robot* raise comparable specters, as does the 2014 film *Ex Machina*. On television, various "Doctor Who," "Star Trek," "Battlestar Galactica," and (now prominently) "Westworld" and "Black Mirror" episodes also explore these themes.

These machine-machinations may look like the kind of consciously hostile conspiracy we naturally fear from aspiring human tyrants. But – as Chapter 3 argued about what causes injustice – they may instead represent the extreme instance of our useful memeplexes spinning out of our control and developing a function that is at once rational to them and insanely wrong to us. For a semi-comic illustrative example proposed by some very distinguished scientists, imagine a software oversight that causes the entire world to be re-manufactured into paper-clips.[2] The latest non-fiction version I have encountered comes from prominent nanotechnology experts, assessing the risk that their project will run amok and turn the earth's surface into grey goo – as if we aren't already gradually doing the same, as Dr. Seuss and others have tried to warn us.

The popular 2008 family film *WALL-E* offers a benign twist on this symptomatic anxiety. Its premise is that a massive corporation called "Buy N Large" has co-evolved with consumerism until the earth becomes an unlivable trash heap, and the obese human race is evacuated onto comfortable starships where they drift through life snacking, as if on an extended sea-cruise vacation. But a single cleanup robot named WALL-E that has been accidentally left functioning on earth gradually develops sentience, emotions, and free will. It begins collecting artifacts of human civilization like a futuristic Indiana Jones, but then finds a single green seedling on the gray earth. In an inversion of archeology, finding something natural amid earth's heaps of ancient artifacts is the transformative miracle, because it means the planet has become habitable again for biological life-forms.

Our species' best strategy may be to induce massive memeplexes – in *WALL-E*, consumer capitalism and the technological singularity – to cancel each other out so we can resume the business of fulfilling our humanity, like the small mammals that were our ancient ancestors weaving around unattended by the massive dinosaurs battling overhead. The singular sentimental piece of robotics called WALL-E is what finally takes the human journey off autopilot and calls our bloated, passive species back to the hard work of being itself. As at the end of *Paradise Lost*, it is a fortunate fall back to a gradually redeemable earth. This reversal also resembles the aforementioned moment in Shakespeare's *The Tempest* when the spirit Ariel remarks that, "were I human," he would take pity on the chastised enemies of his master Prospero (5.1.20) – a comment that appears to divert Prospero from supernaturally domineering revenge on human nature, back to the ordinary burdens of organizing a civil society.

These stories also address a deeper paradox of the human condition. Technological-singularity stories proliferate because they are over-determined, allowing different aspects of our species to express their conflict with each other simultaneously, haunted as such conflicts are by profound guilt and frustration. They mythologize both the synchronic and diachronic struggles between our creaturely and conceptual aspects; that is, they reflect both the fact that we are now uneasily both biological and cultural beings, and the fact that we are on a long arc from the dominance of the former to the dominance of the latter. The stories express quite legitimate fears about runaway technology, from the Industrial Revolution to the nuclear arms race to the digital era, and fears about lost human autonomy in an age of masscult, surveillance, algorithmically targeted advertising, and global culture-war. But these stories also carry our guilty awareness that at some level we ourselves are the disobedient robot, the turncoat android, because the expanded brain, the self-consciousness, the iterative collective learning, and other cultural forces of our species have allowed us to turn against the dictates of our genes. In privileging second-order desires produced at an intellectual level over the urgings of our biology, we become the cyborg-like assemblages that have risen up against our former masters – namely, the drives, logic, and protocols of genetic replication.

The conquest is never complete. From the perspective of our ideational functions and our ethical ideals, our evolved bio-programming is the uncaring and therefore monstrously efficient enemy that is actually already inside us, waiting to burst out (like the horrific hatchings in the *Alien* movies) into phenotype and erase whatever is significant about *Homo sapiens* from the universe. Its signature project is genocide, as a tribal extension of the drive of individual genes to increase their share in the reproductive future, and it often achieves a deadly symbiosis with memeplexes that also seek to monopolize the terrain of the future. This kind of regression is what the conventionally moralistic Duke of Albany fears when human civilization devolves in Shakespeare's *King Lear*: "If that the heavens do not their visible spirits / Send quickly down to tame these vile offences, / It will come, / Humanity must perforce prey upon itself / Like monsters of the deep" (4.2.46–50).

Proud though we are of transcending that predatory biology, part of us also resents and mistrusts the higher-order authorities. Anxiety about the technological singularity speaks for our creaturely side against the memeplex already in place that Freud called the superego: instincts serving collective survival that have become institutionalized as culture, entered our heads, and thereby usurped the body's freedom. The sci-fi fear that mechanical externalizations of our intelligence will subjugate us physically reflects a mostly preconscious anxiety that these moral rules have already subjugated us mentally. They not only frustrate the primal yearnings of the id; they also sublimate the ego into the service of civilization.

Our discontent with those restraints may not be mere selfishness. Dystopic fictions about the technological singularity warn that our triumph over our biochemical instincts (like the triumphs of technology over the biosphere generally) may yet prove a pyrrhic victory. What we have done to our ancestral natural selves may soon be done unto what remains of them in us; the civilized creatures that we have become may be overthrown by the further denaturalized cyborgs we will become.

Having deemed many of our emotional drives and biophysical functions foolish or otherwise disgraceful, and having invented ways to suppress them or conceal them ritually, we now see ourselves as mixed beings that the next phase of the revolution of mind will deem to be also (as our alien enemies in science fiction so often deem us) foolish and obsolete.

Believing ourselves to have conquered many less mindful species, perhaps we are doomed to be conquered someday by an intelligence more artificial than our own. But my theory suggests that we are already becoming slaves of what we have made: socio-cultural systems that have no interest in our sentimental ideas of ourselves (except perhaps as useful sedatives), systems that may appear smart but are also manifestations of a brutal evolutionary logic. The reversion of human society to mere mutual predation – "Nature, red in tooth and claw," as Tennyson called it, in a foreshock of Darwin's insight – which we wrongly thought we had permanently tamed, is certainly always a threat. We fear the vengeance of the pure natural forces, in and around us, that we have disdained and repressed.

The deeper threat is the conversion of human society into memeplexes evolved to be comparably ruthless on behalf of their own reproduction. Engineers worry, rightly, about the danger that hackers will, for their own narrow and inhumane purposes, take over control of our self-driving vehicles, at serious cost to human life. But few seem to recognize a similar betrayal that is already happening.

Sentimental humanism is certainly under attack, and not just by the business-minded forces of neoliberalism. Many evolutionary psychologists and misreaders of Hobbes think we should (in order to be honest and pragmatic), and perhaps inevitably will, revert to the algorithms of mere competition for survival and reproduction – if we ever really left them. The vigorous polymath Howard Bloom based his bestselling 1995 book *The Lucifer Principle*, and his 2010 celebration of capitalism called *The Genius of the Beast*, on that supposition. Bloom believes that a shared idea helps people unify, which makes them powerful, which spreads the idea to the groups they conquer, which is what people are evolutionarily programmed to do, which actually turns out very well. So, he shares my sense that cultures evolve like competing predators, just not my mistrust of the outcome.

But widespread claims that the ancient societies in which human nature evolved were actually packed with violent competition both within and between tribes have been strongly challenged.[3] Not seeing each other as fundamentally competitors might help restore a more loving (and live-and-let-living) relationship to other aspects of our world which are essentially now treated as prey rather than as community companions. I suspect the popularity of videos showing different species of animals nuzzling, protecting, or playing with each other reflects the delight of recognizing that a more peaceful, positive, cooperative vision is not merely a naïve illusion, but a reflection of the fact that life loves life, and – despite the distorted ratio in animal documentaries edited for action-addicted viewers – spends little of its time in combat. Furthermore, many studies confirm that our species "may have been subject to selection promoting both consideration of others and sensitivity to local norms of fairness," in contrast to the rational economic selfishness of chimpanzees and other non-hominins.[4]

Still, many popular television series (say, about Mafiosi, drug dealers, and/or detectives) sell this reductionist view that the most selfish and ruthless behavior is the truest image, the inside story, of how the human world really works. Anyone who believes otherwise is, implicitly, a deluded sucker who can be saved only by a good guy with a gun. The latest season premiere of the immensely popular and brutally violent HBO series *Game of Thrones* (July 16, 2017) directly undermined any effort to question its vision of human life as a constant battle to kill all other people before they can kill you (all in hopes of sitting on what has to be the least comfortable throne, even ergonomically, that has ever existed). The hero Jon Snow tells his sister Sansa that any variation from that grim narrative is just a naive father leaving his children unprepared for "how dirty the world really is." Dickens's *David Copperfield* puts the neoliberal viewpoint in the horrible Mr. Murdstone, who insists on raising David with punishment rather than love, and puts him to work in a factory, telling him, "What is before you, is a fight with the world; and the sooner you begin it, the better" (Chapter 10). Neoliberalism pathologizes altruism. In its claim to deduce essential realities by quantitative algorithms, it even pathologizes imagination. That is a shame.

Against such free-marketeers, fictional literature deploys the Three Musketeers: the pointless panache of a feathered hat, idealism, wit, imagination, courage, and the intricate cooperation that humanity makes possible, and that makes humanity possible. Those defenders of the human experiment are no less needed against this subtler enemy that undoes our human freedom in another way, by memes rather than by genes. Disguised as our liberation from our mere mortal bodies, and demanding not just obedience but reverence, evolving networks of ideas can forestall the fulfillment of our best natures, if we are not vigilant. The reductionist voice is the voice of the villain Iago leading Shakespeare's Othello away from accepting the love of Desdemona as a wonderful human miracle, toward seeing it instead as mere carnal appetite and as (like his acceptance into the white Christian society of Venice) contingent on whether he has earned it – the same mistake Protestantism saw in the Catholic idea of how to achieve salvation. A similar mistake leads Shakespeare's King Lear, no less tragically, into a quantitative measuring of love.

* *

The closer we come to a technological utopia, science fiction warns, the more we risk a dystopia that will sap our humanity. If that happens – and this book argues it is already happening – the humanities may offer suitable territory for some mysterious shared attributes of our species to hide and communicate, like political Resistances and Undergrounds in mountain nooks and safe houses. There, myriad human attributes can take shelter through the reign – temporarily comfortable in some areas but spiritually brutal almost everywhere – of money and technology and other controlling memeplexes to which we have been shortsightedly granting increasing sovereignty over our minds and bodies. Probably it is no coincidence that a prominent version of this story – Ray Bradbury's 1953 novel *Fahrenheit 451*, later filmed by François Truffaut – was written as a protest against the censorship of the Red Scare era, and that its dissident community is built around a collection of books.

Bookish people must protect not only, in our curatorial role, against the loss of civilization, but also, in what we learn from the past about the present and future, against the malfunction of civilization: not just against sliding back, but also against the wrong steps forward. When the memeplexes we have developed to reduce the social and perceptual worlds into manageable forms begin reducing and managing us also, we have to recognize and resist them.

All that can defeat the new overlords, in most of these sci-fi scenarios, is this mysterious quality called humanity, which I think corresponds fairly closely to the professed mission of the humanities: the nearly indomitable spirit, the ability to enter other minds empathetically, the intricate communicative powers of language, the ingenuity of the creative imagination, and respect for the accumulated wisdom of the species. Attempting to out-tech our own tech seems like a trap: we are much less likely to triumph than to slip into either a comfortable or an uncomfortable enslavement. For the humane attributes of our species to prevail, humanistic thinking must find ways to persist.

The fear that undetected memeplexes symbiotic with technology have been usurping human freedom to preserve their own stasis is central to the *Matrix* series of sci-fi films, where super-intelligent machines have turned the human race into mere passive batteries that imagine they are living full sensory and volitional lives – hardly plausible, but an effective metaphor. At the end of the story, guided by the suggestively named Morpheus, the protagonist Neo does what my ideal humanists do in battling memeplexes: he enters into the fictional universe that has his fellow humans in thrall in order to transmute it, and thereby save our species. He will liberate people, not by returning them to a mundane "real world," but by showing them (as artists and other fiction-makers do) "a world where anything is possible." Our choices will lie within the imaginary rather than the material universe – or at least they must come through the imaginary in order to redeem the real. Like Perseus fighting Medusa in ancient Greek mythology, maybe we can bear to see our deadliest enemy only in a mirror, but we can still fight it through reflective representations. The answer to runaway memes is a framed mimesis.

Techno-dystopic stories such as *The Matrix* and *Logan's Run* have a stunningly prescient ancestor in E. M. Forster's 1909 story "The Machine Stops." That Machine functions in much the way I have been arguing our evolved culture functions. It sustains people underground in bland comfort in individual rooms, chatting idly through electronic screens with their friends and family, although

> the Machine did not transmit *nuances* of expression. It only gave a general idea of people – an idea that was good enough for all practical purposes, Vashti thought. The imponderable bloom, declared by a discredited philosophy to be the actual essence of intercourse, was rightly ignored by the Machine, just as the imponderable bloom of the grape was ignored by the manufacturers of artificial fruit.[5]

Otherwise, the closest thing to a human community consists of what are unmistakably massive open online courses (MOOCs), conceived a century before there were any such things:

> it was time to deliver her lecture on Australian music. The clumsy system of public gatherings had been long since abandoned; neither Vashti nor her audience stirred from their rooms. Seated in her armchair she spoke, while they in their armchairs heard her, fairly well, and saw her, fairly well.

Vashti's son Kuno is trying to escape this combination of mental and physical restraints on human potential, clambering up through the infrastructure toward the forbidden and disdained surface of the earth. He tells his horrified mother,

> I did not fear that I might tread upon a live rail and be killed. I feared something far more intangible – doing what was not contemplated by the Machine. Then I said to myself, 'Man is the measure,' and I went, and after many visits I found an opening.

Even if there is no real destination, the quest to get there – the quest to find meanings and values of our own – is a fulfillment of our nature.

As my theory would predict, those who do not serve the Machine are driven out of the co-evolving human gene-pool: "Kuno had lately asked to be a father, and his request had been refused by the Committee. His was not a type that the Machine desired to hand on." As my theory would also predict, the Machine also efficiently and almost invisibly exploits our religious instincts: "The word 'religion' was sedulously avoided, and in theory the Machine was still the creation and the implement of man. But in practice all, save a few retrogrades, worshipped it as divine."

Kuno warns his mother that the Machine made to serve humanity is in fact erasing humanity, making us parts of its own self-serving organism:

> We created the Machine, to do our will, but we cannot make it do our will now. It has robbed us of the sense of space and of the sense of touch; it has blurred every human relation and narrowed down love to a carnal act, it has paralyzed our bodies and our wills, and now it compels us to worship it. The Machine develops – but not on our lines. The Machine proceeds – but not to our goal. We only exist as the blood corpuscles that course through its arteries, and if it could work without us, it would let us die. Oh, I have no remedy – or, at least, only one – to tell men again and again that I have seen the hills of Wessex as Ælfrid saw them when he overthrew the Danes.

The only hope, in other words, is resistance on behalf of independent human perception combined with humanistic learning; specifically, a sympathetic reading of our past through literature.

As the system begins breaking down, new edicts are issued to save faith in the Machine, and they function very much as I have argued the evolving cultural machine is functioning in the 21st century, despite some reflexive assumptions that independent human agency is running that system:

> To attribute these two great developments to the Central Committee is to take a very narrow view of civilization. The Central Committee announced the developments, it is true, but they were no more the cause of them than were the kings of the imperialistic period the cause of war. Rather did they yield to some invincible pressure, which came no one knew whither, and which, when gratified, was succeeded by some new pressure equally invincible. To such a state of affairs it is convenient to give the name of progress. No one confessed the Machine was out of hand. Year by year it was served with increased efficiency and decreased intelligence.

Does such a development really seem unfamiliar to us?

The Selfish Meme and the Deep Self

In science non-fiction, the idea of a "selfish meme" appeared briefly towards the end of Richard Dawkins's transformative 1976 book *The Selfish Gene*. On this point, I think Dawkins has (uncharacteristically) backed down too soon. The cognitive scientist Keith E. Stanovich is also mainly concerned about our struggle against self-serving genes, though he provides a perceptive and eloquent analysis of the possibility that memes are sometimes masters the human race should resist. He asserts that "The fundamental insight triggered by memetic studies is that a belief may spread *without necessarily being true or helping the human being holding the belief in any way.*"[6] I would expand this warning to include the necessity of vigilance against beliefs that help in one way – say, by simplifying an exhaustingly complex ethical and perceptual world – while harming in others. As Stanovich himself points out, memes can be even less kindly to us than genes, which need to help their biological carrier thrive well enough and long enough to reproduce if they are to survive, whereas memes have many other ways to get replicated.[7]

While I admire Stanovich's recognition of the problem, I would amend his proposed cure, which seems to exclude literary functions that seem to address exactly the problems he identifies. If humanity "must aspire to so-called broad rationality – one that critiques the beliefs and desires that go into instrumental calculations," then the humanities must be defended against the rise of the profit-quantifiers. In fact, through most of Stanovich's book, the examples in of evolution-induced malfunctions we must learn to overcome are situations in which people fail to manage money optimally. This may reflect an understandable fascination with the work of Kahneman and others in post-classical economics, but we have to be vigilant (as with sociologist Immanuel Wallerstein's magisterial "world-systems" theory[8]) to make sure the money-meme doesn't outflank our efforts to help us recognize parasites.

Stanovich concludes that "human uniqueness does in fact derive from an architectural feature of the human mind. That feature is the propensity for higher-order representation."[9] Yet, the disciplines richly engaged in analyzing high-order representation are upstaged in his recommendations by the "need to have installed as mindware the tools of rational and scientific thinking." Granted, people utilizing "evaluative memeplexes such as science, logic, and decision theory might begin a process of pruning vehicle-thwarting goals," and "have the potential to create in us a uniquely critical and discerning type of self-reflection," but so do artists, philosophers, literary critics, and historians of many kinds. There can be little room for fiction when one of Stanovich's four basic rules tells us to tolerate only those thoughts "that are true – that is, that reflect the way the world actually is."[10]

Evolution may not be teleological, but perhaps we are. Whatever forces have shaped us and continue to shape us exist on a spectrum from healthy to malignant, depending on what we value, and on a spectrum from visible to invisible, depending on whether we have the will and the tools to see better. At their core, the humanities – and other communities of intellectual resistance – help us weigh those values, and help us widen and sharpen that vision.

Stanovich's admirable plan is unlikely to succeed if he underrates the problems that led people to grant so much power to these memeplexes to begin with. The promise of more extensive analytic thought is an excellent goal, but many people are in flight from thought, and even from objectivity. Is rational scientific inference broad-spectrum enough to identify and extricate the trickier cultural formations that have evolved to resist the tests and controls of human rationality?

Would we even want, could we even bear, entirely rational minds and an entirely rational world anyway? I am not among the critique-all cultural historians who blame the Enlightenment for almost every-thing, as if its rationalist taxonomies had crushed a glowing world of peace, love, and justice. But optimism that science will, alone and automatically, blend increased information and revered rationality into collective liberation is hard to reconcile with the history, political and cultural, of the intervening centuries. Perhaps we need other, less direct and less positivistic ways of coming at the truth, and ways of carrying it home in containers that have handles, insulation, and decoration.

Years after writing that last sentence, I found a similar conclusion, in Michael Pollan's latest book, about what is necessary to make the insights provided by psychedelic drugs tolerable: "these powerful medicines can be dangerous – both to the individual and to the society – when they don't have a sturdy social container: a steadying set of rules and rituals" and the guidance of a shamanistic figure, together offering "a cultural vessel of some kind" for "these powerful, anarchic medicines … a kind of Apollonian counterweight to contain and channel their sheer Dionysian force."[11]

Alternatives are especially essential if the absence of teleology in the modern scientific view empties life of anything that feels like transcendent meaning, leaving us nothing to set against death. We are again like Hamlet, walking through a graveyard strewn with the skulls of those (like the clown Yorick who kissed and entertained Hamlet in his childhood) who loved us and made us laugh; how then do we push on with our life's work? Ask Siri about that on an iPhone and see whether technology offers a more adequate answer than Shakespeare's.

The compelling critique, in recent decades, of science's claim to be value-free and outside of culture means that science too must consider what cause it is seeking to serve, perhaps by asking itself some human-istic questions, even while humanists must try (as I have tried in this book) to see what science can do to explain and combat our social and spiritual problems. Pitirim Sorokin's grand synthetic theory of socio-cultural cycles was already warning, before World War II, that the hu-man race may be in a Sensate phase, where material reality is deemed to be the ultimate reality, and the individual consumer's pleasure is assumed to be the highest good; and in the decadent phase of that phase, such that revolutionary and technological violence and selfish sensualism have "begun to menace the further existence of humanity," leading to a yearning for some renewal of spiritual meaning.[12]

In Western societies, for a very long time, the escape from materialism has mostly resided in the concept of a soul, but there are different ways of framing that concept. Clearly, most human beings have higher-order aspirations for themselves. Even the villains of Shakespearean tragedy, such as Claudius, Edmund, Macbeth, and Aufidius, wish they could wish better wishes so they could be better people. Matthew B. Crawford, a researcher at the Institute for Advanced Study of Culture, observes that

> Animals are guided by appetites that are fixed, and so are we, but we can also form a second-order desire, 'a desire for a desire,' when we entertain some picture of the sort of person we would *like* to be – a person who is better not because she has more self-control, but because she is moved by worthier desires. Acquiring the tastes of a serious person is what we call education. Does it have a future? The advent of engineered, hyperpalatable mental stimuli compels us to ask the question.[13]

The very category of self-actualization, the ability to have it as a conscious goal, and the multiple adjacent layers of consciousness necessary to produce these internal debates are probably unique to our species, and make us meaningfully unique and valuable as individuals. This claim is an iteration of Pico della Mirandola's deduction (in his 1486 "Oration on the Dignity of Man") that the human need to manufacture ourselves – for example, with garments and tools – where other creatures come ready-made indicates that we alone are destined for the burdens and opportunities of free will, and hence endowed with a soul.

That soul may be secular, consisting of whatever in our nature and consciousness is able to resist the bio-programming protocols on behalf of some other chosen value, whether for good or for ill. "Spiritual" need not be a euphemism for "religious." We are in the grasp, but not necessarily in the thrall, of genetic controllers and somewhat less recognized cultural controllers. That situation confers on us what I consider a moral obligation to think about which of those forces to obey, which to resist, and which to redirect, with a kind of socio-cultural judo, toward the advantage of what we consider the best parts of ourselves as participants in life. The goal is what classical philosophy called *eudaimonia*: a good life, likely to combine durable pleasures with philosophical guidance and political engagement. Free from corruption by parasitic systems and other pathologies, the quest for *eudaimonia* will lead toward *arête*: wisdom, fortitude, generosity, and other virtues coinciding to produce the fulfillment of human potential.

The old subgenre called a dialogue between soul and body remains relevant, although I would recast it as between, on the one side, a broad, wakeful, loving consciousness, and on the other side a creature playing out the algorithms of mindlessly self-perpetuating systems, whether of genes or of memes. The work of the humanistic educator, all the way from Plato into the 21st century, therefore includes something like the work of the clergy: helping that soul discover a valid good (rather than the clever, meretricious simulator of good, or the mere soother of the moment), and showing how and why to embrace it. Although our inmost and most intricate moral consciousness may not connect us to an immortal deity, it is evidently what mostly separates us from the rest of mortal life. We are thus a singularity, and (like Adam and Eve in exile from Edenic innocence) have to find our own way, and help others find theirs. We may be unique in this mission not only as a contemplative species but also as a recent phase of contemplation: only as educated human beings living in the post-Darwin era are we truly able to plan the mission. But what might a guidebook look like, if who we are and how we travel matters more than the final destination?

We could start by remembering how that journey begins. Nearly all children come into the world hoping for love, wishing to learn how to speak and think, and even how to feel, spouting an inexhaustible fountain of questions, and determined above all to live, as a self among others. At the risk of sounding pathetically romantic, in either the general or the historical sense of "pathetic" and "romantic," what higher learning in the humanities ideally tries to do is to sustain those projects, and the hunger that drives them, against a thousand forces that conspire to discourage them and divert them into narrow, dead-end paths. Young people have more synaptic plasticity (the ability to intensify or diminish connections between neurons) than adults, and they can pass that attribute along to any society whose institutions have become too effective, in their own defense, at suppressing it.

Plato, with his intensely conservative ideal of government, feared that potential, arguing that

> when the programme of games is prescribed and secures that the same children always play the same games and delight in the same toys in the same way and under the same conditions, it allows the real and serious laws also to remain undisturbed; but when these games vary and suffer innovations, amongst other constant alterations the children are always shifting their fancy from one game to another, so that neither in respect of their own bodily gestures nor in respect of their equipment have they any fixed and acknowledged standard of propriety and impropriety; but the man they hold in special honour is he who is always innovating or introducing some novel device in the matter of form or colour or something of the sort; whereas it would be perfectly true to say that a State can have no worse pest than a man of that description.[14]

William Wordsworth is one of many poets and novelists who, in contrast, regularly employ a child's perspective to critique the diseases of their society, presumably because children are not yet fully invested in the dominant culture and indoctrinated by it. This idealization of children as sacred innocents to be protected may not have been as common in pre-Renaissance Western societies,[15] but at least since the mid-17th century, it has become pervasive and intense. Thomas Traherne played the wide-eyed, generous-hearted child so that he could more effectively inveigh against the conformist consumerism that was decimating both the imagination and nature, as art became overwhelmingly Neoclassical and natural philosophy became science. William Blake joined Wordsworth in a similar protest against the results of that Neoclassical culture, and against the nascent Industrial Revolution. Lewis Carroll used the misprisions of childhood to show that the domineering Victorian culture, so proud of its correctness and mature good sense, could be seen as largely insane. Charles Dickens used young protagonists to show that Victorian adults were cruel and hypocritical at exactly the moments they supposed themselves benevolent and systematically right-minded. Against the cold-heartedness of some northern European cultures, German post-Holocaust literature (such as Günter Grass's *The Tin Drum*) and Scandinavian cinema (especially as directed by Ingmar Bergman and Lasse Hallström) have made similar use of the child's-eye view. So, too, it is worth noting, do many of the poets of 21st-century Islamic jihad.[16]

Unless they are schooled out of it, children can help us register the diseases of society and the possibility of affection across conventional social divisions, even across species. Inexpert in the practices of culture, children are the stem cells of the body-politic, closer to the shared sources of life, and therefore still capable of developing toward many different kinds of functions – including bad ones, as recent campaigns against bullying and books such as *Lord of the Flies* seek to alert us. Their imaginations offer an exuberant escape from the memeplex we are herded into for a screening of our mass-produced fantasy life. Allowing toddlers to be sucked into the narrow channels of most iPad programs (and literal channels of Disney) seems a waste of that potential: just the kind of recapture a self-protective socio-economic system would encourage. The quality of their education is therefore absolutely crucial. The question is how to improve it.

Quantifying Educational Quality

From the late-19th through the mid-20th centuries, John Dewey repeatedly warned that pedagogical malpractice was producing passive minds, and warned against the assumption that human learning consists primarily of accumulating data: the same mistake I am attributing to the Information Age as a whole. Masses of data can displace the human instinct – dangerous to the powers that be – to seek knowledge, to see deeply enough to distinguish illusory goods from real ones. It is a diverted appetite, where more is easily mistaken for better, like pornography instead of more humane forms of desire and response.

But the pressures of the Cold War steered American schools back away from Dewey, and toward training competitive technologists. Now the shock-doctrines of economic crisis are exerting the same regressive influence, audible even in President Obama's 2013 State of the Union address, which targeted funding to "classes that focus on science, technology, engineering and math – the skills today's employers are looking for to fill the jobs that are there right now and will be there in the future."

While many humanities professors insist that our field needs to become more technological and careerist because the public no longer values what we offer, the facts suggest otherwise, and the discrepancy is revealing. What may be wiser to do instead is to begin breaking the spell of technophilic consumer-capitalism, by encouraging our fellow citizens to recognize something that they already understand, but have been taught to dismiss, ignore, or repress. Naturally we want our children to have good prospects for employment, and will encourage those children to achieve that through their education. Yet, like millions of other parents, I pay large sums for higher education that is not a vocational-technology program. We know perfectly well that there is more to our children than the sum of their SAT scores, and that their happiness and fulfillment will depend on more than their salaries.

Many of us also recognize that, in a world changing ever more rapidly, the rote learning of specific facts and technologies (encouraged by the current fixation on test-based education) is a superhighway to obsolescence. The "No Child Left Behind" policies, ironically, mean no childhood left: no time for either bodies or minds to play freely. The only durable knowledge will be that which provides adaptability, helps assimilate complexity, and refines the skill of interpretation rather than memorization – another reason allowing children to explore their natural environment should be valued more highly in education.[17]

At a recent conference on the future of literary study, an earnest and intelligent Professor of English from an elite university urged us to defend ourselves against a coming onslaught of assessment-driven funding by developing a taxonomy of the skill-sets our fields provide, and systems to quantify students' improvement in these marketable mental functions during their undergraduate years. My counter-suggestion was that entering students in all majors should be required to write an hour-long essay on a topic such as, "How do you cope with the fundamentally tragic aspects of human existence?" and then to do so again as they approached graduation, so we could see what valuable skills each major had developed. Everyone seemed to assume I was joking.

Whatever develops a creative but disciplined mind, a heart open to other people, and a voice capable of communicating with them and with oneself is almost certain to produce a better life. In fact, with technologies and economies transforming as quickly as they do these days, and with cultures in such critical collisions, those may be the only skills we can be confident are going to be valuable, wherever and whenever that student runs into an opportunity or a crisis. Looking far backwards as well as ahead, the greatest advantage of the expanded human brain was (recent studies of creativity suggest) not its deductive or computational power, but instead its "greater ability to free-associate."[18] Marcel Proust's novels, exploring at great length the complexities of his own mind and his perception of and interaction with others, are not a decadent modern waste of our time; they epitomize and reinforce the qualities that have driven our evolution since the origin of our species.

The notion that expected earnings are the only reasonable goal and reliable gauge of the worth of any enterprise is widespread, but there are treasures buried deeper than that bottom line, and they are not written in numbers. That pleasure is presumed not to be a profit is itself a symptom of a neoliberal work-for-money ethic. To adapt a point made by Stefan Collini,[19] would many people complete the following half-dozen sentences in something like the following way? Looking back at my life, my happiest moments were ... the times I generated the most profit for my corporation's stockholders. I love my children because ... they are going to be job-creators and active consumers to keep the economy growing. I'm so glad I took them to play at the beach and the amusement park because ... the tourist industry is crucial to California's tax-base. In fact, my family really enjoys beach trips because ... they might help the kids find work someday as oceanographers. Sometimes it's good to sit around with a few friends and have some laughs because ... the ads on sitcoms help us decide what to buy. It's still great listening to the Beatles because ... their records repeatedly helped Capitol Records surpass its quarterly sales projections. Yet that is the way many politically and financially powerful people and organizations seem to think we think, or ought to think. My home university has been considering funding its research centers along the model of the Browne Report that is already subjugating my British colleagues to an elaborate, faux-quantitative, "rational," market-driven financial hierarchy which would starve the humanities. Meanwhile, the British government is pushing even further in this direction, bringing teaching as well as research under this regimen, via a document ironically called "Fulfilling Our Potential" – another document Collini has critiqued brilliantly.[20]

Professors in the humanities, as in other academic areas, have been successful in fields where competition for jobs is overwhelming. Most were near the top of their college classes, and so could probably have earned more money elsewhere; the tenured ones could certainly keep their jobs with very little effort. Yet, the vast majority of my academic friends regularly work far beyond business hours, for love of teaching and research, the latter of which they do in synergistic cooperation with colleagues worldwide, as well as performing, from a sense of duty, countless administrative tasks and student services they could safely refuse.

What then is the advantage of turning this profession into a zero-sum business of institutional competition, to be evaluated and funded, not by people who actually understand it and care about it, but instead by converting it into crude quantitative rather than qualitative measures? That shift is especially misguided because it encourages more crude quantity and less quality of publication, to the disadvantage of the entire project of scholarship, since it leaves us wading through work that exists not because someone was excited to share a good idea backed by good evidence, but instead because the dean who handles promotions needed a higher unit-publications score.

All these metrics do is allow administrators to pretend they know, with scientific certainty, which work is worth supporting, whereas in fact they are only able to create that supposed information by blinding themselves to the full complexity of the issue. They submit the work to a narrow and artificial external algorithm, a memeplex everyone in academia repeatedly serves at great expense of time and morale. It is proverbially miserable to work for someone stupider than you are, yet we are being drawn into an effort to invent a boss much stupider than the current system of peer-review.

Universities and especially humanities programs are increasingly being required to show that we have "impact" on society, and that we know exactly how we are achieving that impact. We are also required to avow – from the political rather than the business flank of the right wing – that we intend no impact on society. Is it shocking that we often fail to meet those mutually exclusive criteria? We value literature largely because quantitative measures are gravely inadequate to human experience; we are then assigned to find quantitative measures of how well we have taught that.

This kind of program is a quest for artificial unintelligence: an attempt to create a machine that will be conveniently incapable of registering and responding to complexity as a human mind does. This is an epitome of the counterproductive human response to cognitive overload generally, and it revives the problem discussed earlier in terms of digital signals replacing analog. Would obliging Da Vinci to convert the Mona Lisa to paint-by-numbers outlines and then to fill them back in neatly have yielded a better painting than the *sfumato* version in the Louvre, allowing us to see more clearly the "real" picture? (Figures 11 and 12).

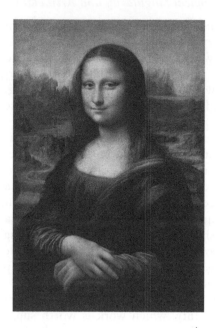

Figure 11 "Mona Lisa" by Leonardo da Vinci (early 16th century).

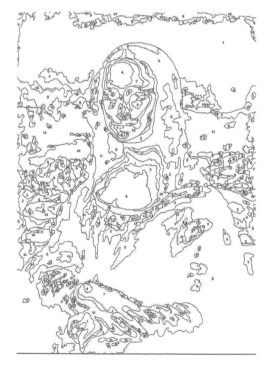

Figure 12 "Mona Lisa" for painting by numbers.

A prominent recent critique of quantitative sociology has revealed the same kind of problem: coding attributes into simple categories and numbers produces clarity that masks itself as both science and insight, but often merely reflects back the deficiencies and biases of the original coding, not a heretofore hidden truth about the societies under study.[21] What, aside from a highly questionable claim to exact and unbiased information, is gained by rendering the data crude enough to count and then reassembling it stripped of the nuance that is a key talent of our species?

And what is gained, except the power of politicians and of the self-perpetuating meme of bureaucracy, by turning academia into a market of goods damaged by their conversion into commodities, and thereby convincing scholars to shape their careers by cynical calculation rather than by the impractical passion that is actually their practical value to the species? Several studies of contemporary professions have shown that

> There is really no substitute for the integrity that inspires people to do good work because they want to do good work. And the more we rely on incentives as substitutes for integrity, the more we will need to rely on them as substitutes for integrity.[22]

Specifically regarding universities, "the case has never been properly made for why the professional autonomy of academics should be mistrusted and bureaucratic formalism preferred."[23] Subjugating the humanities to a business-consultancy model is like attempting a "Moneyball" strategy for a game in which how to play must always be indeterminate, and winning is not the point.

It is much as if the government were to issue the following press release to its citizenry:

> In these difficult financial times, our society can no longer afford to indulge the fuzzy and antiquated practice of choosing friends by "feelings." Instead, we will utilize proven modern scientific principles of management. You will rank everyone you know on our Affinity Census grid, which our software will then match to a set of your personal performance goals. Multiplying the correlations by the number of things in listed categories that each friendship-applicant has done for you lately will identify your actual friends.
>
> You will offer each of these amity-partners a monthly payment (minus a nominal fee to MateMetrics, the private corporation hired to oversee this process), scaled to their private-sector earning power, as incentives to remain among your social clients.

Those who accept will be assigned, as your "Co-Efficients," to spend a specified amount of time with you on impactful friendship-related activities, audited by tracking your smartphones and supplemented by mandatory monthly online reports specifying exactly what each friend has done to improve the life-actualization of each other friend, and how those outcomes have been publicized and monetized.

We anticipate some whining from people who will claim that these rational measures constitute a philistine assault on their cozy traditions of friendship. They will claim to have access to subtle and complex aspects of their friendships which only they may recognize: aspects so deep, so nuanced, and so protean that they cannot be adequately articulated on a checklist. That, however, is always the posture of elitists who consider themselves too good and sensitive for the genius of the market and the hard facts of the real world.

It is easy to doubt that such a program would really produce more and better friendship. Defenders of the humanities in the 21st century must remind people – students, parents, and (other) funders alike – of what justifies that doubt.

Medical care is now undergoing a similar degradation: humane motives and complex human skills of recognition are being curtailed to better serve the demands of computer systems and corporate profit. UCLA Medical Center, where I receive my care, is one of countless such places around the country that are increasingly obliging physicians to convert their notes on patients into a system of numerical codes that simplify records and thereby facilitate billing. Rather than being encouraged to prioritize and contextualize items to communicate effectively with each patient and the patient's other professional caregivers by addressing the interlocking aspects of the problems and possible solutions, physicians are being pressured to check off a swarm of diagnoses and associated tests so that the hospital can charge insurers more – costs then passed along (with added overhead) to the insured and the taxpayers.[24] Metrics can help measure the relative efficiency of various treatments (including no treatment) and target resources for broad population-health efforts, but the immediate beneficiary will be the financial-managerial functions of large corporations – and medical care in the United States has already been badly compromised by subjugating to a profit model a commodity whose customers' demand is largely inelastic to price (the same can be said of the privatizing of other indispensable public services). The coding system will also make it difficult for physicians to convey the nuances that are the essence of helpful communication among diagnosticians.

The arts of observation of the complicated realities of health will thus, like so many other areas of human life lately, be converted into something cruder and less salubrious for two reasons: to make us more manageable for digital processing, and especially to allow more efficient and extensive billing for modularized units. The prestigious *New England Journal of Medicine* reports that "software developers have been oriented toward providing documentation needed to satisfy auditors rather than developing important functions such as clinical decision support that would improve patient care," and "medical groups and hospitals commonly use [Medicare Fee Schedule]-based relative value units to assess physicians' productivity ... codes that don't reflect what physicians actually do – or should do – for patients." The reimbursement guidelines "specify the required contents of the medical record in excruciating – and often irrelevant – detail ... The detailed guidelines often cause clinicians to overdocument, making the medical record an ineffective source of communication."[25] Again, in other words, our society mistakes for progress what is in fact a self-serving, self-preserving function that has evolved in the memeplexes we created – a function that actively disserves our human talents and our human values.

In a more brutally direct instance of the alliance of metrics and money overriding the interests of patients and the doctors trying to care for those patients, some US Veterans Affairs hospitals have (according to a 2018 report in the *New York Times*) been turning away the most seriously ill patients despite having many open beds, and administrators have been refusing to authorize somewhat risky but medically necessary surgeries and designating people for hospice care only, even while they remained potentially curable, all in an effort to improve quality-of-care metrics that are damaged by deaths in the hospital (which damage also damages hospital administrators' bonuses). Diagnoses are misrepresented, compromising future care, to avoid falling into categories the system believes show neglected preventative care.[26] The metrics improve and the patients deteriorate.

The shortcomings of metrics have sent economies tumbling all over the world. As Michael Lewis's book *The Big Short* and the movie based on it make clear, the 2008 financial collapse resulted not only from greed, but specifically from the sorting of reality (in this case, real estate) into codes: mortgage derivatives and their ratings, numbers based on other numbers, while the managerial structure of various institutions kept everyone feeding the system by discouraging them from looking beyond the illusory immediate profits. Like the misguided sports pundits of the last Interchapter, they trusted the statistics instead of taking perspective on the physical and human realities the statistics claimed to reflect but actually concealed.

The acute problem with neoliberalism is not the existence of market competition itself, but rather the assumption that such competition produces an absolute truth, in the form of financial outcomes, that we must obviously obey. The capitalist functions my earlier chapters have been decrying are therefore closely allied to the over-valuation of quantitative measures of value I am critiquing now. This is an instance of the arbitrary "regime of veridiction" Michel Foucault warned against in his strikingly prescient *Birth of Biopolitics* lectures in the late 1970s.

Marching directly toward happiness and prosperity, and counting on sheer numbers to get us there, is like Pickett's Confederate army charging toward imagined victory at Gettysburg, or the Redcoats marching in formation into the sniper fire of the American colonists on Breed's Hill. Even if we win some battles, we lose the war. What we need instead is asymmetrical warfare on some cultural juggernauts, on behalf of some great traditions of liberty. This chapter has touched on a few areas where I have encountered the artificial unintelligence imposed on us by the false and jealous god Quantification; anyone seeking a wider view of the problem as it distorts life in the 21st century and worsens injustice should read Cathy O'Neil's lucid *Weapons of Math Destruction*.

Harari's equally lucid overview of the history of our species concludes that "The most important impact of script on human history is precisely this: it has gradually changed the way humans think and view the world. Free association and holistic thought have given way to compartmentalization and bureaucracy."[27] But, just as the culture called fiction enables resistance to the fiction called culture, so the writing of a novel or a tragedy can undo some of the narrowing that has been steadily imposed by the invention of writing itself.

Famous Last Words

If a principal task of human beings, and especially of scholars in the humanities, is the selective transmission of culture, rendering the good audible and the bad questionable, then we first have to try to understand what culture is good for: how it brings us together while also protecting some valuable differences.

That is certainly no straightforward task. This book has argued that seemingly mysterious and sinister actions of human society can be understood not only as a conspiracy of human villains but also as the product of several interrelated phenomena: partly as the playing-out of a set of relatively simple behavioral rules over multiple iterations, partly as a distribution of roles by a collective human brain that has evolved to balance stability with innovation, and partly as our interaction with selfish memes that have developed their own strategic mechanisms for survival.

Yet, these are not finally incompatible explanations under the rubric of co-evolution, and I have tried to draw them together comprehensibly. As highly self-conscious rather than purely instinctive beings, we can think many things (including crushingly about our own mortality). We can perceive reality and duty in nearly infinite different ways, and can therefore choose any kind of behavior. But, we are also a species that survives only in communities. So, culture has to take over the tasks (dictated biochemically in most other creatures) of providing a coherent set of instructions and beliefs, and giving shape to the overwhelming data offered by the internal and external worlds. Culture is, for that as well as other more obviously practical reasons, a reflexively conservative force.

Since humanity's reactionary tendencies reinforce the control that memeplexes can exercise for their own survival and reproduction, cultural conservatism has to be balanced by dissidence and creativity that allow culture to evolve so we can adapt to changing physical and mental environments. This matches the amalgamation of dutiful copying (to take advantage of wisdom accumulated in a relevant past) and bold trial-and-error experimentation (to be ready for change) that has been fundamental to humanity's co-evolution with our cultures. Formal arts are a safe mode for creating those mutations, as the fiction-function provides a device for testing alternative choices without having to spend actual lives on them. Humanistic scholarship offers a device for testing them outside the local pressures of tribal politics and short-term advantage. And higher education helps to create individuals who can carry independent judgments out into society in surprisingly transformative ways. Richerson and Boyd observe that

> we organize institutions from a simple tribal council to highly complex modern ones, such as the research university and the political party, that are designed to direct the course of cultural evolution .... With a reasonable picture of cultural evolution in hand, we could begin to understand how we might humanize processes that often exact savage costs in the currency of human misery.[28]

Certainly something has to help a society sort fruitful innovation from mere aberration, in a prudent manner informed by both immediate circumstance and distant perspective, and unprejudiced by powerful memeplexes whose self-interest might disguise what actually serves the collective long-term human interest. Throughout my exposition of these ideas, I have tried to be clear that I am using the sciences in support of some humanistic values rather than claiming my own work is scientific, and I hope the range of my examples – which obliges me to keep them brief – indicates that putting a few broad ideas together in this new way renders a variety of cultural phenomena, past and present, coherently intelligible.

I suspect that the widespread loyalty to the arts and to liberal-arts education derives not only from an aspiration to designated objects of cultural prestige and therefore upward mobility but also from an intuitive understanding that these allegedly impractical practices actually defend us against more selfish aggregations of memes: viruses in the body-cultural whose disservice to humanity is often initially recognizable only by a feeling that they are ugly. The aesthetic response serves the mind much as taste serves the body: as an instinctual early-warning system about what to ingest and what to expel. The fact that many readings "are pursued for mental pleasure," as commentators as far back as Cicero have noted, may thus refute rather than validate the warnings of those same commentators against "reading fiction, from which no utility can be extracted."[29]

Instead of allowing the value of artistic creativity and humanistic education to be eclipsed by such criteria, perhaps we should ask, non-rhetorically, why anyone would doubt that value. If Aristotle and his heir Ficino are correct that creatures achieve goodness, joy, and fulfillment by exercising their characteristic abilities, and if evolution has given *Homo sapiens* unique faculties for language, imagination, subtlety, and community, then the arts and humanities are essential to our well-being. Those who scoff at the uselessness of these studies and those who celebrate their benign neglect of utility share the modern illusion that anything lacking a quantifiable economic benefit is, for worse or better, essentially without purpose.[30] Yet anything that – along with its many indirect benefits – can offer us a perspective outside of a self-perpetuating memeplex such as consumer capitalism is surely precious. Pricelessness is priceless.

What should be the legacy of one generation to the next? A primary obligation is certainly a healthy biosphere, but there are other inheritances as well. It is widely supposed (though I think far from established) that the successes of the human species have reduced its genetic evolution.[31] A notable exception is deliberate DNA engineering that erases errors in the code and (more often than not) passes along the healthiest attributes of each generation to the next. But, we already have some wonderful and proven technologies for such desirable corrections and transmissions – and they work on cultural drivers, not just biological ones. One is called a story, or a book; another is called a school, or a university (Figures 13–15).

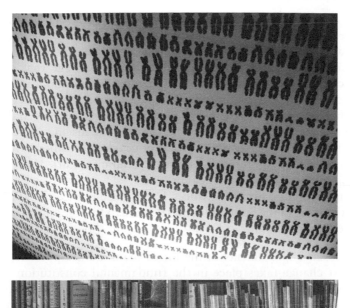

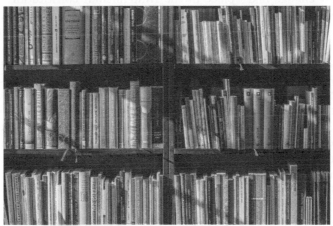

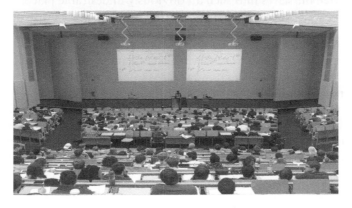

Figure 13–15 Chromosomes, library shelf, and lecture hall.

The choice between archival and activist models of the university is therefore a false one. Without the archive (including the equivalent of what was, until quite recently, mistakenly dismissed as "junk" non-coding DNA), we would lack the ancient heritage that provides perspective and that we can activate when needed. Without the activist impulse, we would lack the motive to decide which parts of that heritage, and what departures from it, are required by our current and future environments.[32] Edward Said asserts that for the disempowered to expose and resist injustice requires "what Foucault once called 'a relentless erudition,' scouring alternative sources, exhuming buried documents, reviving forgotten (or abandoned) histories."[33]

Let me therefore give four voices from that heritage the last words about the value of the humanities for the human future. John Stuart Mill became convinced that

> no great improvements in the lot of mankind are possible, until a great change takes place in the fundamental constitution of their modes of thought. The old opinions in religion, morals, and politics, are so much discredited in the more intellectual minds as to have lost the greater part of their efficacy for good, while they have still life enough in them to be a powerful obstacle to the growing up of any better opinions on those subjects. When the philosophic minds of the world can no longer believe its religion, or can only believe it with modifications amounting to an essential change of its character, a transitional period commences, of weak convictions, paralysed intellects, and growing laxity of principle, which cannot terminate until a renovation has been effected ... and when things are in this state, all thinking or writing which does not tend to promote such a renovation, is of very little value beyond the moment.[34]

Mill's close contemporary Ralph Waldo Emerson understood why we have gotten ourselves into such an obviously undesirable place, and how we can move beyond it. His mesmerizing essay "Circles" warns,

> Beware when the great God lets loose a thinker on this planet. Then all things are at risk. It is as when a conflagration has broken out in a great city, and no man knows what is safe, or where it will end. There is not a piece of science, but its flank may be turned to-morrow; there is not any literary reputation, not the so-called eternal names of fame, that may not be revised and condemned. The very hopes of man, the thoughts of his heart, the religion of nations, the manners and morals of mankind, are all at the mercy of a new generalization.

Two paragraphs later, Emerson observes that

> all nature is the rapid efflux of goodness executing and organizing itself. Much more obviously is history and the state of the world

at any one time directly dependent on the intellectual classification then existing in the minds of men. The things which are dear to men at this hour are so on account of the ideas which have emerged on their mental horizon, and which cause the present order of things as a tree bears its apples. A new degree of culture would instantly revolutionize the entire system of human pursuits.[35]

And, almost exactly 50 years ago as I write this, Martin Luther King Jr.'s first public speech against the Vietnam War packed his sharp new message in the reassuring Ciceronian symmetries derived from his old-fashioned education. He warned about the same dangers of allied meme-plexes I am warning about, and saw hope in similar forms of resistance:

> surely this is the first time in our nation's history that a signifi-cant number of its religious leaders have chosen to move beyond the prophesying of smooth patriotism to the high grounds of a firm dissent based upon the mandates of conscience and the reading of history. Perhaps a new spirit is rising among us.... I am convinced that if we are to get on to the right side of the world revolution, we as a nation must undergo a radical revolution of values. We must rapidly begin ... the shift from a thing-oriented society to a person-oriented society. When machines and computers, profit mo-tives and property rights are considered more important than peo-ple, the giant triplets of racism, extreme materialism, and militarism are incapable of being conquered.[36]

To that it is hard to add anything but "Amen."

At the heart of evolution is a tension between replication and innova-tion. We are able, in small but potentially consequential ways, to decide what to preserve and what to alter – especially in the influential area of culture, if we recognize that we must direct it to serve our ideals rather than its own reproduction. Practices that at once stabilize our best traditions and give us the ability to test other pathways at low cost are immensely valuable, especially as they oblige our rational discipline and our imagination to cooperate productively, and allow us to model a world that is, both physically and ethically, more fluid and complex than our mental lassitude and shortsighted practicality usually allow us to consider. Playing and dreaming are not mere escape, but rehearsals for a better and freer rendition of life and participation in its myriad glories. Nor is suspended certainty a failure of the mind. The last word therefore goes to the beautiful and enigmatic last words of Stevens's *The Man with the Blue Guitar*, solemnly celebrating "The moments when we choose to play / The imagined pine, the imagined jay."

Notes

Chapter 1

1 bell hooks, *Writing Beyond Race: Living Theory and Practice* (New York: Routledge, 2013), 37. Reproduced with permission through the Copyright Clearance Center.

2 Kurt Vonnegut, *Player Piano* (New York: Dial Press, 1999), 315. Copyright 1952, 1980 by Kurt Vonnegut. Used by permission of Laurel-Leaf, an imprint of Random House Children's Books, a division of Penguin Random House LLC. All rights reserved.

3 Joseph Henrich, *The Secret of Our Success* (Princeton, NJ: Princeton University Press, 2015) offers a highly convincing and reader-friendly argument for the fundamental importance of transmitted culture.

4 Steven Pinker, *How the Mind Works* (New York: Norton, 1997), 211–98, explores the relationship between our binocular vision and the way we cognize external reality. His page 241 considers how "Stereo vision" offers "a paradigm of how other parts of the mind might work," which is very much how I am using it.

5 Anne Burdick et al., *Digital_Humanities* (Cambridge, MA: MIT, 2012), 37.

6 George Eliot, *Middlemarch*, (Berlin: Asher & Co., 1871–2), bk. 2, 351.

7 Henry Plotkin, *Evolutionary Worlds without End* (Oxford: Oxford University Press, 2010), 164, in reference to the important work of Kevin Laland, describes the plausible correlation between West African yam cultivation and the sickle-cell S allele. See also Chapter 3 of William H. Durham, *Coevolution: Genes, Culture, and Human Diversity* (Stanford: Stanford University Press, 1991). On the protective functions that may have allowed the Tay-Sachs mutation to survive, see Isabelle C. Withrock et al., "Genetic diseases conferring resistance to infectious diseases," in *Genes & Diseases*, Vol. 2, # 3, September 2015, 247–54; doi:10.1016/j.gendis.2015.02.008.

8 Aneri Pattani, "They Were Shorter and at Risk for Arthritis, but They Survived an Ice Age," *New York Times*, July 6, 2017. The original study, viewable at www.nature.com/articles/ng.3911, acknowledges that the correlation with colder parts of the world could have other causes.

9 Cf. Clifford Geertz, "The Impact of the Concept of Culture on the Concept of Man," *Bulletin of the Atomic Scientists* 22, no. 4 (1966):

> culture is best seen not as complexes of concrete behavior patterns ... but as a set of control mechanisms—plans, recipes, rules, instructions (what computer engineers call 'programs')—for the governing of behavior .... man is precisely the animal most desperately dependent upon such extra-genetic, outside-the-skin control mechanisms, such cultural programs, for ordering his behavior .... One of the most significant facts about us may finally be that we all begin with the natural equipment to live a thousand kinds of life but end in the end having lived only one.

10 Ernest Gellner, *Plough, Sword and Book: The Structure of Human History* (London: Collins Harvill, 1988), 14.

11 All quotations from Shakespeare's plays will be based on *The Riverside Shakespeare*, ed. G. B. Evans, 2nd edition (Boston, MA: Houghton Mifflin, 1997), with the act, scene, and line numbers in parentheses.

12 John Tooby and Leda Cosmides, "The Psychological Foundations of Culture," in *The Adapted Mind: Evolutionary Psychology and the Generation of Culture*, eds. Jerome H. Barkow, Leda Cosmides, and John Tooby (New York: Oxford University Press, 1992), 103, note that this "frame problem" constitutes "an implacable problem facing every problem-solving computational system. ... in developmental psychology, it is called the 'need for constraints on induction' ... in perception, they say that the stimulus array 'underdetermines' the interpretation." My point is that culture augments the aspects of psychology that attack this problem.

13 Sheldon Klein, "The Invention of Computationally Plausible Knowledge Systems in the Upper Paleolithic," in *The Origins of Human Behaviour*, ed. R. A. Foley (London: Unwin Hyman, 1991), 67.

14 Philip Lieberman, *The Unpredictable Species* (Princeton, NJ: Princeton University Press, 2013), 112–13. Jonathan Metzl, *The Protest Psychosis: How Schizophrenia Became a Black Disease* (Boston, MA: Beacon Press, 2010), 30, records efforts by apologists for slavery to claim that high levels of schizophrenia-like symptoms in liberated slaves proved them more suitable to captivity.

15 Peter J. Richerson and Robert Boyd, *Not by Genes Alone: How Culture Transformed Human Evolution* (Chicago: University of Chicago Press, 2005), 135, observe that, considering the massive metabolic requirements of human brains, as well as the dangers they add to the process of birth, the complications that can occur in their development, and the time needed to load them with information, "all animals are under stringent selection pressure to be as stupid as they can get away with." And that is before considering the psychic burdens of an elaborate consciousness that this chapter is emphasizing.

16 Our retinas have receptors that fire at certain peak wavelengths, and our minds evidently deploy an elaborate system of correction to permit us to see a single-color object as single-colored when parts of it are in varied light, and to see it as the same color at different times of day when the spectral effects would tell us otherwise. Still, the fact that a discussion of "Possible Adaptive Functions of a Categorical Organization of Colors" focuses on the value of communicating better about colors, and does not entertain the possibility that this system serves the need to simplify experience typifies the neglect of cognitive load in analyses of cultural evolution; see Roger N. Shepard, "The Perceptual Organization of Colors," in *The Adapted Mind*, eds. J. L. Barkow, L. Cosmides, and J. Tooby, 523–24.

17 Henrich, *Secret of Our Success*, 321; his page 240 also explores these cultural variations.

18 Joseph Henrich, Steven J. Heine, and Ara Norenzayan, "The Weirdest People in the World?" Abstract, *Behavioral and Brain Sciences*, 2010.

19 Susan McKinnon, *Neo-Liberal Genetics: The Myths and Moral Tales of Evolutionary Psychology* (Chicago, IL: Prickly Paradigm Press, 2005), 26.

20 Cf. Robin I. M. Dunbar, "Brain Cognition in Evolutionary Perspective," in *Evolutionary Cognitive Neuroscience*, eds. Steven Platek, Todd Shackelford, and Julian Keenan (Cambridge, MA: MIT Press, 2007), 41:

> Barrett et al. (2003) have suggested that the only defining feature of hominoids as a group relative to simians is that great ape (and human)

social groups tend to be dispersed over much larger geographical areas ... the computational demands of having to factor virtual individuals (those not physically present) into their calculations about relationship with individuals that are physically present may have been the trigger that precipitated the hominoid trajectory.

There seems to be a strong correlation in primates between the size of brains and the degree of a species' sociability; see Joan B. Silk, Susan C. Alberts, and Jeanne Altmann, "Social Bonds of Female Baboons Enhance Infant Survival," *Science* 302, no. 5648 (2003): 1231–34.

21 Richerson and Boyd, *Not by Genes*, 15 and 129.
22 Carl Zimmer, "The Purpose of Sleep? To Forget, Scientists Say," *New York Times*, February 2, 2017, www.nytimes.com/2017/02/02/science/sleep-memory-brain-forgetting.html accessed February 26, 2017.
23 Zhenzhong Cui et al., "Increased NR2A:NR2B Ratio Compresses Long-Term Depression Range and Constrains Long-Term Memory," *Scientific Reports* 3, no. 1036 (January 8, 2013), doi:10.1038/srep01036.
24 Dunbar, "Brain Cognition," 41.
25 Li-Hung Chang et al., "Age-Related Declines of Stability in Visual Perceptual Learning," *Current Biology* 24, no. 24 (December 15, 2014): 2926–29, doi:10.1016/j.cub.2014.10.041.
26 Pam Belluck, "Study Finds That Brains With Autism Fail to Trim Synapses as They Develop," *New York Times*, August 21, 2014, www.nytimes.com/2014/08/22/health/brains-of-autistic-children-have-too-many-synapses-study-suggests.html:

> Experts said the fact that young children in both groups had roughly the same number of synapses suggested a clearing problem in autism rather than an overproduction problem. 'More is not better when it comes to synapses, for sure, and pruning is absolutely essential,' said Lisa Boulanger, a molecular biologist at Princeton who was not involved in the research .... Dr. Sulzer's team also found biomarkers and proteins in the brains with autism that reflected malfunctions in the system of clearing out old and degraded cells, a process called autophagy.

See also Guomei Tang et al., "Loss of mTOR-Dependent Macroautophagy Causes Autistic-like Synaptic Pruning Deficits," *Neuron* 83, no. 5 (September 3, 2014): 1131–43, doi:10.1016/j.neuron.2014.07.040.
27 Jorge Luis Borges, *Ficciones* (New York: Grove Press, 1962), 114: Ireneo Funes

> was, let us not forget, almost incapable of general, platonic ideas. It was not only difficult for him to understand that the generic term *dog* embraced so many unlike specimens of differing sizes and different forms; he was disturbed by the fact that a dog at three-fourteen (seen in profile) should have the same name as the dog at three-fifteen (seen from the front).

28 For a modern meditation on this idea, see Bill McKibben, *The Age of Missing Information* (New York: Random House, 2006), which compares the input from nearly a hundred television channels with that from sitting on a mountain over the same 24 hours.
29 Daniel J. Levitin, *The Organized Mind* (New York: Penguin, 2014) calculates this by estimating 5–7 bits of information processed per apperception, with each apperception taking 1/15th of a second; he argues that the burdensome inputs have increased sharply in modern society. In *Silicon Dreams: Information, Man, and Machine*, Robert Lucky posits that the conscious mind cannot process more than 50 bits per second (New York: St. Martins, 1989).

On the website Quora, Brian Roemmele estimates 50, drawing loosely on the work of the great Claude Shannon, www.quora.com/Does-the-mind-record-everything-that-comes-through-our-five-physical-senses; accessed September 7, 2015. See also Marcus E. Raichle, "Two Views of Brain Function," *Trends in Cognitive Sciences* 14, no. 4 (April 2010): 180–90, doi:10.1016/j.tics.2010.01.008, with special emphasis on the processing of visual information.

30 Mihaly Csikszentmihalyi, *Flow and the Foundations of Positive Psychology* (Dordrecht: Springer, 2014), xvi.

31 Alexis de Tocqueville, *Democracy in America*, trans. George Lawrence (New York: Harpers, 2000), 605; vol. 3 ch. 14.

32 Burdick et al., *Digital_Humanities*, 25, briefly discusses the "outsourcing of memory." Among the optimistic recent arguments are Gary Small et al., "Your Brain on Google: Patterns of Cerebral Activation during Internet Searching," *The American Journal of Geriatric Psychiatry* 17, no. 2 (February 2009): 116–26, and Clay Shirky, *Cognitive Surplus: Creativity and Generosity in a Connected Age* (New York: Penguin, 2010); Shirky believes that technology has generated a "cognitive surplus" that could be put to charitable uses. This liberated and hence liberating capacity may help explain the increased tendency toward toleration of differences in clothing, sexuality, and religion indicated by recent surveys of young people in populations with good access to informational technology, although that may be simply an effect of normalizing exposure. In any case, it seems to me questionable whether minds neither trained by memorization nor accessing memories through internally spontaneous associations will in fact be more cognitively productive.

33 Clifford Geertz, "The Growth of Culture and the Evolution of Mind," in *The Interpretation of Cultures: Selected Essays* (New York: Basic Books, 1973), 67.

34 On the Greek crisis of social mobility, see George Thompson, *Aeschylus and Athens* (1941; repr. London: Beekman, 1980), 2.

35 Plato, *Laws;* trans. R. G. Bury; Loeb Classical Library Vol. 187 (Cambridge, MA: Harvard University Press, 1926), 363; bk. 5, 739b–d.

36 Robert Boyd and Peter J. Richerson, *The Origin and Evolution of Cultures* (Oxford University Press, 2005), 380.

37 Alex Mesoudi, *Cultural Evolution: How Darwinian Theory Can Explain Human Culture and Synthesize the Social Sciences* (Chicago: University of Chicago Press, 2011), 5–6. Mesoudi's more recent work explores some interesting variations within, and even contradictions of, this tendency.

38 Richard E. Nisbett and Dov Cohen, *Culture of Honor: The Psychology of Violence in the South* (Boulder, CO: Westview Press, 1996). This tendency may be connected to something in Scotch-Irish heritage, but since the tendency doesn't appear in Scotch-Irish populations elsewhere in the United States, its roots are cultural rather than simply genetic.

39 Robert M. Sapolsky, "Rich Brain, Poor Brain," *Los Angeles Times*, October 18, 2013, www.latimes.com/opinion/op-ed/la-oe-sapolsky-cognitive-load-poverty-20131018-story.html.

40 Cathy O'Neil, *Weapons of Math Destruction: How Big Data Increases Inequality and Threatens Democracy* (New York: Crown, 2016), 69–82.

41 For a good exposition of this claim, see Ellen Condliffe Lagemann, *Liberating Minds: The Case for College in Prison* (New York: Free Press, 2016).

42 Max Weber, *The Protestant Ethic and the Spirit of Capitalism* (London: Unwin Hyman, 1905).

43 For a social-scientific rather than novelistic explication of this problem, see Erving Goffman's classic *The Presentation of Self in Everyday Life* (New York: Anchor, 1959).

44 Writing this paragraph required resigning myself to accusations of transphobia. But assuming that psychopathology is the only reason anyone would question the latest version of an ever-shifting dogma seems a facile *ad hominem* evasion. Many transgender persons certainly recognize that binary genders may be illusory; see Julie L Nagoshi *et alia*, "Deconstructing the complex perceptions of gender roles, gender identity, and sexual orientation among transgender individuals," in *"Feminism & Psychology*, October 10, 2012; http://journals.sagepub.com/doi/abs/10.1177/0959353512461929?-journalCode=fapa; accessed June 6, 2018.

45 Howard Bloom, *The Lucifer Principle: A Scientific Expedition into the Forces of History* (New York: Atlantic Monthly Press, 1997), 147, citing various sources.

46 Brandy Smith and Sharon Home, "Gay, Lesbian, Bisexual and Transgendered Experiences with Earth-Spirited Faith," *Journal of Homosexuality* 52 (2007), 235–48. Ian Waisler and Rhea Wolf, *Queer Astrology Anthology*, 2013, I.ix, asserts that "gays and feminists long found a kinship with astrology and astrological studies." Bonnie J. Morris, *The Disappearing L: Erasure of Lesbian Spaces and Culture*, (Albany, NY: SUNY Press, 2017), 157, comments on lesbians "who self-identified as witches and Tarot readers." See also www.outinperth.com/styleaid-tarot/.

47 Michael Suk-Young Chwe, *Rational Ritual: Culture, Coordination, and Common Knowledge* (Princeton, NJ: Princeton University Press, 2001), 89.

48 Robyn Creswell and Bernard Haykel, "Battle Lines," *The New Yorker*, June 8 and 15, 2015.

49 Robyn Creswell, "Hearing Voices," *The New Yorker*, December 18 and 25, 2017, 107.

50 Robert N. Watson, *Back to Nature* (Philadelphia: University of Pennsylvania Press, 2006), 137–65.

51 James C. Scott, *Weapons of the Weak: Everyday Forms of Peasant Resistance* (New Haven, CT: Yale University Press, 1985).

52 Michael Pollan, *How to Change Your Mind: What the New Science of Psychedelics Teaches Us about Consciousness, Dying, Addiction, Depression, and Transcendence* (New York: Penguin, 2018) describes such an array in the treatment-rooms of the guides for his "trips."

53 Bob Dylan, "I Threw It All Away," *Nashville Skyline*, Columbia Records, 1969.

54 "The Idea of Order at Key West," and "The Man with the Blue Guitar" are quoted from *The Collected Poems of Wallace Stevens* by Wallace Stevens, copyright © 1954 by Wallace Stevens and copyright renewed 1982 by Holly Stevens. Used by permission of Alfred A. Knopf, an imprint of the Knopf Doubleday Publishing Group, a division of Penguin Random House LLC. All rights reserved.

55 Daniel Lord Smail, *On Deep History and the Brain* (Berkeley: University of California Press, 2008), 172.

56 Sigmund Freud, *Civilization and its Discontents*, 1930, trans. James Strachey (New York: Norton, 1962), 33. Near the end of that book (91), Freud flirts with an expansion of this theory in the direction this book takes it:

> If the development of civilization has such a far-reaching similarity to the development of the individual and if it employs the same methods, may we not be justified in reaching the diagnosis that, under the influence of cultural urges, some civilizations, or some epochs of civilization—possibly the whole of mankind—have become 'neurotic'?

57 Freud, *Civilization*, 34.
58 Quoted by Geoffrey Galt Harpham, *The Humanities and the Dream of America* (Chicago: University of Chicago Press, 2011), 86.
59 Cf. Howard Bloom's assertion that "Like genes, memes do not operate in solo, but interlock in the mosaics that form *Weltanshauungs*, worldviews ... generally a vast grid of metaphors starting with the creation of the universe and designed to answer every mystery in life"; *Lucifer Principle*, 131. Bloom, however, assumes that these memeplexes – especially capitalism – are both benign and irresistible.
60 Karl Popper, *The Open Society and its Enemies*, 2nd ed. rev. (Princeton, NJ: Princeton University Press, 1950), 314, makes a similar point.
61 Richerson and Boyd, *Not by Genes*, 167.
62 Morten L. Kringelbach and Kent C. Berridge, "New Pleasure Circuit Found in the Brain," *Scientific American* 307, August, 2012; https://www.scientificamerican.com/article/new-pleasure-circuit-found-brain.
63 Marion Blute, *Darwinian Social Evolution: Solutions to Dilemmas in Cultural and Social Theory* (Cambridge: Cambridge University Press, 2010), 8–9 offers a characteristically wise overview of the many different terms used, in various disciplines, for what is transmitted culturally.

Interchapter: Modern Medievalism

1 Gillian R. Brown and Peter J. Richerson, "Applying Evolutionary Theory to Human Behaviour: Past Differences and Current Debates," *Journal of Bioeconomics* 16, no. 2 (July 2014): 105, doi:10.1007/s10818-013-9166-4, observes that, "Human Behavioural Ecologists start with the expectation that behaviour will be optimal, while Evolutionary Psychologists emphasize cases of 'mis-match' between modern environments and domain-specific, evolved psychological mechanisms."
2 Tocqueville, *Democracy*, 49; vol. 1, Chapter 2.
3 William Deresiewicz, *Excellent Sheep: The Miseducation of the American Elite and the Way to a Meaningful Life* (New York: Free Press, 2014).
4 Geoffrey Hosking, *The First Socialist Society: A History of the Soviet Union from Within* (Cambridge: Harvard University Press, 1985), 168–9.
5 Creswell and Haykel, "Battle Lines."
6 Carol Symes, "Medievalism, White Supremacy, and the Historian's Craft," *AHA Today* (blog), November 2, 2017, http://blog.historians.org/2017/11/medievalism-white-supremacy-historians-craft/.

Chapter 2

1 Stanislaw Lem, *Imaginary Magnitude*, trans. Mark E. Heine (New York: Harcourt Brace, 1984), 130–31. Copyright 1981 by Stanislaw Lem, Krakow. English translation copyright 1984 by Houghton Mifflin Harcourt Publishing Company. All rights reserved.
2 Justin L. Barrett, "Exploring the Natural Foundations of Religion," *Trends in Cognitive Sciences* 4, no. 1 (January 2000): 29–34, cited in Daniel C. Dennett, *Breaking the Spell: Religion as a Natural Phenomenon* (New York: Penguin, 2007), 109.
3 Brian Boyd, *On the Origin of Stories: Evolution, Cognition, and Fiction* (Cambridge, MA: Harvard University Press, 2009), 137; see also Stewart Guthrie, *Faces in the Clouds: A New Theory of Religion* (New York: Oxford University Press, 1995), on the underlying causes of anthropomorphizing reflexes, especially in religion.

4 For example, *The Hand That Rocks the Cradle*, dir. Curtis Hanson (1992), *My Daughter's Keeper*, dir. Heinrich Dahms, and *Don't Tell Mom the Babysitter's Dead*, dir. Stephen Herek (both 1991 – a year that also featured the similarly themed video game *The Adventures of Willy Beamish*), *The Guardian*, dir. William Friedkin (1990), *Postcards from the Edge*, dir. Mike Nichols (1990), *Fatal Attraction*, dir. Adrian Lyne (1987), *Baby Boom*, dir. Charles Shyer (1987), and *Mr. Mom*, dir. Stan Dragoti (1983).

5 Hugh Wilford, *The Mighty Wurlitzer: How the CIA Played America* (Cambridge, MA: Harvard University Press, 2009).

6 This should not be confused with Jung's "collective unconscious," which, contrary to popular belief, was a structural theory of personal psychology akin to Kant's theory of human epistemology.

7 Thomas Picketty, *Capital in the Twenty-First Century* (Cambridge, MA: Belknap, 2013).

8 This history was exposed by a front-page investigative piece in the *Los Angeles Times*; Sara Jerving et al., "What Exxon Knew about Warming in the Arctic," *Los Angeles Times*, October 11, 2015.

9 Popper, *Open Society*, 287–88, provides a strong critique of the widespread belief that social malfunctions are "the result of the direct design by some powerful individuals and groups"; Popper acknowledges that conspiracies do occur, but notes that most of them fail.

10 Dennett, *Breaking the Spell*, 78.

11 Michel Foucault, *Discipline and Punish: The Birth of the Prison*, trans. Alan Sheridan (New York: Pantheon, 1977).

12 Despite the allure of the acronym "ANT," I will not pursue this claim into Actor Network Theory, which rightly sees the world as intricately interactive, but compromises the sense of agency necessary to making differences on behalf of our values. Julian Jaynes's engagingly ambitious *The Origin of Consciousness in the Breakdown of the Bicameral Mind* (1976; Boston: Mariner, 2000) speculates that, until some 3,000 years ago, human beings heard – as absolute external authority – a voice of instruction in one side of their brains that was actually produced in the other side. The instructions of culture camouflaged as fundamental truth still seem to me to reach most human minds in a comparable way.

13 Robert Dorit, "All Things Small and Great," *The American Scientist* 96, no. 4 (July–August 2008): 284–86. Earlier studies had indicated about ten non-self cells for every self cell; see Ron Sender, Shai Fuchs, and Ron Milo, "Are We Really Vastly Outnumbered? Revisiting the Ration of Bacterial to Host Cells in Humans," *Cell* 164, no. 3 (January 2016): 337–40, doi:10.1016/j.cell.2016.01.013.

14 A century ago, Alfred Kroeber's description of human society as a determinative "superorganism" drew cogent objections from Alexander Goldenweiser, "The Autonomy of the Social," and Edward Sapir, "The Status of Washo," in *American Anthropologist* 19, no. 3 (July–September 1917): 447–50. See also the work of Alfred Schütz, as he attempts a phenomenological reading of human experience that mediates the individual and the collective.

15 Boyd, *Origin of Stories*, 161.

16 Karen Armstrong, *Fields of Blood: Religion and the History of Violence* (New York: Anchor, 2014), mounts a strong defense of religion against the charge that it has been the main source of warfare. The evidence that religion has been at least a key rationale for a lot of sectarian violence remains strong, however.

17 Richerson and Boyd, *Not by Genes*, 211.

18 McKinnon, *Neo-Liberal Genetics*, 124–26, is typical of this dismissiveness, choosing simplistic, sexist, and wildly universalizing statements by a few evolutionary psychologists as her straw-men, and mocking (in a manner

disquietingly reminiscent of Cartesian vivisectionists) as revealingly anthro-pomorphic the application of terms such as "decide," "solves the problem," and "preferences," to a female weaverbird's mate selection, without explaining what other language would justly describe these acts of sexual selection.

19 This distinction has been studied under the concept of "r/K selection," although the notion of a neat binary between the two strategies has been effectively challenged. The technical term for offspring needing such extended nurture is "altricial."

20 Bert Hölldobler and E. O. Wilson, *The Superorganism: The Beauty, Elegance, and Strangeness of Insect Societies* (New York: Norton, 2009), 58.

21 Hölldobler and Wilson, *The Superorganism*, 136.

22 Hölldobler and Wilson, *The Superorganism*, 250.

23 Hölldobler and Wilson, *The Superorganism*, 80.

24 Kathleen D. Vohs et al., "Decision Fatigue Exhausts Self-Regulatory Resources", www.psychologytoday.com/sites/default/files/attachments/584/decision200602-15vohs.pdf.

25 For a lively philosophical and historical critique of what he calls (on p. 42) "this twelve-thousand-year machine called *agrilogistics*," see Timothy Morton, *Dark Ecology: For a Logic of Future Coexistence* (New York: Columbia University Press, 2016), 38–59.

26 Thomas D. Seeley, *The Wisdom of the Hive: The Social Physiology of Honey Bee Colonies* (Cambridge, MA: Harvard University Press, 1995), 263–65. See also Olli J. Loukola et al., "Bumblebees Show Cognitive Flexibility by Improving on an Observed Complex Behavior," *Science* 355, no. 6327 (February 24, 2017): 833–36, doi:10.1126/science.aag2360.

27 Freud, *Civilization*, 43.

28 Hölldobler and Wilson, *The Superorganism*, 58.

29 Richard Dawkins, *The Selfish Gene* (New York: Oxford University Press, 1989).

30 Alfred Kroeber is the classic voice for the view that cultures create geniuses, rather than vice versa. See Dean Keith Simonton, *Greatness: Who Makes History and Why* (New York: The Guilford Press, 1994).

31 Thomas Schelling, "Dynamic Models of Segregation," *Journal of Mathematical Sociology* 1, no. 2 (1971): 143–86.

32 Jonathan Rauch, "Seeing Around Corners," *The Atlantic*, April, 2002. Evolutionary biologists such as Regis Ferrière (at the University of Arizona) have undertaken a major research project based on understanding cells as a population, and thence constructing models of the co-evolution of animals and their ambient ecology. My thought-experiment here is almost the converse: understanding a population as cells.

33 Richard Rothstein, *The Color of Law: A Forgotten History of How Our Government Segregated America* (New York: Liveright, 2017).

34 For a current political affirmation of this function, see Amanda Taub, "How 'Islands of Honesty' Can Crush a System of Corruption," *New York Times*, December 9, 2016.

35 Kim Lane Scheppele, "Responses and Discussion," in *The Humanities and Public Life*, eds. Peter Brooks with Hilary Jewett (New York: Fordham University Press, 2014), 124.

36 James C. Scott, *Domination and the Arts of Resistance* (New Haven, CT: Yale University Press, 1990), 198–204.

37 This is wonderfully explicated in Dana Cairns Watson, *Gertrude Stein and the Essence of What Happens* (Nashville, TN: Vanderbilt University Press, 2005), 153–62.

38 David L. Hull, "Taking Memetics Seriously: Memetics Will Be What We Make It," in *Darwinizing Culture: The Status of Memetics as a Science*, ed. Robert Aunger (New York: Oxford University Press, 2001), 61.

39 David Quammen, *Spillover: Animal Infections and the Next Human Pandemic* (New York: Norton, 2012), 518–19.
40 Martha C. Nussbaum, *Not for Profit: Why Democracy Needs the Humanities* (Princeton: Princeton University Press, 2010), 41, citing the work of Solomon Asch.
41 David Zucchino, "An Afghan Uprising of One," *Los Angeles Times*, June 2, 2013, 1.
42 Hannah Arendt, *The Human Condition*, 2nd ed. (Chicago, IL: University of Chicago Press, 1998), 190.
43 "Biological Altruism," *Stanford Encyclopedia of Philosophy*, last revised July 21, 2013, http://plato.stanford.edu/entries/altruism-biological/.
44 Eliot, *Middlemarch*; bk. 8; 371.
45 Cass R. Sunstein, "Social Norms and Social Roles," *Program in Law and Economics Working Paper*, no. 36 (1996), doi:10.2307/1123430.
46 Walt Whitman, from *The Complete Prose Works of Walt Whitman* (New York: Knickerbocker Press, 1902), Vol. 2, 82.

Interchapter: Software is Hard on Humanity

1 Philip Cordes and Michael Hülsman, "Self-Healing Supply Networks: A Complex Adaptive Systems Perspective," in *Supply Chain Safety Management: Security and Robustness in Logistics*, eds. Michael Eßig, Michael Hülsmann, Eva-Maria Kern, and Stephan Klein-Schmeink (Heidelberg: Springer, 2013), 227; see also 218, on the way Complex Adaptive Logistics Systems "enable logistics objects to interact with each other and to render decisions on their own, without having to ask a central management"; so "self-organizing logistics system structures can be created, which might contribute to trigger self-healing processes and hence, increase the system's robustness." Such systems are increasingly designed to enable their "autonomous recovery after the supply network faces a targeted attack or random damage" (219).

Chapter 3

1 Freud, *Civilization*, 88. Reproduced by permission of The Marsh Agency Ltd on behalf of Sigmund Freud Copyrights, for electronic distribution, and by permission of W.W. Norton & Company, Inc., for print distribution.
2 It is important to remember that "Cultural systems are ... functionally integrated entities, and they occupy a middle ground between a super-organism and an aggregate, a locus that is difficult to conceptualize if one is wedded to a traditional population-genetics-based metaphor"; Yuval Laor and Eva Jablonka, "The Evolution and Development of Culture," review of *Cultural Evolution: How Darwinian Theory Can Explain Human Culture and Synthesize the Social Sciences*, by Alex Mesoudi, *History and Theory* 52, no. 2 (May 2013): 295.
3 Charles Darwin, *The Descent of Man, and Selection in Relation to Sex* (London: J. Murray, 1871; repr. Princeton University Press, 2008), 1:166. Cf. Julian H. Steward, *Theory of Culture Change: The Methodology of Multilinear Evolution* (Urbana: University of Illinois Press, 1955), 37:

> Cultures do, of course, tend to perpetuate themselves, and change may be slow .... But over the millennia cultures in different environments have changed tremendously, and these changes are basically traceable to new adaptations required by changing technology and productive arrangements.

4 http://theconversation.com/natural-selection-in-black-and-white-how-industrial-pollution-changed-moths-43061; accessed June 3, 2018.

5 Kathleen McAuliffe, *This Is Your Brain on Parasites: How Tiny Creatures Manipulate Our Behavior and Shape Society* (Boston, MA: Houghton Mifflin, 2016), 5.

6 Zimmer, Carl, "Our Microbiome May Be Looking Out for Itself," *New York Times*, August 14, 2014. www.nytimes.com/2014/08/14/science/our-microbiome-may-be-looking-out-for-itself.html.

7 Albert Einstein, "What Life Means to Einstein: An Interview by George Sylvester Viereck," *The Saturday Evening Post* (October 26, 1929), 117. Yuval Noah Harari, *Sapiens: A Brief History of Humankind* (New York: HarperCollins, 2015), 243, comments that

> postmodernist thinkers describe nationalism as a deadly plague that spread throughout the world in the nineteenth and twentieth centuries, causing wars, oppression, hate and genocide. The moment people in one country were infected with it, those in neighbouring countries were also likely to catch the virus. The nationalist virus presented itself as being beneficial for humans, yet it has been beneficial mainly to itself.

8 Timothy Snyder, *Bloodlands: Europe between Hitler and Stalin* (New York: Basic Books, 2012).

9 Yascha Mounk, *The People versus Democracy: Why Our Freedom Is in Danger and How to Save It* (Cambridge, MA: Harvard University Press, 2018).

10 William E. Connolly, *A World of Becoming* (Durham, NC: Duke University Press, 2011), 172.

11 Arlie Russell Hochschild, *Strangers in Their Own Land: Anger and Mourning on the American Right* (New York: The New Press, 2016) reports amazing interviews of this kind: Southern working-class conservatives who have been painfully forced to recognize environmental horrors and claim to care about them, but refuse to endorse any government control of the polluters.

12 Lynn Stout, *The Shareholder Value Myth: How Putting Shareholders First Harms Investors, Corporations, and the Public* (San Francisco, CA: Berrett-Koehler, 2012).

13 Andrew Jacobs and Matt Richtel, "How Big Business Got Brazil Hooked on Junk Food," *New York Times*, September 17, 2017.

14 Lee Drutman, *The Business of America Is Lobbying: How Corporations Became Politicized and Politics Became More Corporate* (New York: Oxford University Press, 2016), makes this case compellingly.

15 Martin Gilens and Benjamin I. Page, "Testing Theories of American Politics: Elites, Interest Groups, and Average Citizens," Abstract. *Perspectives on Politics* 12, no. 3 (September 2014): 564–81.

16 Jane Mayer, *Dark Money: The Hidden History of the Billionaires Behind the Rise of the Radical Right* (New York: Doubleday, 2016).

17 David Hawkes, *Idols of the Marketplace: Idolatry and Commodity Fetishism in English Literature, 1580–1680* (New York: Palgrave, 2001).

18 Richerson and Boyd, *Not by Genes*, 151.

19 M. Berdoy, J. P. Webster, and D. W. Macdonald, "Fatal Attraction in Rats Infected with *Toxoplasma gondii*," *Proceedings of the Royal Society B: Biological Sciences* 267, no. 1452 (August 2000): 1591–94, doi:10.1098/rspb.2000.1182.

20 Smail, *Deep History*, 170–71.

21 Bob Yirka, "Evidence suggests Neanderthals took to boats before modern humans," https://phys.org/news/2012-03-evidence-neanderthals-boats-

modern-humans.html; accessed June 10, 2018. Also, www.pbs.org/wgbh/nova/evolution/defy-stereotypes.html; and www.smithsonianmag.com/smart-news/neanderthals-may-have-practiced-the-ancient-art-of-interior-design-180948094/.

22 McAuliffe, *This Is Your Brain*, 14.

23 Brown and Richerson, "Applying Evolutionary Behaviour," 111.

24 Stephen Shennan, *Genes, Memes and Human History: Darwinian Archaeology and Cultural Evolution* (London: Thames and Hudson, 2002), 46, observes that "in the field of fashion in particular, 'viral marketing' is now being adopted as a sales tool, with attractive individuals being seeded as points of contagion."

25 Mark Edmundson suggests this perspective in *Self and Soul: A Defense of Ideals* (Cambridge, MA: Harvard University Press, 2015) although elsewhere he takes a more positive view of football.

26 Smail, *Deep History*, argues that Christianity forbids some self-soothing behaviors such as masturbation and alcohol consumption because they reduce the church's power to command loyalty as the one source for such stress-relief. My book is complementary to Smail's. He is mostly interested in retrieving pre-history, whereas I am mostly interested in explaining the past 500 years of human history. He is focused on the ways human history is shaped by the craving for new stimulations. I am looking at the opposite factor: the way human history is shaped by an aversion to exciting novelties.

27 Scott Atran, *In Gods We Trust: The Evolutionary Landscape of Religion* (New York and Oxford: Oxford University Press, 2002).

28 Scott Atran, *Talking to the Enemy: Sacred Values, Violent Extremism, and What It Means to Be Human* (New York: Penguin, 2011), xiii.

29 Karl Marx, "The German Ideology" in *Knowledge and Postmodernism in Historical Perspective*, ed. Joyce Oldham Appleby et al. (Hove: Psychology Press, 1996), 184.

30 Popper, *Open Society*, 1.

31 See Johann Hari, "What's Really Causing the Prescription Drug Crisis," *Los Angeles Times*, January 15, 2017, A18.

32 Margaret Talbot, "The Addicts Next Door," *The New Yorker*, June 5 & 12, 2017.

33 The main commonalty among Americans who become Islamic jihadis is a "need for stability," according to Showtime's 2017 documentary. Terrorism expert and former FBI special agent Ali Soufan points out that military defeats of ISIS only deflect the jihad into terrorism in other regions "If we don't change the narrative or kill the ideology"; Ali Lorraine, "Inside the Minds of U.S. Jihadis," *Los Angeles Times*, March 25, 2017, E1 and E8.

34 Kimberlé W. Crenshaw, "Mapping the Margins: Intersectionality, Identity Politics, and Violence against Women of Color," *Stanford Law Review* 43, no. 6 (July 1991): 1241–99.

35 The term was coined by William H. Calvin, "The Brain as a Darwin Machine," *Nature* 330 (1987): 33–34, to describe non-biological entities that nonetheless develop through a competition among multiple variants for survival and reproduction.

36 On this and other aspects of women's liberation that seem to have played into the hands of neoliberal capitalism, see Nancy Fraser, "How Feminism Became Capitalism's Handmaiden – And How to Reclaim It," *The Guardian*, October 14, 2013, www.theguardian.com/commentisfree/2013/oct/14/feminism-capitalist-handmaiden-neoliberal.

37 Neil Postman, *Amusing Ourselves to Death: Public Discourse in the Age of Show Business* (New York: Penguin, 1986), vii and 111.

38 Tocqueville, *Democracy*, 691; bk. 4, ch. 6.

39 Oscar Wilde, "The Soul of Man under Socialism," in *Collected Works of Oscar Wilde* (Ware, Hertfordshire: Wordsworth Editions, 2007), 1049.

40 Herbert Marcuse, *One-Dimensional Man* (1964; rpt. New York: Routledge Classics, 2002), 3–16.

41 Richard W. Byrne and Andrew Whiten, *Machiavellian Intelligence: Social Expertise and the Evolution of Intellect in Monkeys, Apes, and Humans* (New York: Oxford University Press, 1988), 9; quoted in Michael Carrithers, "Why Humans Have Cultures," *Man*, n. s., 25, no. 2 (June 1990): 195.

42 McAuliffe, *This Is Your Brain*, 36, describes the way parasites who need to get into the gut of egrets make a killifish "so mellow that it doesn't get anxious in a situation that should make the animal fearful." Digger wasps paralyze the crickets on which their offspring will eventually feed: the crickets become their own preservative.

43 Carl Zimmer, "Our Microbiome." Michael Pollan, *The Omnivore's Dilemma: A Natural History of Four Meals* (New York: Penguin, 2006). See also Harari, *Sapiens*, 80, on the way "a handful of plant species, including wheat, rice and potatoes ... domesticated *Homo sapiens*, rather than vice versa."

44 "The Thing" by William Carlos Williams, from THE COLLECTED POEMS: VOLUME II, 1939–1962, copyright 1948, 1962 by William Carlos Williams. Reprinted by permission of New Directions Publishing Corp.

45 Jaron Lanier, *You Are Not a Gadget* (New York: Knopf, 2011), 128.

46 Alexander Stille, "Holy Orders," *New Yorker*, September 14, 2015, 60.

47 Widely practiced religions such as Hinduism and Buddhism instead offer reincarnation and/or a suggestion that personal extinction is ultimately desirable.

48 Joseph Henrich, Edward Slingerland, and Ara Norenzayan, "The Evolution of Prosocial Religions," in *Cultural Evolution: Society, Technology, Language, and Religion*, ed. Peter J. Richerson and Morten H. Christiansen (Cambridge, MA: MIT Press, 2013), 340 and 336–340.

49 Henrich, Slingerland, and Norenzayan, "Evolution of Prosocial Religions," 340.

50 On ecological stabilization, see the work of Roy Rappaport. On the subjugation of the Dinka, see Raymond C. Kelly, *The Nuer Conquest: The Structure and Development of an Expansionist System* (Ann Arbor: University of Michigan Press, 1985).

51 Durham, *Coevolution*.

52 Robert Boyd, Peter J. Richerson, and Joseph Henrich, "The Cultural Evolution of Technology: Facts and Theories," in Richerson and Christiansen, *Cultural Evolution*, 127.

53 Kevin N. Laland, *Darwin's Unfinished Symphony: How Culture Made the Human Mind* (Princeton, NJ: Princeton University Press, 2017), 215–16, and Richerson and Boyd, *Not by Genes*, 191–92.

54 Kim Sterelny, *The Evolved Apprentice: How Evolution Made Humans Unique* (Cambridge, MA: MIT Press, 2012), offers a deep analysis of this process. It is also the "secret" of Henrich's *Secret of Our Success*.

55 Cf. Brown and Richerson, "Applying Evolutionary Theory," 119–20: "social institutions usually include a system of rewards that favour those who conform to the institution and punishments for those who don't, damping down individual-level variation within groups."

56 Gellner, *Plough, Sword and Book*, 253.

57 The philosopher Robert Brandon argues that "No Darwinian account of the evolution of any lineage of organisms entirely escapes being a how-possibly explanation," and so the evolutionary biologists scoffing at "just-so stories" are vulnerable to the *tu quoque* reply — the ancient version of "I know you are, so what am I?"; see Richerson and Boyd, *Not by Genes*, 127.

58 Anthony Gottlieb, "It Ain't Necessarily So," *The New Yorker*, September 17, 2012, 87.

59 Gottlieb, "It Ain't Necessarily So," 89.

60 Dennett, *Breaking the Spell*, 170.

61 David Sloan Wilson, *Darwin's Cathedral: Evolution, Religion, and the Nature of Society* (Chicago: University of Chicago Press, 2002), explores this balance perceptively. J. A. Coyne, "They Shall Have Their Rewards on Earth, Too," *Times Literary Supplement*, November 1, 2002, 31, challenges Wilson's argument on the grounds that many religious practices seem unlikely to serve even the group-selection version of evolution on which Wilson's claim depends. I believe that the selfishness of meme-complexes can explain these seemingly maladaptive aspects of cultural institutions.

62 Compare George Plimpton's recurrent description, in *The Bogey Man: A Month on the PGA Tour* (New York: HarperCollins, 1968), of an over-coached American golfer trying to achieve a natural swing while hearing Japanese admirals screaming a cacophony of commands in his head.

63 "Cultural adaptations, like all adaptations, can, and perhaps usually eventually do, become maladaptive"; Roy Rappaport, quoted by Brian Hoey and Tom Fricke, "From Sweet Potatoes to God Almighty: Roy Rappaport on Being a Hedgehog," *American Ethnologist* 34, no. 3 (2007): 581–99.

64 The ground for Mesoudi's work in this regard was prepared by the technical research in Luigi Luca Cavalli-Sforza and Marcus W. Feldman, *Cultural Transmission and Evolution: A Quantitative Approach* (Princeton: Princeton University Press, 1991) and Robert Boyd and Peter J. Richerson, *Culture and the Evolutionary Process* (Chicago, IL: University of Chicago Press, 1985).

65 Laor and Jablonka, "Evolution and Development of Culture," 290–99; see also Robert Boyd, "Cultural Evolution Comes of Age," review of *Cultural Evolution: How Darwinian Theory Can Explain Human Culture and Synthesize the Social Sciences*, by Alex Mesoudi; *Trends in Ecology & Evolution* 27, no. 8 (August 2012): 419.

66 In addition to scholars cited elsewhere, and with apologies to those whose work I have wrongly neglected, consider the work of Lisa Zunshine and Simon Kirby.

67 Joseph Fracchia and Richard Lewontin, "Does Culture Evolve?" *History and Theory* 38 (1999): 52–78; see also the clarifying responses of Garry Runciman in the same journal.

68 On the Darwinian aspects of the evolution of languages, see for example William Croft, "Evolutionary Linguistics," *Annual Review of Anthropology* 37 (2008): 219–34; and Roger Lass, *How Languages Emerge* (Cambridge: Cambridge University Press, 2006).

69 Morten H. Christiansen and Nick Chater, "Language as Shaped by the Brain," *Behavioural and Brain Sciences* 31 (2008): 489–558; quoted in Plotkin, *Evolutionary Worlds*, 116.

70 Darwin, *Descent of Man*, 1:59–61.

71 Christopher Shea, "The New Science of the Birth and Death of Words," *Wall Street Journal*, March 17, 2012; based on Alexander M. Petersen et al., "Statistical Laws Governing Fluctuations in Word Use from Word

Birth to Word Death," *Scientific Reports* 2, no. 313 (2012), doi:10.1038/srep00313.

72 Robert N. Watson, "Shakespeare's New Words," *Shakespeare Survey* 65 (2012): 358–77, and "Coining Words on the Elizabethan and Jacobean Stage," *Philological Quarterly* 88 (2009): 49–75.

73 Gary Taylor, *Cultural Selection: Why Some Achievements Survive the Test of Time and Others Don't* (New York: Basic Books, 1996).

74 Fracchia and Lewontin, "Does Culture Evolve?" 63–64.

75 Hull, 49:

> I want to encourage memeticists to ignore the in-principle objections that have been raised to memetics no matter how cogent they may turn out to be and proceed to develop their theory in the context of attempts to test it.

76 Shennan, *Genes, Memes and Human History*, 56–57.

77 Shennan, *Genes, Memes and Human History*, 264.

78 Richerson and Boyd, *Not by Genes*, 51.

79 Richerson and Boyd, *Not by Genes*, 53.

80 Richerson and Boyd, *Not by Genes*, 60.

81 Richerson and Boyd, *Not by Genes*, 203–4.

82 Dan Sperber, *Explaining Culture: A Naturalistic Approach* (Oxford: Blackwell, 1996).

83 Joseph Carroll, *Reading Human Nature: Literary Darwinism in Theory and Practice* (Albany, NY: SUNY Press, 2001), 45.

84 Richerson and Boyd, *Not by Genes*, 156–57, 189, and 201.

85 Henrich, *Secret of Our Success*, 144.

86 Friedrich Nietzsche, *Beyond Good and Evil* (1886), trans. Walter Kaufman (New York: Vintage, 1989): 203.

87 Louis Menand, *The Metaphysical Club: A Story of Ideas in America* (New York: Farrar, Straus, 2002), xi–xii.

88 Colin McGinn, "The Problem of Philosophy," *Philosophical Studies* 76 (1994): 133–56.

89 Sigmund Freud, *Standard Edition of the Complete Psychological Works of Sigmund Freud*, eds. James Strachey et al. (London: Hogarth Press, 1953–74), 17:261.

90 Harari, *Sapiens*, 166.

91 Marshall McLuhan, *From Cliché to Archetype* (New York: Penguin, 1970), 9.

92 Bill McKibben, *The End of Nature* (1989; repr., New York: Random House, 2006).

93 On gossip as a social body's defense mechanism, see David Sloan Wilson, *Evolution for Everyone: How Darwin's Theory Can Change the Way We Think about Our Lives* (New York: Delta, 2007), 160. On "digital Maoism," see Lanier, 79–80.

94 McKinnon, *Neo-Liberal Genetics*, 30–31, discusses the flaws in many such claims.

95 Ralph J. Hexter, "Conquering Obstacles to Kingdom and Fate: The Ethics of Reading and the University Administrator," in Brooks, 89.

96 Kevin N. Laland and John Odling-Smee, "The Evolution of the Meme," in Aunger, *Darwinizing Culture*, 129.

97 Michelle Scalise Sugiyama, "Narrative Theory and Function: Why Evolution Matters," *Philosophy and Literature* 25, no. 2 (2001): 238 and 233–50 passim.

98 Brown and Richerson, "Applying Evolutionary Theory," 113–14.

99 David Sloan Wilson, "Evolutionary Social Constructivism," in *The Literary Animal: Evolution and the Nature of Narrative*, eds. Jonathan Gottschall, David Sloan Wilson, E. O. Wilson and Frederick C. Crews (Evanston, IL: Northwestern University Press, 2005), 27.

100 Matthew Fisher, *Scribal Authorship and the Writing of History in Medieval England* (Columbus: Ohio State University Press, 2012), has painstakingly shown that medieval scribes were not mere copyists, but imposed ideological choices on their selections and alterations of received texts.

101 Bernice Eiduson, *Scientists: Their Psychological World* (New York: Basic, 1962). Quoted in Richard Rhodes, *The Making of the Atomic Bomb* (New York: Simon and Schuster, 2012), 151.

102 Charles Perreault, "The Pace of Cultural Evolution," *PLoS ONE* 7, no. 9 (2012): e45150. doi:10.1371/journal.pone.0045150; www.plosone.org/article/info%3Adoi%2F10.1371%2Fjournal.pone.0045150.

103 Elizabeth Culotta, "Did Modern Humans Get Smart or Just Get Together?" *Science* 328, no. 5975 (April 9, 2010): 164, doi:10.1126/science.328.5975.164. H. Clark Barrett, via personal communication, passed along current research findings concerning the Shuar people. Joseph Henrich's research on Tasmania suggests that some version of genetic drift reduces the diversity of ideas in small populations.

104 Boyd and Richerson, *Origin and Evolution*, 379.

105 Barkow, Tooby, and Cosmides, *The Adapted Mind*, 24.

106 Bradd Shore, *Culture in Mind: Cognition, Culture, and the Problem of Meaning* (New York: Oxford University Press, 1996), studies an impressive range of instances in support of his integrative theory.

107 Kim Sterelny, *Thought in a Hostile World: The Evolution of Human Cognition* (London: Blackwell, 2003).

108 Brown and Richerson, "Applying Evolutionary Theory," 116.

109 Plotkin, *Evolutionary Worlds*, 110.

110 Max Ehrenfreund, "A Majority of Millennials Now Reject Capitalism, Poll Shows," *The Washington Post*, April 26, 2016, www.washingtonpost.com/news/wonk/wp/2016/04/26/a-majority-of-millennials-now-reject-capitalism-poll-shows/; Chris McGreal, "'The S-word': How Young Americans Fell in Love with Socialism," *The Guardian*, September 2, 2017, www.theguardian.com/us-news/2017/sep/02/socialism-young-americans-bernie-sanders.

111 https://jacobinmag.com/2018/06/millennials-unions-corporations-opinion-class-struggle.

Interchapter: The Crow Tribe in Flight

1 Jonathan Lear, *Radical Hope: Ethics in the Face of Cultural Devastation* (Cambridge, MA: Harvard University Press, 2006), 16–17.

2 Lear, *Radical Hope*, 38.

3 Lear, *Radical Hope*, 32.

4 Lear, *Radical Hope*, 51.

5 Lear, *Radical Hope*, 70–71.

Chapter 4

1 Cf. Gellner, *Plow, Sword and Book*, 246: "In a society based on a generalized, school-transmitted 'high' (literate) culture, a man's capacity to identify with communities defined by such high cultures becomes the most important factor in his life."

2 Harari, *Sapiens*, 27.

3 Ian Tattersall, *The Monkey in the Mirror: Essays on the Science of What Makes Us Human* (New York: Mariner Books, 2003), 126. Harari, 34, similarly argues that the Neanderthals would have won a battle of the bodies, but were beaten by this aspect of Cro-Magnon mentalities.

4 Walt Whitman, *Democratic Vistas*, in *Complete Prose Works* (Boston: Small, Maynard & Company, 1902), 231, 202, 200.

5 Harari, *Sapiens*, 27.

6 Calvert Watkins, *How to Kill a Dragon: Aspects of Indo-European Poetics* (New York: Oxford University Press, 1995).

7 Seamus Heaney, *The Government of the Tongue* (New York: Farrar Straus, 1990), 107.

8 Gerald M. Edelman and Vernon B. Mountcastle, *The Mindful Brain: Cortical Organization and the Group-Selective Theory of Higher Brain Function* (Cambridge, MA: MIT Press, 1978).

9 J. R. R. Tolkien, *The History of Middle-earth*, ed. Christopher Tolkien, vol. 10, *Morgoth's Ring* (Boston, MA: Houghton, 1993), 396.

10 William E. Connolly, *Neuropolitics: Thinking, Culture, Speed* (Minneapolis: University of Minnesota Press, 2002), 64. Cf. William James, *Principles of Psychology* (New York: Dover, 1890), 1:288. See also Arthur F. Kinney, *Shakespeare and Cognition: Aristotle's Legacy and Shakespearean Drama* (New York: Routledge, 2006), 16, which notes that only about 10% of data received by the eye is actually transmitted to the active mind.

11 Pollan, *How to Change*.

12 Cf. Morton's more poetic formulation: "Dark ecology thinks the truth of death, a massive cognitive relief that if integrated into social form would embody nonviolence," *Dark Ecology*, 161.

13 Matthew Hutson, "What Is Art?" *The Atlantic*, July/August 2014, 28; citing Landau et al., "Windows Into Nothingness," *Journal of Personality and Social Psychology* 90, no. 6 (June 2006): 879–92.

14 This is the view of Lactantius in the 4th century AD, drawing on Lucretius, and Augustine came to support it, as did Aquinas and most modern commentators, although a tradition from Cicero prefers an etymology through *relegere*, meaning, to treat carefully, with a nod toward the re-reading of sacred texts.

15 Tocqueville, *Democracy*, 445; bk. 1, ch. 5.

16 Gellner, *Plow, Sword and Book*, 107.

17 Gellner, *Plow, Sword and Book*, 75.

18 Popper, *Open Society*, makes clear that scientists no less than people in the arts and humanities can be forces for a healthy kind of open consciousness. The classic statement of this imperative for cooperation is C. P. Snow's 1959 *The Two Cultures*, more recently picked up by E. O. Wilson's 1998 *Consilience*.

19 John Tooby and Leda Cosmides, "Does Beauty Build Adapted Minds?" in *Evolution, Literature, and Film: A Reader*, eds. Brian Boyd, Joseph Carroll, and Jonathan Gottschall (New York: Columbia University Press, 2010), 183.

20 Mark Swed, "Is Streaming a Threat to Music?" *Los Angeles Times*, August 9, 2015, F5. David Levitin, *This Is Your Brain on Music* (New York: Dutton, 2006), explores this in more depth.

21 On these functions of neuroplasticity, Lisa Wong and Robert Viagas, *Scales to Scalpels: Doctors Who Practice the Healing Arts of Music and Medicine* (New York: Pegasus, 2012).

22 Cf. Arnold H. Modell, *Imagination and the Meaningful Brain* (Boston, MA: MIT Press, 2006), on the way music and temporality bond mothers and children, and 168–69 on the contribution of music and dance to the building of life-long communities. See also Wilson, *Evolution for Everyone*, 182–85.

23 Karl Popper, "Natural Selection and the Emergence of Mind" (lecture, Darwin College, Cambridge, November 8, 1977), www.informationphilosopher. com/solutions/philosophers/popper/natural_selection_and_the_emergence_ of_mind.html.

24 R. A. Foley, "How Useful Is the Culture Concept in Early Hominid Studies?" in *Human Behaviour*, ed. Foley, 31, notes that "The principal advantage of a simulation programme is that it answers 'what if' questions very rapidly and at very low cost and risk."

25 Derek Parfit, *Reasons and persons* (Oxford: Oxford University Press, 1986).

26 Maja Djikic, Keith Oatley, and Mihnea C. Moldoveanua, "Opening the Closed Mind: The Effect of Exposure to Literature on the Need for Closure," *Creativity Research Journal* 25, no. 2 (2013): 150.

27 Elaine Scarry, "Poetry, Injury, and the Ethics of Reading," in *Humanities*, ed. Brooks, 41; citing Steven Pinker, *The Better Angels of Our Nature: Why Violence Has Declined* (New York: Penguin, 2011).

28 Keith Oatley, Raymond A. Mar, and Maja Djikic, "The Psychology of Fiction: Present and Future," in *Cognitive Literary Studies: Current Themes and New Directions*, eds. Isabel Jaén and Julien Jacques Simon (Austin: University of Texas Press), 242–44.

29 Scheppele, "Responses and Discussion," 146.

30 Mitchum Huehls, *After Critique: Twenty-First-Century Fiction in a Neoliberal Age* (New York: Oxford University Press, 2016), describes a "neoliberal circle" in which attempts to criticize that system find themselves relying on values that the system has already subsumed.

31 Naomi Klein, *This Changes Everything: Capitalism vs. the Climate* (New York: Simon & Schuster, 2014), makes this point compellingly.

32 John Muir, "The Hetch Hetchy Valley," *Sierra Club Bulletin* 6, no. 4 (1908).

33 Brian Boyd, *Why Lyrics Last: Evolution, Cognition, and Shakespeare's Sonnets* (Cambridge, MA: Harvard University Press, 2012).

34 See, for example, the work of Rappaport, as discussed by Richard Parmentier, "Untitled," *Chicago Journals* 43, no. 2 (2003): 162–64.

35 Vernon Watkins, *Poems for Dylan* (Wales: Gomer Press, 2003), ix and vii ix, reprinting the obituary published in the *Times* November 10, 1953.

36 Kay Redfield Jamison, *Robert Lowell: Setting the River on Fire: A Study of Genius, Mania, and Character* (New York: Knopf, 2017). Jamison, a distinguished professor of psychiatry at Johns Hopkins, asserts that correlation here and elsewhere. She also quotes the poet Lowell describing his agonizing life-long manic-depression as "a character made up of stiffness and disorder" or, elsewhere, "instinct and conscience" (19). This seems to me to verify my sense that the balance between restricting and releasing consciousness is a dangerously delicate one, matching the dilemma of human beings as bodies and souls, and suggests that bipolar illness might enable artistry by making the sufferer register the depths and limitations of the two extremes that artistic creation must navigate.

37 Caitlin Flanagan, "Hysteria and the Teenage Girl," www.nytimes.com/ 2012/01/29/opinion/sunday/adolescent-girl-hysteria.html.

38 Another version of this mixture is the use of "memory palaces" to permit recall of vast amounts of material: the practitioner imagines a castle, and then creates a narrative moving through it.

39 Carrithers, "Why Humans Have Cultures," 200.

40 Boyd, *Origin of Stories*, 405.

41 Laurent Dubreuil, "On Experimental Criticism: Cognition, Evolution, and Literary Theory," *Diacritics* 39, no. 1 (Spring 2009): 17.

42 Mark Edmundson, "Humanities Past, Present — and Future," *New Literary History* 36, no. 1 (2005): 43–46, nicely articulates how *Walden* had this kind of effect on him.

43 McAuliffe, *This Is Your Brain*, 163; her 182–83 observe the ethically dubious broader effects of such aversion.

44 Pollan, *How to Change*, 321.

45 Ralph Waldo Emerson, "Circles," in *The Prose Works* (Boston: Fields, Osgood, & Co., 1870), vol. 1, 379.

46 Neuroscience News, "How LSD Affects Language," August 22, 2016, http://neurosciencenews.com/language-lsd-neuroscience-4883/.

47 E. O. Wilson, "How to Unify Knowledge," *Annals of the New York Academy of Sciences* 935 (2001): 16.

48 For a somewhat absurdly detailed mathematical study of these ratios, see Kurt Gray et al., "The Science of Style"; http://journals.plos.org/plosone/article?id=10.1371/journal.pone.0102772.

49 Hutson, "What Is Art?" 28; citing Wijnand Adriaan Pieter van Tilburg and Eric Raymond Igou, "From Van Gogh to Lady Gaga: Artist Eccentricity Increases Perceived Artistic Skill and Art Appreciation," *European Journal of Social Psychology* (2014), doi:10.1002/ejsp.1999.

50 Hutson, "What Is Art?" 28; citing Meskin et al., "Mere Exposure to Bad Art," *British Journal of Aesthetics* 53, no. 2 (April 2013): 139–64.

51 Joseph Bulbulia et al., "The Cultural Evolution of Religion," in *Cultural Evolution*, eds. Richerson and Christiansen, 389. See also Henrich, *Secret of Our Success*, 159. See also Walter Freeman, "A Neurobiological Role of Music in Social Bonding," in *The Origins of Music*, eds. Nils L. Wallin, Björn Merker, and Steven Brown (Cambridge, MA: MIT Press, 2000), 420–21.

52 Bulbulia et al., "Cultural Evolution of Religion," 390.

53 Henrich, *Secret of Our Success*, 131 and 136.

54 Yann Martel, *The Life of Pi* (New York: Houghton Mifflin, 2002), 40–41.

55 Pollan, *How to Change*, 122–24.

Interchapter: Party Politics

1 "Chained to the Rhythm," by Katy Perry, Max Martin, Ali Payami, Sia, and Skip Marley, from the album *Witness*; the video was directed by Matthew Cullen and released on Vevo.

Chapter 5

1 Lem, *Imaginary Magnitude*, 131–32.

2 Susan L. Brinson, *The Red Scare, Politics, and the Federal Communications Commission, 1941–1960* (London: Praeger, 2004), 71.

3 Quoted by Brinson, *The Red Scare*, 73. For more details of this campaign, see John A. Salmond, *The Conscience of a Lawyer: Clifford J. Durr and American Civil Liberties, 1899–1975* (Tuscaloosa: University of Alabama Press, 1990), 102–3.

4 Jonathan C. Hagel, "In Search of the 'Racist White Psyche': Racism and the Psychology or Prejudice in American Social Thought, 1930–1960" (PhD diss., Brown University, 2001), 285.

5 See Bill Cooke, "The Kurt Lewin-Goodwin Watson FBI/CIA Files: A 60th Anniversary Then-and-There of the Here-and-Now," *Human Relations* 60, no. 3 (March 2007): 455:

> The file also notes that Watson chaired the Westchester Committee for Human Rights, which denounced as 'a whitewash' a June 1950 report of a Grand Jury inquiry into the infamous Peekskill riots, where thousands of American Legion veterans attacked a Paul Robeson concert .... Watson is also recorded as chairing a dinner in honour of Harvard social scientist and Pan-Africanist, W.E.B. DuBois, also named as a 'concealed Communist.'

6 John Dewey and Goodwin Watson, "A Forward View: A Free Teacher in a Free Society," in *John Dewey: The Later Works, 1925–1953*, ed. Jo Anne Boydston, vol. 11, 1935–1937 (Carbondale: Southern Illinois University Press, 1987), 536–37, 544.

7 Dewey and Watson, "A Forward View," 537, 559, 549.

8 Brinson, *The Red Scare*, 88.

9 Chanthou Boua, trans., "The Party's Four-Year Plan to Build Socialism in All Fields," in *Pol Pot Plans the Future: Confidential Leadership Documents from Democratic Kampuchea, 1976–1977*, trans. and eds. David P. Chandler, Ben Kiernan and Chanthou Boua (New Haven, CT: Yale University Press, 1988), 49; quoted by Daniel Cottom, *Why Education Is Useless* (Philadelphia: University of Pennsylvania Press, 2003), 196.

10 Foster Klug, "Rohingya Say Myanmar Targeted the Educated in Genocide," June 6, 2018, https://apnews.com/3a486e94ea7e48d1bfa5a5e0e1bf0518; accessed June 26, 2018.

11 "About Us," Professor Watchlist, www.professorwatchlist.org/about-us/; accessed November 25, 2016.

12 Robert C. Harvey, *The Art of the Comic Book: An Aesthetic History* (Jackson: University Press of Mississippi, 1996), 43.

13 Edward W. Said, *Humanism and Democratic Criticism* (New York: Columbia University Press, 2004), 80; quoted by Harpham, *Humanities*, 44.

14 "Gorbachev on 1989," interview by Katrina vanden Heuvel and Stephen F. Cohen, *The Nation*, October 28, 2009, www.thenation.com/article/gorbachev-1989/.

15 Edward W. Said, *Representations of the Intellectual* (New York: Vintage, 1996), 23.

16 Quoted by Stephen Greenblatt, *The Swerve: How the World Became Modern* (New York: Norton, 2011), 239.

17 Plato, "The Apology of Socrates," in *The Apology, Phaedo, and Crito of Plato*, vol. 2, trans. and eds. Benjamin Jowett, Hastings Crossley, and George Long (New York: Collier, 1909), 18. On the gadfly role of modern professors of the Humanities, see Helen Small's nicely measured and careful overview in *The Value of the Humanities* (Oxford: Oxford University Press, 2013), especially p. 137 on its relevance to political systems.

18 Robert Milder, "The Radical Emerson?" in *Cambridge Companion to Ralph Waldo Emerson*, eds. Joel Porte and Saundra Morris (Cambridge: Cambridge University Press, 1999), 55. Part of this passage is quoted in Andrew Delbanco, *College: What It Was, Is, and Should Be* (Princeton, NJ: Princeton University Press, 2012).

19 Modell, *Imagination*, 140.

20 Adam Kuper, "If Memes Are the Answer, What Is the Question?" in *Darwinizing Culture*, ed. Robert Aunger (Oxford: Oxford University Press, 2001), 184.

21 Tony Judt, *Ill Fares the Land: A Treatise on Our Present Discontents* (London: Penguin, 2010), 171.

22 Louis Menand, *The Marketplace of Ideas: Reform and Resistance in the American University* (New York: Norton, 2010), 104.

23 Stephen J. Gould, *Bully for Brontosaurus: Reflections in Natural History* (New York: Norton, 1991), 429–30.

24 Michael Bérubé, *What's Liberal about the Liberal Arts* (New York: Norton, 2006), 26–65, and Russell Jacoby, *Dogmatic Wisdom* (New York: Anchor, 1995), 29–58, each reveal how the supposed outrages most widely circulated in the right-wing media bore little resemblance to the facts that eventually emerged.

25 Stefan Collini, *What Are Universities For?* (London: Penguin, 2012), 5, observes that "in many parts of continental Europe, universities ... are directly under the control of the national or regional minister for education. Such institutions are seen as direct instruments of government policy ..." Collini, 33–35, traces the still-continuing decline of British universities as they are forcibly transformed from mostly autonomous institutions based on peer-review to government-controlled institutions based on economic valuations.

26 See Pat Rynard, "Senator Mark Chelgren Aims to Purge Democrats from Iowa Universities," *Iowa Starting Line*, February 20, 2017, http://iowastartingline.com/2017/02/20/senator-chelgren-aims-purge-democrats-iowa-universities/.

27 Quoted by Cottom, *Why Education Is Useless*, 195.

28 Quoted by Virginia Woolf, in note 19 to Part One of her *Three Guineas* (London: Hogarth Press, 1938).

29 Quoted by Cottom, *Why Education Is Useless*, 6.

30 Harpham, *Humanities*, 40, observes that the advances sought through interdisciplinary work "can only be made if the disciplines remain strong. Committed to partial knowledge and limited vision, the disciplines represent indispensable guardrails against runaway amateurism and what Menand called aimless eclecticism."

31 Jeffrey Herf, "How the Culture Wars Matter," in *Higher Education under Fire: Politics, Economics, and the Crisis of the Humanities*, eds. Michael Bérubé and Cary Nelson (London: Routledge, 1994), 159–60.

32 For evidence of how narrowing the orthodoxies on such points can become, even in the hands of longtime liberation-minded academic paradigm-stretchers at elite universities, see Jesse Singal, "This Is What a Modern-Day Witch Hunt Looks Like," *New York Magazine*, May 2, 2017, http://nymag.com/daily/intelligencer/2017/05/transracialism-article-controversy.html.

33 For a larger perspective on the way asking authorities to provide protection reinforces their ability to impose injustice, see Wendy Brown, *States of Injury: Power and Freedom in Late Modernity* (Princeton, NJ: Princeton University Press, 1995).

34 L. Gordon Crovitz, "Information Age: Chicago School of Free Speech," *Wall Street Journal*, November 23, 2015, www.wsj.com/articles/chicago-school-of-free-speech-1448231860. The "Disinvited Speakers" link in a widely cited Vox article on the supposed illiberalism of liberal campuses cited three cases: those two plus that of Robert Birgeneau, who also chose to cancel his appearance when controversy arose: see Libby Nelson, "Yale's Big Fight over Sensitivity and Free Speech, Explained," *Vox*, November 7, 2015, www.vox.com/2015/11/7/9689330/yale-halloween-email.

35 www.nytimes.com/2016/08/27/us/university-of-chicago-strikes-back-against-campus-political-correctness.html; accessed June 11, 2018.

36 https://csl.uchicago.edu/news/office-lgbtq-student-life%E2%80%99s-safe-space-program-launches-over-summer, accessed June 12, 2018.

37 Courtney Coelho, "Tendency to Fear is Strong Political Influence," *News from Brown*, February 5, 2013, http://news.brown.edu/pressreleases/2013/02/fear; based on Peter K. Hatemi et al., "Fear as a Disposition and an Emotional State: A Genetic and Environmental Approach to Out-Group Political Preferences," *American Journal of Political Science* 57, no. 1 (April 2013): 279–93. doi:10.1111/ajps.12016.

38 Daniel M. T. Fessler, Anne C. Pisor, and Colin Holbrook, "Political Orientation Predicts Credulity Regarding Putative Hazards," *Psychological Science* 28, no. 5 (May 2017): 651–60, doi:10.1177/0956797617692108.

39 Thomas Frank, *What's the Matter with Kansas?* (New York: Metropolitan Books, 2004). See similarly Jared Diamond, *Guns, Germs, and Steel: The Fates of Human Societies* (New York: Norton, 1997), 276: "Why do commoners tolerate the transfer of the fruits of their hard labor to kleptocrats? This question, raised by political theorists from Plato to Marx, is raised anew by voters in every modern election." Perhaps memetics can augment the more overtly political answers to that question.

40 While there are certainly progressive aspects of Modi's campaign pledges, relative to the recent history of Indian politics, his populist Hindu nationalism aligns him in several ways with the regressive forces I am describing.

41 Henrich, *Secret of Our Success*, 325.

42 Debra Bradley Ruder, "The 'Water Cooler' Effect," *Harvard Magazine*, May–June 2011. Hull, "Taking Memetics Seriously," 62, also shows that the most successful research teams tend to be small groups that are part of a larger intellectual community.

43 Jonah Lehrer, "Groupthink: The Brainstorming Myth," *The New Yorker*, January 30, 2012.

44 Sherry Turkle, "Stop Googling. Let's Talk," www.nytimes.com/2015/09/27/opinion/sunday/stop-googling-lets-talk.html?smid=nytcore-ipad-share&smprod=nytcore-ipad&_r=0, describes a massive drop among empathy responses among college students in recent decades, and plausibly links it to the displacement of in-person conversation by texting and other online exchanges.

45 These qualifying clauses are what differentiate universities from ancient monasteries. Contrary to a common assumption among scholars dedicated to exposing the hegemonic power of ruling institutions, Christianity was often an enclave of resistance to social injustice, as Debora Shuger and others have shown. Yet universities must be far more receptive to heresies than institutional Christianity has generally been.

46 Samuel Beckett, *Proust* (London: Chatto and Windus, 1930), 8.

47 Collini, *What Are Universities For?*, 56–57.

48 Watson, *Back to Nature*, 257–96.

49 Chwe, *Rational Ritual*, 27.

50 Chwe, *Rational Ritual*, 30–33.

51 Harari, *Sapiens*, 118.

52 Penelope Murray and Peter Wilson, *Music and the Muses: The Culture of "mousikē" in the Classical Athenian City* (New York: Oxford University Press, 2004), 271.

53 Peter Schjeldahl, "The Anti-Modernists," *The New Yorker*, March 24, 2014, 96–97.

54 On the wastefulness of for-profit education, see Christopher Newfield, *The Great Mistake: How We Wrecked Public Universities and How We Can Fix Them* (Baltimore, MD: Johns Hopkins University Press, 2016).

55 Carrithers, "Why Humans Have Cultures," 197–8.

56 Thomas Bender, "Politics, Intellect, and the American University, *1945–1995*," *Daedalus* 126, no. 1 (Winter 1997): 1–38; cited by Menand, *Marketplace*, 75.

57 Cooke, "FBI/CIA Files," 458.

58 Brinson, *The Red Scare*, 88–89.

59 Tawney, Richard Henry, *Religion and the Rise of Capitalism* (New York: Harcourt Brace, 1926).

60 The same discomfort may explain why the US military concealed the millions of dollars it paid to professional sports teams for what a report called "paid patriotism," in the form of various ceremonies honoring the military, welcoming soldiers home, allowing members of the military to perform the national anthem, etc.; Marcus E. Howard, "Senators Detail 'Paid-For Patriotism,'" *Los Angeles Times*, November 5, 2015, D1.

61 Examples include the Bass family donations that Yale could not finally accept, and the financial pressure brought to bear by conservative alumni groups, often in alliance with the National Association of Scholars.

62 Collini, *What Are Universities For?*, 39; the response Collini quotes (48) from Cardinal Newman's famous *The Idea of the University* from the 1850s seems hardly less applicable today.

63 Jerry Z. Muller, "The Tyranny of Metrics," *Chronicle of Higher Education*, January 21, 2018.

64 Nussbaum, *Not For Profit*, 138, quotes this portion of Obama's 2009 speech: Barack Obama, "Remarks of the President to the United States Hispanic Chamber of Commerce," March 10, 2009, http://obamawhitehouse.archives.gov/the-press-office/remarks-president-united-states-hispanic-chamber-commerce.

65 Quoted by Cottom, *Why Education Is Useless*, 50.

66 Delbanco, *College*, 150–62; p. 143 lists a number of studies of the ways monetary incentives have been corrupting higher education.

67 Andrew Leonard, "Conservatives Declare War on College," *Salon*, February 22, 2013, www.salon.com/2013/02/22/conservatives_declare_war_on_college/.

68 Valerie Strauss, "How Gov. Walker Tried to Quietly Change the Mission of the University of Wisconsin," *Washington Post*, February 5, 2015, accessed online June 26, 2018.

69 Scott Walker, "UW Flexible Degree," Office of the Governor, State of Wisconsin, June 2012, www.uwgb.edu/sofas/structures/governance/senate/agendas/Flexible%20Degree%20Proposal%20Packet1.pdf.

70 Robert N. Watson, "The Humanities Really Do Produce A Profit," *Chronicle of Higher Education*, March 21, 2010. A similar argument was made more extensively in Christopher Newfield's excellent *Unmaking the Public University* (Cambridge, MA: Harvard University Press, 2008), 208–19.

71 Zöe Carpenter, "How a Right-Wing Political Machine Is Dismantling Higher Education in North Carolina," *The Nation*, June 8, 2015, www.thenation.com/article/how-right-wing-political-machine-dismantling-higher-education-north-carolina/.

72 Adam Smith, *An Inquiry into the Nature and Causes of the Wealth of Nations*, ed. J. R. McCulloch (Edinburgh: Adam and Charles Black, 1863), 347.

73 Sharon Rider, "The Future of the European University: Liberal Democracy or Authoritarian Capitalism?" *Culture Unbound* 1 (2009): 83–104, www.cultureunbound.ep.liu.se/v1/a07/cu09v1a07.pdf.

74 Lorraine Daston, "Can Liberal Education Save the Sciences?" *The Point*, 2016, https://thepointmag.com/2016/examined-life/can-liberal-education-save-the-sciences.

75 In February of 2016, the Republican majority in the US House of Representatives passed a bill (H.R. 3293) insisting that National Science Foundation grants be given only to projects that show how they will benefit the national interest. Much of the research indispensable toward many of modern science's most valuable discoveries would never have been able to satisfy that short-term instrumentalist criterion.

76 Chris Lorenz, "If You're So Smart, Why Are You under Surveillance? Universities, Neoliberalism, and New Public Management," *Critical Inquiry* 38, no. 3 (Spring 2012): 603.

77 Lorenz, "If You're So Smart," 609.

78 Harari, *Sapiens*, 174.

79 Harari, *Sapiens*, 316–18.

80 Edward E. Baptist, *The Half Has Never Been Told: Slavery and the Making of American Capitalism* (New York: Basic Books, 2014).

81 Tocqueville to Ernest de Chabrol, New York, June 9, 1831, in *The Tocqueville Reader: A Life in Letters and Politics*, eds. Olivier Zunz and Alan S. Kahan (Oxford: Blackwell, 2002), 41.

82 Karl Polanyi, "The Essence of Fascism," in *Christianity and the Social Revolution*, eds. John Lewis, Karl Polanyi, and Donald K. Kitchin (London: Victor Gollancz Ltd, 1935), 392.

83 Samuel E. Abrams, "The Right and Wrong Business Lessons for Schools," *Los Angeles Times*, January 8, 2017, A18, offers data supporting these perspectives. He directs the National Center for the Study of Privatization in Education at my father's employer during his long Red-Scare ordeal: Teachers College at Columbia University.

84 John Colet, *The sermo[n] of doctor Colete, made to the conuocacion at Paulis* (1512; London: Thomas Berthelet, 1530); NSTC 5550; in *Religion in Tudor England: An Anthology of Primary Sources*, eds. Debora Shuger and Ethan Shagan (Waco, TX: Baylor University Press, 2016); modernized spelling.

85 Pope Francis, "Address to the New Non-Resident Ambassadors to the Holy See: Kyrgyzstan, Antigua and Barbuda, Luxembourg and Botswana," *Clementine Hall*, May 16, 2013, www.vatican.va/holy_father/francesco/speeches/2013/may/documents/papa-francesco_20130516_nuovi-ambasciatori_en.html. The quotations in these closing paragraphs are all from this speech.

Interchapter: Digital Humanities

1 For an excellent defense of the potential of Digital Humanities to intervene against malfunctions of the "soft infrastructure" of society, see Alan Liu, "Drafts for *Against the Cultural Singularity* (book in progress)," May 2, 2016, http://liu.english.ucsb.edu/drafts-for-against-the-cultural-singularity.

2 Robert N. Watson, "Coriolanus and the 'Common Part,'" *Shakespeare Survey* 69 (2016): 181–97; and "Lord Capulet's Lost Compromise: Editing and the Binary Dynamics of *Romeo and* Juliet," *Renaissance Drama* 43, no. 1 2015: 53–83.

Chapter 6

1 William Johnson Cory, *Eton Reform*, vol. 2 (London: Spottiswoode and Co., 1861), 5–7.

2 The main plot of the 2015 James Bond movie *Spectre* turns on the same point.

3 Thomas Kuhn, *The Structure of Scientific Revolutions* (Chicago, IL: University of Chicago Press, 1962).

4 Robert N. Watson, "Protestant Animals: Puritan Sects and English Animal-Protection Sentiment, 1550–1650," *ELH* 81, no. 4 (2014): 1111–48.

5 Watson, *Back to Nature*, 166–225.

6 Daniel C. Dennett, *Darwin's Dangerous Idea: Evolution and the Meanings of Life* (New York: Touchstone, 1995), 516, imagines this as a cultural version of preserving biodiversity.

7 Harpham, *Humanities*, 11–12, drawing on Francis Oakley's *Community of Learning: The American College and the Liberal Arts Tradition* (Oxford: Oxford University Press, 1992), and Bruce Kimball's *Orators and Philosophers* (New York: Teachers College Press, 1986).

8 Henrich, *Secret of Our Success*, 97–100.

9 John Dewey, *Democracy and Education: An Introduction to the Philosophy of Education* (New York: Macmillan, 1916), 52; quoted by Michael Roth in his unflinchingly cogent *Beyond the University: Why Liberal Education Matters* (New Haven, CT: Yale University Press, 2014), 167.

10 Susan Blackmore, "The Evolution of Meme Machines," in *Ontopsychology and Memetics*, eds. Antonio Meneghetti et al. (Rome: Psicologica Editrice, 2003), 233–40.

11 Robert N. Watson, "*Midsummer Night's Dream* and the Ecology of Human Being," in *Ecocritical Shakespeare*, eds. Lynne Bruckner and Dan Brayton (London: Routledge, 2011), 33–56.

12 Watson, "Coriolanus."

13 Michael Pollan, "Some of My Best Friends Are Bacteria," *New York Times Sunday Magazine*, May 12, 2013.

14 Pollan, "Some."

15 Djikic, Oatley, and Moldoveanua, "Opening," 149.

16 Emerson, "Circles," 380–81.

17 Modell, *Imagination*, 5.

18 Nicholasa Mohr, *Growing Up Inside the Sanctuary of My Imagination* (New York: Simon and Schuster, 1994), 45.

19 Rolf Jensen, *The Dream Society: How the Coming Shift from Information to Imagination Will Transform Your Business* (New York: McGraw-Hill, 2001). Graeme Wood, "Anthropology Inc.," *The Atlantic*, March, 2013, 49, leads with a similar discovery about how vodka culture shapes its sales: "the host puts it in the freezer, and listens to the story of where the bottle came from." Across a variety of test cities, "What mattered most, to the partygoers and their hosts, were the narratives that accompanied the drinks."

20 Catherine Rampell, "A reason to major in the humanities," https://economix. blogs.nytimes.com/2012/02/09.

21 Jamie Holmes, *Nonsense: The Power of Not Knowing* (New York: Crown/ Penguin, 2015).

22 Djikic, Oatley, and Moldoveanua, "Opening," 153, makes this observation and cites Jeremy L. Warner, Robert M. Najarian, and Lawrence M. Tierney, Jr., "Uses and Misuses of Thresholds in Diagnostic Decision Making," *Academic Medicine* 85 (2010): 556–68.

23 Arabella L. Simpkin, and Richard M. Schwartzstein, "Tolerating Uncertainty — The Next Medical Revolution?" *New England Journal of Medicine* 375 (November 3, 2016): 1713–15.

24 Frank Rich, "Karl Rove Beats the Democrats Again," *New York Times*, June 18, 2006.

25 Quoted by Melissa Deckman, *Tea Party Women* (New York: New York University Press, 2016), 228.

26 Bulbulia et al., "Cultural Evolution of Religion," in Richerson and Christiansen, *Cultural Evolution*, 402.

27 William Easterly, *The White Man's Burden: Why the West's Efforts to Aid the Rest Have Done So Much Ill and So Little Good* (New York: Penguin, 2007).

28 Katherine Lepani, *Islands of Love, Islands of Risk: Culture and HIV in the Trobriands* (Nashville, TN: Vanderbilt University Press, 2012).

29 This accusation has been pushed most prominently by Milford Bateman; see, for example, "Has the Microfinance Bubble Really Burst?" *From Poverty to Power* (blog), April 20, 2011, www.oxfamblogs.org/fp2p/?p=5161. For a more moderate view, see Ben Casselman, "Microloans Don't Solve Poverty," *FiveThirtyEight*, December 8, 2015, http://fivethirtyeight.com/features/microloans-dont-solve-poverty/.

30 Kai Hammerich and Richard D. Lewis, *Fish Can't See Water: How National Culture Can Make or Break Your Corporate Strategy* (Chichester: Wiley, 2013).

31 Ron Suskind, "Faith, Certainty, and the Presidency of George W. Bush," *The New York Times Magazine*, October 17, 2004.

32 Jared Diamond, *Collapse: How Societies Choose to Fail or Succeed* (New York: Penguin, 2011), 21. Smail finds similar examples explored in Charles Redman, *Human Impact on Ancient Environments* (Tucson: University Arizona Press, 1999) and Brian M. Fagan, *Floods, Famines, and Emperors* (New York: Basic Books, 1999).

33 Patt Morrison, "We Couldn't Save Cecil the Lion, but Can We Save the Planet?" *Los Angeles Times*, August 12, 2015, www.latimes.com/opinion/op-ed/la-oe-morrison-kareiva-20150812-column.html. For a more fully scholarly anthropological study of the effects of cultural difference on environmental sustainability, see Scott Atran and Douglas L. Medin, *The Native Mind and the Cultural Construction of Nature* (Cambridge, MA: MIT Press, 2008).

34 Atran and Medin, *The Native Mind*, 16.

35 Keith E. Stanovich, *The Robot's Rebellion: Finding Meaning in the Age of Darwin* (Chicago, IL: University Chicago Press, 2004), 122–23. On some of the risks of applying neuroscience in criminal proceedings, see Dominique J. Church, "Neuroscience in the Courtroom: An International Concern," *William and Mary Law Review* 53, no. 5; Rev. 1825 (2012): 1826–53, http://scholarship.law.wm.edu/wmlr/vol53/iss5/8.

36 William Edward Burghardt Du Bois, "The Talented Tenth," in *The Negro Problem* (New York: James Pott & Co., 1903), 31–76.

37 Judt, *Ill Fares the Land*, 53.

38 John Dewey, *Art as Experience* (New York: Penguin, 1934), 336.

39 Nicholas K. Humphrey, "The Social Function of Intellect," in *Growing Points in Ethology*, eds. P. P. G. Bateson and R. A. Hinde (Cambridge: Cambridge University Press, 1976), 309; quoted by Carrithers, "Why Humans Have Cultures," 193.

40 Quoted by Elizabeth D. Samet, "Mouse-Boys, Literate Spiders, and the Security of Imagination," in *What Is Education*, eds. Lee Oser and Rosanna Warren (Boston, MA: ALSCW, 2012), 15.

41 Amos Funkenstein, *Theology and the Scientific Imagination* (Princeton, NJ: Princeton University Press, 1986), 163.

42 Funkenstein, *Theology*, 157.

43 Funkenstein, *Theology*, 11; see also Edward Grant, *A History of Natural Philosophy from the Ancient World to the Nineteenth Century* (Cambridge: Cambridge University Press, 2007), 283: "Medieval natural philosophers … often showed that ideas thought impossible by Aristotle were in fact possible under certain conditions that could be produced supernaturally.

They did this by the assumption of counterfactual conditions and thought experiments."

44 Funkenstein, *Theology*, 178.

45 Readers of contemporary social theorists may recall that Jean-François Lyotard raises a similar objection to Jürgen Habermas's pursuit of norms.

46 Theodor Adorno, *Negative Dialectics*, trans. E. B. Ashton (London: Routledge, 1973), 242–43; quoted by Cottom, *Why Education Is Useless*, 24.

47 Hubert Zapf, *Literature as Cultural Ecology* (London: Bloomsbury, 2016), 90 and 92.

48 Barbara B. Watson, "On Power and the Literary Text," *Signs* (Autumn, 1975), 112

49 Cooke, "FBI/CIA Files," 460.

50 Herf, "Culture Wars," 152.

51 Theodor Adorno et al., *The Authoritarian Personality* (New York: Harper, 1950).

52 Max Horkheimer, "Traditional and Critical Theory," in *Critical Theory: Selected Essays*, trans. Matthew J. O'Connell (New York: Continuum, 1972), 219.

53 Eugéne Ionesco, *Rhinoceros and Other Plays*, trans. Derek Prouse (New York: Grove Press, 1960), 107.

54 Neil Postman and Charles Weingartner, *Teaching as a Subversive Activity* (New York: Delacorte, 1969), 3–4.

55 Djikic, Oatley, and Moldoveanua, "Opening," 149. Walter Roach, a long-time expert in market research, reports (by personal communication) that

> Focus group moderators have seen this too: very often client observers in the back room, eager for confirmation of their particular perspective on the issue at hand (especially if it is highly political), will seize on the one participant out of ten who happens to agree with them – ignoring the other nine who disagree.

56 Maggie E. Toplak and Keith E. Stanovich, "Associations between Myside Bias on an Informal Reasoning Task and Amount of Post-Secondary Education," *Applied Cognitive Psychology* 17, no. 7 (2003): 851–60, https://doi.org/10.1002/acp.915. Kate Distin, Cultural Evolution (Cambridge: Cambridge University Press, 2011), 179–80, observes that "a longer time spent in university" increased the ability of the experimental subjects to step outside their existing beliefs.

Interchapter: Why Aristotle Would Have Won Plenty of Drachmae Betting on College Football Bowl Games

1 David Wharton, "Poll Vaulting," *Los Angeles Times*, September 7, 2016; citing Ed Feng's PowerRank website.

2 www.rand.org/pubs/research_reports/RR2242.html; accessed June 26, 2018.

Chapter 7

1 Excerpt from Frantz Fanon, *BLACK SKIN, WHITE MASKS*, 180; English translation copyright © 2008 by Richard Philcox. Used by permission of Grove/Atlantic, Inc. Any third party use of this material, outside of this publication, is prohibited.

2 Andrew Martin, "The Scientific A-Team Saving the World from Killer Viruses, Rogue AI and the Paperclip Apocalypse," *The Guardian*, August 30, 2014, www.theguardian.com/technology/2014/aug/30/saviours-universe-four-unlikely-men-save-world.

3 Douglas P. Fry and Patrik Söderberg, "Myths about Hunter-Gatherers Redux: Nomadic Forager War and Peace," *Journal of Aggression, Conflict and Peace Research* 6, no. 4 (2014): 255–66, doi:10.1108/JACPR-06-2014-0127. For a more extensive version of this argument, see Douglas P. Fry, *The Human Potential for Peace: An Anthropological Challenge to Assumptions about War and Violence* (New York: Oxford University Press, 2006) and David Stannard, *American Holocaust: The Conquest of the New World* New York: (Oxford University Press, 1993).

4 Laland, *Darwin's Unfinished Symphony*, 20.

5 Forster's story is reprinted in *The Science Fiction Century*, vol. 1, ed. David G. Hartwell (New York: Tom Doherty Associates, 2006); the passages quoted here appear on 135–49.

6 Stanovich, *Robot's Rebellion*, xii; see also his 176.

7 Stanovich, *Robot's Rebellion*, 192.

8 See the discussion of Wallerstein's work by Nicholas Abercrombie, Stephen Hill, and Bryan Turner in the *Dictionary of Sociology*, 5th ed. (London: Penguin, 2006).

9 Stanovich, *Robot's Rebellion*, xiv.

10 Stanovich, *Robot's Rebellion*, 184, 202, 201, 186.

11 Pollan, *How to Change*, 215, 230.

12 Pitirim Sorokin, *Society, Culture, and Personality: Their Structure and Dynamics* (New York: Cooper Square, 1969), 706.

13 Matthew B. Crawford, *The World Beyond Your Head: On Becoming an Individual in an Age of Distraction* (New York: Farrar Straus, 2015), 19–20.

14 Plato, *Laws*, 797a–c; vol. 7, 33.

15 Philippe Ariès, *Centuries of Childhood: A Social History of Family Life*, trans. Robert Baldick (New York: Random House, 1962). Charlotte Scott, *The Child in Shakespeare* (Oxford: Oxford University Press, 2018), offers an illuminating alternative to the conventional view that Shakespeare's works took little interest in children.

16 Creswell and Haykel, "Battle Lines," observe that "Many jihadi poems use the conceit of a child speaker; it provides them with a figure of innocence and truthfulness."

17 Richard Louv's best-selling and award-wining *Last Child in the Woods* (New York: Algonquin, 2005), makes this important argument extensively.

18 Heather Pringle, "The Origins of Creativity," *Scientific American*, March, 2013: 42.

19 Collini, *What Are Universities For?* 144.

20 Stefan Collini, "Who Are the Spongers Now?" *London Review of Books*, January 21, 2016.

21 Richard Biernacki, *Reinventing Evidence in Social Inquiry: Decoding Facts and Variables* (London: Palgrave, 2012).

22 Barry Schwartz, *Why We Work* (New York: Simon and Schuster, 2015), building on William Sullivan's *Work and Integrity: The Crisis and Promise of Professionalism in America* (Stanford, CA: Jossey-Bass, 2004).

23 Lorenz, "If You're So Smart," 607.

24 Abraham Vergese, Professor of Internal Medicine at Stanford University, observes that "our daily progress notes have become bloated cut-and-paste monsters that are inaccurate and hard to wade through," but they serve to

"make it possible to bill at the highest level for that encounter"; "Machine Medicine," *New York Times Magazine*, May 20, 2018: 59.

25 Robert A. Berenson, Peter Basch, and Amanda Sussex, "Revisiting E&M Visit Guidelines — A Missing Piece of Payment Reform," *New England Journal of Medicine* 364, no. 20 (May 19, 2011): 1892–95, doi:10.1056/NEJMp1102099.

26 Dave Philipps, "At Veterans Hospital in Oregon, a Push for Better Ratings Puts Patients at Risk, Doctors Say," *New York Times*, January 1, 2018, www.nytimes.com/2018/01/01/us/at-veterans-hospital-in-oregon-a-push-for-better-ratings-puts-patients-at-risk-doctors-say.html.

27 Harari, *Sapiens*, 130.

28 Richerson and Boyd, *Not by Genes*, 253.

29 Cicero, *De Finibus Bonum et Malorum*, trans. H. Rackham (Cambridge, MA: Harvard University Press, 1931), 453.

30 For a list of nine studies, performed 2006–2011, that demonstrate the usefulness of reading literary fictions, see Jaén and Simon, *Cognitive Literary Studies*, 21.

31 On whether technology has slowed human evolution, see Jay T. Stock, "Are Humans Still Evolving?" *EMBO Reports* 9 (2008): S51–S54, doi:10.1038/embor.2008.63.

32 Smail argues that stratifying social behaviors evolved to fit some conditions of the Paleolithic period became latent, then revived when they proved reproductively beneficial under conditions that no longer required the egalitarianism of hunter-gatherer functions.

33 Said, *Representations*, xviii.

34 John Stuart Mill, *Autobiography* (London, 1873; repr. Oxford: Oxford University Press, 1924), ch. 7, 202–3.

35 Emerson, "Circles," 379.

36 Martin Luther King, Jr., "Beyond Vietnam," Riverside Church, New York, NY, April 4, 1967; quoted in *Voices of a People's History of the United States*, 2nd ed., ed. Howard Zinn and Anthony Arnove (New York: Seven Stories Press, 2004), 423–26.

Bibliography

Abercrombie, Nicholas, Stephen Hill, and Bryan Turner. *Dictionary of Sociology*. 5th ed. London: Penguin, 2006.

Abrams, Samuel E. "The Right and Wrong Business Lessons for Schools." *Los Angeles Times*, January 8, 2017.

Adorno, Theodor. *Negative Dialectics*. Translated by E. B. Ashton. London: Routledge, 1973.

Adorno, Theodor. *Philosophy of New Music*. Minneapolis: University of Minnesota Press, 2006.

Adorno, Theodor, Else Frenkel-Brunswik, Daniel J. Levinson, and Nevitt Sanford. *The Authoritarian Personality*. New York: Harper, 1950.

Arendt, Hannah. *The Human Condition*. 2nd ed. Chicago, IL: University of Chicago Press, 1998.

Ariès, Philippe. *Centuries of Childhood: A Social History of Family Life*. Translated by Robert Baldick. New York: Random House, 1962.

Aristotle, Poetics.

Armstrong, Karen. *Fields of Blood: Religion and the History of Violence*. New York: Anchor, 2014.

Atran, Scott. *In Gods We Trust: The Evolutionary Landscape of Religion*. New York and Oxford: Oxford University Press, 2002.

Atran, Scott. *Talking to the Enemy: Sacred Values, Violent Extremism, and What It Means to Be Human*. New York: Penguin, 2011.

Atran, Scott, and Douglas L. Medin. *The Native Mind and the Cultural Construction of Nature*. Cambridge, MA: MIT Press, 2008.

Aunger, Robert, ed. *Darwinizing Culture: The Status of Memetics as a Science*. Oxford: Oxford University Press, 2001.

Baptist, Edward E. *The Half Has Never Been Told: Slavery and the Making of American Capitalism*. New York: Basic Books, 2014.

Barkow, Jerome H., Leda Cosmides, and John Tooby, editor. *The Adapted Mind: Evolutionary Psychology and the Generation of Culture*. New York: Oxford University Press, 1992.

Barrett, Justin L. "Exploring the Natural Foundations of Religion." *Trends in Cognitive Sciences* 4, no. 1 (January 2000): 29–34.

Bateman, Milford. "Has the Microfinance Bubble Really Burst?" *From Poverty to Power* (blog), April 20, 2011, www.oxfamblogs.org/fp2p/?p=5161.

Beane, Silas. "Are We Living in a Simulation?" Interview by *BBC Focus* magazine, March 2013.

Beckett, Samuel. *Proust*. London: Chatto and Windus, 1930.

Belluck, Pam. "Study Finds That Brains with Autism Fail to Trim Synapses as They Develop." *New York Times*, August 21, 2014. www.nytimes.com/2014/08/22/health/brains-of-autistic-children-have-too-many-synapses-study-suggests.html.

Bender, Thomas. "Politics, Intellect, and the American University, 1945–1995." *Daedalus* 126, no. 1 (Winter 1997): 1–38.

Berdoy, M., Joanne P. Webster, and David W. Macdonald. "Fatal Attraction in Rats Infected with *Toxoplasma Gondii*." *Proceedings of the Royal Society B: Biological Sciences* 267, no. 1452 (August 2000): 1591–94. doi:10.1098/rspb.2000.1182.

Berenson, Robert A., Peter Basch, and Amanda Sussex. "Revisiting E & M Visit Guidelines—A Missing Piece of Payment Reform." *New England Journal of Medicine* 364, no. 20 (May 19, 2011): 1892–95. doi:10.1056/NEJMp1102099.

Bérubé, Michael. *What's Liberal about the Liberal Arts*. New York: Norton, 2006.

Biernacki, Richard. *Reinventing Evidence in Social Inquiry: Decoding Facts and Variables*. London: Palgrave, 2012.

Blackmore, Susan. "The Evolution of Meme Machines." In *Ontopsychology and Memetics*, edited by Antonio Meneghetti et al., 233–40. Rome: Psicologica Editrice, 2003.

Bloom, Howard. *The Genius of the Beast*. Amherst, NY: Prometheus Books, 2009.

Bloom, Howard. *The Lucifer Principle: A Scientific Expedition into the Forces of History*. New York: Atlantic Monthly Press, 1997.

Blumenberg, Hans. *Work on Myth*. Translated by Robert M. Wallace. Boston: MIT Press, 1985.

Blute, Marion. *Darwinian Social Evolution: Solutions to Dilemmas in Cultural and Social Theory*. Cambridge: Cambridge University Press, 2010.

Borges, Jorge Luis. *Ficciones*. New York: Grove Press, 1962.

Boua, Chanthou, trans. "The Party's Four-Year Plan to Build Socialism in All Fields." In *Pol Pot Plans the Future: Confidential Leadership Documents from Democratic Kampuchea, 1976–1977*. Translated and Edited by David P. Chandler, Ben Kiernan, and Chanthou Boua, 36–118. New Haven, CT: Yale University Press, 1988.

Boyd, Brian. *On the Origin of Stories: Evolution, Cognition, and Fiction*. Cambridge, MA: Harvard University Press, 2009.

Boyd, Brian. *Why Lyrics Last: Evolution, Cognition, and Shakespeare's Sonnets*. Cambridge, MA: Harvard University Press, 2012.

Boyd, Robert. "Cultural Evolution Comes of Age." Review of *Cultural Evolution: How Darwinian Theory Can Explain Human Culture and Synthesize the Social Sciences*, by Alex Mesoudi. *Trends in Ecology & Evolution* 27, no. 8 (August 2012): 419.

Boyd, Robert, and Peter J. Richerson. *Culture and the Evolutionary Process*. Chicago, IL: University of Chicago Press, 1985.

Boyd, Robert, and Peter J. Richerson. *The Origin and Evolution of Cultures*. New York: Oxford University Press, 2005.

Boyd, Robert, Peter J. Richerson, and Joseph Henrich. "The Cultural Evolution of Technology: Facts and Theories." In *Cultural Evolution*, edited by Richerson and Christiansen, 119–42. Cambridge, MA: MIT Press, 2013.

Brinson, Susan L. *The Red Scare, Politics, and the Federal Communications Commission, 1941–1960*. London: Praeger, 2004.

Brooks, Peter, ed. *The Humanities and Public Life*. With Hilary Jewett. New York: Fordham University Press, 2014.

Brown, Gillian R., and Peter J. Richerson. "Applying Evolutionary Theory to Human Behaviour: Past Differences and Current Debates." *Journal of Bioeconomics* 16, no. 2 (July 2014): 105–28. doi:10.1007/s10818-013-9166-4.

Brown, Wendy. *States of Injury: Power and Freedom in Late Modernity*. Princeton, NJ: Princeton University Press, 1995.

Bulbulia, Joseph, Armin W. Geertz, Quentin D. Atkinson, Emma Cohen, Nicholas Evans, Pieter François, Herbert Gintis, et al. "The Cultural Evolution of Religion." In *Cultural Evolution*, edited by Richerson and Christiansen, 381–404. Cambridge, MA: MIT Press, 2013.

Burdick, Anne, Johanna Drucker, Peter Lunenfeld, Todd Presner, and Jeffrey S. Schnapp. *Digital_Humanities*. Cambridge, MA: MIT Press, 2012.

Byrne, Richard W., and Andrew Whiten. *Machiavellian Intelligence: Social Expertise and the Evolution of Intellect in Monkeys, Apes, and Humans*. New York: Oxford University Press, 1988.

Calvin, William H. "The Brain as a Darwin Machine." *Nature* 330 (1987): 33–34.

Capellini, Terence D., Hao Chen, Jiaxue Cao, Andrew C. Doxey, Ata M. Kiapour, Michael Schoor, and David M Kingsley. "Ancient Selection for Derived Alleles at a GDF5 Enhancer Influencing Human Growth and Osteoarthritis Risk." *Nature Genetics* 49 (July 3, 2017): 1202–10.

Carpenter, Zöe. "How a Right-Wing Political Machine Is Dismantling Higher Education in North Carolina." *The Nation*, June 8, 2015. www.thenation.com/article/how-right-wing-political-machine-dismantling-higher-education-north-carolina/.

Carrithers, Michael. "Why Humans Have Cultures." *Man*, n. s., 25, no. 2 (June 1990): 189–207.

Carroll, Joseph. *Reading: Literary Darwinism in Theory and Practice*. Albany, NY: SUNY Press, 2001.

Carson, Rachel. *The Silent Spring*. Boston, MA: Houghton Mifflin, 1962.

Casselman, Ben. "Microloans Don't Solve Poverty." *FiveThirtyEight*, December 8, 2015. http://fivethirtyeight.com/features/microloans-dont-solve-poverty/.

Cavalli-Sforza, Luigi Luca, and Marcus W. Feldman. *Cultural Transmission and Evolution: A Quantitative Approach*. Princeton, NJ: Princeton University Press, 1991.

Certeau, Michel de. *The Practice of Everyday Life*. Translated by Steven Rendall. Berkeley: University of California Press, 2011.

Chang, Li-Hung, Kazuhisa Shibata, George J. Andersen, Yuka Sasaki, and Takeo Watanabe. "Age-Related Declines of Stability in Visual Perceptual Learning." *Current Biology* 24, no. 24 (December 15, 2014): 2926–29. doi:10.1016/j.cub.2014.10.041.

Christiansen, Morten H., and Nick Chater. "Language as Shaped by the Brain." *Behavioural and Brain Sciences* 31 (2008): 489–558.

Church, Dominique J. "Neuroscience in the Courtroom: An International Concern." *William and Mary Law Review* 53, no. 5; Rev. 1825 (2012): 1826–53. http://scholarship.law.wm.edu/wmlr/vol53/iss5/8.

Chwe, Michael Suk-Young. *Rational Ritual: Culture, Coordination, and Common Knowledge*. Princeton, NJ: Princeton University Press, 2001.

Cicero. *De Finibus Bonum et Malorum*. Translated by H. Rackham. Cambridge, MA: Harvard University Press, 1931.

Coelho, Courtney. "Tendency to Fear Is Strong Political Influence." *News from Brown*, February 5, 2013, http://news.brown.edu/pressreleases/2013/02/fear.

Colet, John. *The sermo[n] of doctor Colete, made to the conuocacion at Paulis*. London: Thomas Berthelet, 1530. NSTC 5550. In *Religion in Tudor England: An Anthology of Primary Sources*, edited by Debora Shuger and Ethan Shagan. Waco, TX: Baylor University Press, 2016.

Collini, Stefan. *What Are Universities For?* London: Penguin, 2012.

Collini, Stefan. "Who Are the Spongers Now?" *London Review of Books*, January 21, 2016.

Connolly, William E. *Neuropolitics: Thinking, Culture, Speed*. Minneapolis: University of Minnesota Press, 2002.

Connolly, William E. *A World of Becoming*. Durham, NC: Duke University Press, 2011.

Cooke, Bill. "The Kurt Lewin-Goodwin Watson FBI/CIA Files: A 60th Anniversary Then-and-There of the Here-and-Now." *Human Relations* 60, no. 3 (March 2007): 435–62.

Cordes, Philip, and Michael Hülsman. "Self-Healing Supply Networks: A Complex Adaptive Systems Perspective." In *Supply Chain Safety Management: Security and Robustness in Logistics*, edited by Michael Eßig, Michael Hülsmann, Eva-Maria Kern, and Stephan Klein-Schmeink, 217–30. Heidelberg: Springer, 2013.

Cory, William Johnson. *Eton Reform*. Vol. 2. London: Spottiswoode and Co., 1861.

Cottom, Daniel. *Why Education Is Useless*. Philadelphia: University of Pennsylvania Press, 2003.

Coyne, J. A. "They Shall Have Their Rewards on Earth, Too." *Times Literary Supplement*, November 1, 2002.

Crawford, Matthew B. *The World Beyond Your Head: On Becoming an Individual in an Age of Distraction*. New York: Farrar Straus, 2015.

Crenshaw, Kimberlé W. "Mapping the Margins: Intersectionality, Identity Politics, and Violence against Women of Color." *Stanford Law Review* 43, no. 6 (July 1991): 1241–99.

Creswell, Robyn. "Hearing Voices." *The New Yorker*, December 18 & 25, 2017.

Creswell, Robyn, and Bernard Haykel. "Battle Lines." *The New Yorker*, June 8 and 15, 2015.

Croft, William. "Evolutionary Linguistics." *Annual Review of Anthropology* 37 (2008): 219–34.

Crovitz, L. Gordon. "Information Age: Chicago School of Free Speech." *Wall Street Journal*, November 23, 2015, www.wsj.com/article_email/chicago-school-of-free-speech-1448231860-lMyQjAxMTI1NzI3MzEyNDM2Wj.

Csikszentmihalyi, Mihaly. *Flow and the Foundations of Positive Psychology*. Dordrecht: Springer, 2014.

Cui, Zhenzhong, Ruiben Feng, Stephanie Jacobs, Yanhong Duan, Huimin Wang, Xiaohua Cao, and Joe Z. Tsien. "Increased NR2A:NR2B Ratio Compresses

Long-Term Depression Range and Constrains Long-Term Memory." *Scientific Reports* 3, no. 1036 (January 8, 2013). doi:10.1038/srep01036.

Culotta, Elizabeth. "Did Modern Humans Get Smart or Just Get Together?" *Science* 328, no. 5975 (April 9, 2010): 164. doi:10.1126/science. 328.5975.164.

Darwin, Charles. *The Descent of Man, and Selection in Relation to Sex*. 2 vols. London: J. Murray, 1871. Photoreproduction. Princeton, NJ: Princeton University Press, 2008.

Daston, Lorraine. "Can Liberal Education Save the Sciences?" *The Point*, 2016, https://thepointmag.com/2016/examined-life/can-liberal-education-save-the-sciences.

Dawkins, Richard. *The Selfish Gene*. New York and Oxford: Oxford University Press, 1989.

Deckman, Melissa. *Tea Party Women*. New York: New York University Press, 2016.

Delbanco, Andrew. *College: What It Was, Is, and Should Be*. Princeton, NJ: Princeton University Press, 2012.

Dennett, Daniel C. *Breaking the Spell: Religion as a Natural Phenomenon*. New York: Penguin, 2007.

Dennett, Daniel C. *Darwin's Dangerous Idea: Evolution and the Meanings of Life*. New York: Touchstone, 1995.

Deresiewicz, William. *Excellent Sheep: The Miseducation of the American Elite and the Way to a Meaningful Life*. New York: Free Press, 2014.

Dewey, John. *Art as Experience*. New York: Penguin, 1934.

Dewey, John. *Democracy and Education: An Introduction to the Philosophy of Education*. New York: Macmillan, 1916.

Dewey, John, and Goodwin Watson. "A Forward View: A Free Teacher in a Free Society." In *John Dewey: The Later Works, 1925–1953*. Vol. 11, *1935–1937*, edited by Jo Anne Boydston, 535–47. Carbondale: Southern Illinois University Press, 1987.

Diamond, Jared. *Collapse: How Societies Choose to Fail or Succeed*. New York: Penguin, 2011.

Diamond, Jared. *Guns, Germs, and Steel: The Fates of Human Societies*. New York: Norton, 1997.

Diamond, Jared. *The Third Chimpanzee*. New York: Harpers, 2006.

Distin, Kate. *Cultural Evolution*. Cambridge: Cambridge University Press, 2011.

Djikic, Maja, Keith Oatley, and Mihnea C. Moldoveanua. "Opening the Closed Mind: The Effect of Exposure to Literature on the Need for Closure." *Creativity Research Journal* 25, no. 2 (2013): 149–54.

Dorit, Robert. "All Things Small and Great." *The American Scientist* 96, no. 4 (July–August 2008): 284–86.

Drutman, Lee. *The Business of America Is Lobbying: How Corporations Became Politicized and Politics Became More Corporate*. New York: Oxford University Press, 2016.

Du Bois, William Edward Burghardt. "The Talented Tenth." In *The Negro Problem*, 31–76. New York: James Pott & Co., 1903.

Dubreuil, Laurent. "On Experimental Criticism: Cognition, Evolution, and Literary Theory." *Diacritics* 39, no. 1 (Spring 2009): 3–23.

Dunbar, Robin I. M. "Brain Cognition in Evolutionary Perspective." In *Evolutionary Cognitive Neuroscience*, edited by Steven Platek, Todd Shackelford, and Julian Keenan, 21–46. Cambridge, MA: MIT Press, 2007.

Durham, William H. *Coevolution: Genes, Culture, and Human Diversity.* Stanford, CA: Stanford University Press, 1991.

Dutton, Denis. *The Art Instinct.* London: Bloomsbury, 2010.

Easterly, William. *The White Man's Burden: Why the West's Efforts to Aid the Rest Have Done So Much Ill and So Little Good.* New York: Penguin, 2007.

Edelman, Gerald M., and Vernon B. Mountcastle. *The Mindful Brain: Cortical Organization and the Group-Selective Theory of Higher Brain Function.* Cambridge, MA: MIT Press, 1978.

Edmundson, Mark. "Humanities Past, Present – and Future." *New Literary History* 36, no. 1 (2005): 43–46.

Edmundson, Mark. *Self and Soul: A Defense of Ideals.* Cambridge, MA: Harvard University Press, 2015.

Ehrenfreund, Max. "A Majority of Millennials Now Reject Capitalism, Poll Shows." *The Washington Post*, April 26, 2016, www.washingtonpost.com/news/wonk/wp/2016/04/26/a-majority-of-millennials-now-reject-capitalism-poll-shows/.

Eiduson, Bernice. *Scientists: Their Psychological World.* New York: Basic, 1962.

Einstein, Albert. "What Life Means to Einstein: An Interview by George Sylvester Viereck." *The Saturday Evening Post*, October 26, 1929.

Eliot, George. *Middlemarch.* Berlin: Asher and Co., 1871–72.

Emerson, Ralph Waldo. "Circles." In *The Prose Works.* Boston: Fields, Osgood, & Co., 1870.

Fagan, Brian M. *Floods, Famines, and Emperors.* New York: Basic Books, 1999.

Fellman, Bruce. "Born-Again Brains." *Yale Alumni Magazine*, May/June, 2013.

Ferrari, Massimo. "Sources for the History of the Concept of Symbol from Leibniz to Cassirer." In *Symbol and Physical Knowledge: On the Conceptual Structure of Physics*, edited by Massimo Ferrari and Ion-Olimpiu Stamatescu, 3–32. Berlin: Springer, 2002.

Fessler, Daniel M. T., Anne C. Pisor, and Colin Holbrook. "Political Orientation Predicts Credulity Regarding Putative Hazards." *Psychological Science* 28, no. 5 (May 2017): 651–60. doi:10.1177/0956797617692108.

Fisher, Matthew. *Scribal Authorship and the Writing of History in Medieval England.* Columbus: Ohio State University Press, 2012.

Flanagan, Caitlin. "Hysteria and the Teenage Girl." www.nytimes.com/2012/01/29/opinion/sunday/adolescent-girl-hysteria.html.

Foley, R. A., "How Useful Is the Culture Concept in Early Hominid Studies?" In *The Origins of Human Behaviour.* Edited by R. A. Foley. 25–38.

Foley, R. A., ed. *The Origins of Human Behaviour.* London: Unwin Hyman, 1991.

Forster, E. M. "The Machine Stops." In *The Science Fiction Century*, vol. 1, edited by David G. Hartwell, 135–46. New York: Tom Doherty Associates, 2006.

Foucault, Michel. *Discipline and Punish: The Birth of the Prison.* Translated by Alan Sheridan. New York: Pantheon, 1977.

Fracchia, Joseph, and Richard Lewontin. "Does Culture Evolve?" *History and Theory* 38 (1999): 52–78.

Francis, Pope. "Address to the New Non-Resident Ambassadors to the Holy See: Kyrgyzstan, Antigua and Barbuda, Luxembourg and Botswana." Clementine Hall, May 16, 2013, www.vatican.va/holy_father/francesco/speeches/2013/may/documents/papa-francesco_20130516_nuovi-ambasciatori_en.html.

Frank, Arthur. *The Wounded Storyteller: Body, Illness, and Ethics*. Chicago, IL: University of Chicago Press, 1995.

Frank, Thomas. *What's the Matter with Kansas?* New York: Metropolitan Books, 2004.

Frankl, Viktor. *Man's Search for Meaning*. 1946; rpt. Boston, MA: Beacon Press, 2006.

Fraser, Nancy. "How Feminism Became Capitalism's Handmaiden – And How to Reclaim It." *The Guardian*, October 14, 2013, www.theguardian.com/commentisfree/2013/oct/14/feminism-capitalist-handmaiden-neoliberal.

Freeman, Walter. "A Neurobiological Role of Music in Social Bonding." In *The Origins of Music*, edited by Nils L. Wallin, Björn Merker, and Steven Brown, 411–24. Cambridge, MA: MIT Press, 2000.

Freud, Sigmund. *Civilization and Its Discontents*. 1930. Translated by James Strachey. New York: Norton, 1962.

Freud, Sigmund. *Standard Edition of the Complete Psychological Works of Sigmund Freud*. Edited by James Strachey, Anna Freud, Carrie Lee Rothgeb, and Angela Richards. 24 vols. London: Hogarth Press, 1953–74.

Fry, Douglas P. *The Human Potential for Peace: An Anthropological Challenge to Assumptions about War and Violence*. New York: Oxford University Press, 2006.

Fry, Douglas P., and Patrik Söderberg. "Myths about Hunter-Gatherers Redux: Nomadic Forager War and Peace." *Journal of Aggression, Conflict and Peace Research* 6, no. 4 (2014): 255–66, doi:10.1108/JACPR-06-2014-0127.

Funkenstein, Amos. *Theology and the Scientific Imagination*. Princeton, NJ: Princeton University Press, 1986.

Geertz, Clifford. "The Growth of Culture and the Evolution of Mind." In *The Interpretation of Cultures: Selected Essays*, 55–83. New York: Basic Books, 1973.

Geertz, Clifford. "The Impact of the Concept of Culture on the Concept of Man." *Bulletin of the Atomic Scientists* 22, no. 4 (1966): 2–8.

Gellner, Ernest. *Plough, Sword and Book: The Structure of Human History*. London: Collins Harvill, 1988.

Gilens, Martin, and Benjamin I. Page. "Testing Theories of American Politics: Elites, Interest Groups, and Average Citizens." Abstract. *Perspectives on Politics* 12, no. 3 (September 2014): 564–81.

Goffman, Erving. *The Presentation of Self in Everyday Life*. New York: Anchor, 1959.

Goldenweiser, Alexander. "The Autonomy of the Social." *American Anthropologist* 19, no. 3 (July–September 1917): 447–49.

Gorbachev, Mikhail. "Gorbachev on 1989." By Katrina vanden Heuvel and Stephen F. Cohen. *The Nation*, October 28, 2009. www.thenation.com/article/gorbachev-1989/.

Gottlieb, Anthony. "It Aint Necessarily So." *The New Yorker*, September 17, 2012.

Gould, Stephen J. *Bully for Brontosaurus: Reflections in Natural History*. New York: Norton, 1991.

Grant, Edward. *A History of Natural Philosophy from the Ancient World to the Nineteenth Century*. Cambridge: Cambridge University Press, 2007.

Gray, Kurt et al. "The Science of Style." http://journals.plos.org/plosone/article?id=10.1371/journal.pone.0102772.

Greenblatt, Stephen. *The Swerve: How the World Became Modern*. New York: Norton, 2011.

Greenblatt, Stephen. "Why Holiday Stories Matter." *The New York Times*, December 20, 2017.

Guthrie, Stewart. *Faces in the Clouds: A New Theory of Religion*. New York and Oxford: Oxford University Press, 1995.

Hagel, Jonathan C. "In Search of the 'Racist White Psyche': Racism and the Psychology or Prejudice in American Social Thought, 1930–1960." PhD diss., Brown University, 2001.

Hammerich, Kai, and Richard D. Lewis. *Fish Can't See Water: How National Culture Can Make or Break Your Corporate Strategy*. Chichester: Wiley, 2013.

Harari, Yuval Noah. *Sapiens: A Brief History of Humankind*. New York: HarperCollins, 2015.

Hari, Johann. "What's Really Causing the Prescription Drug Crisis." *Los Angeles Times*, January 15, 2017.

Harpham, Geoffrey Galt. *The Humanities and the Dream of America*. Chicago, IL: University of Chicago Press, 2011.

Harvey, Robert C. *The Art of the Comic Book: An Aesthetic History*. Jackson: University Press of Mississippi, 1996.

Hatemi, Peter K., Rose McDermott, Lindon J. Eaves, Kenneth S. Kendler, and Michael C. Neale. "Fear as a Disposition and an Emotional State: A Genetic and Environmental Approach to Out-Group Political Preferences." *American Journal of Political Science* 57, no. 1 (April 2013): 279–93. doi:10.1111/ajps.12016.

Hawkes, David. *Idols of the Marketplace: Idolatry and Commodity Fetishism in English Literature, 1580–1680*. New York: Palgrave, 2001.

Heaney, Seamus. *The Government of the Tongue*. New York: Farrar Straus, 1990.

Henrich, Joseph. *The Secret of Our Success*. Princeton, NJ: Princeton University Press, 2015.

Henrich, Joseph, Edward Slingerland, and Ara Norenzayan. "The Evolution of Prosocial Religions." In *Cultural Evolution*, edited by Richerson and Christiansen, 335–48. Cambridge, MA: MIT Press, 2013.

Henrich, Joseph, Steven J. Heine, and Ara Norenzayan. "The Weirdest People in the World?" Abstract. *Behavioral and Brain Sciences* 33, no. 2–3 (2010): 61–83. doi:10.1017/S0140525X0999152X.

Herf, Jeffrey. "How the Culture Wars Matter." In *Higher Education under Fire: Politics, Economics, and the Crisis of the Humanities*, edited by Michael Bérubé and Cary Nelson, 149–62. London: Routledge, 1994.

Hexter, Ralph J., and Craig Buckwald. "Conquering Obstacles to Kingdom and Fate: The Ethics of Reading and the University Administrator." In *The Humanities and Public Life*. Edited by Peter Brooks, with Hilary Jewett, 83–91. New York: Fordham University Press, 2014.

Hochschild, Arlie Russell. *Strangers in Their Own Land: Anger and Mourning on the American Right*. New York: The New Press, 2016.

Hoey, Brian, and Tom Fricke. "From Sweet Potatoes to God Almighty: Roy Rappaport on Being a Hedgehog." (Includes an interview with Roy Rappaport.) *American Ethnologist* 34, no. 3 (2007): 581–99.

Hölldobler, Bert, and E. O. Wilson. *The Superorganism: The Beauty, Elegance, and Strangeness of Insect Societies*. New York: Norton, 2009.

Holmes, Jamie. *Nonsense: The Power of Not Knowing*. New York: Crown/ Penguin, 2015.

hooks, bell. *Writing Beyond Race: Living Theory and Practice*. New York: Routledge, 2013.

Hosking, Geoffrey. *The First Socialist Society: A History of the Soviet Union from Within*. Cambridge, MA: Harvard University Press, 1985.

Howard, Marcus E. "Senators Detail 'Paid-For Patriotism.'" *Los Angeles Times*, November 5, 2015.

Huehls, Mitchum. *After Critique: Twenty-First-Century Fiction in a Neoliberal Age*. New York: Oxford University Press, 2016.

Hugo, Victor. Les Misérables. Translated by Isabel F. Hapgood. New York: Thomas Y. Crowell, 1887.

Hull, David L. "Taking Memetics Seriously: Memetics Will Be What We Make It." In *Darwinizing Culture*, edited by Aunger, 43–68. Oxford: Oxford University Press, 2001.

Humphrey, Nicholas K. "The Social Function of Intellect." In *Growing Points in Ethology*, edited by Paul Patrick Gordon Bateson and R. A. Hinde, 303–17. Cambridge: Cambridge University Press, 1976.

Hutson, Matthew. "What Is Art?" *The Atlantic*, July/August, 2014.

Ionesco, Eugéne. *Rhinoceros and Other Plays*. Translated by Derek Prouse. New York: Grove Press, 1960.

Jaén, Isabel, and Julien Jacques Simon, eds. *Cognitive Literary Studies: Current Themes and New Directions*. Austin, TX: University of Texas Press, 2012.

Jacobs, Andrew, and Matt Richtel. "How Big Business Got Brazil Hooked on Junk Food." *New York Times*, September 17, 2017.

Jacoby, Russell. *Dogmatic Wisdom*. New York: Anchor, 1995.

James, William. *Principles of Psychology*. 2 vols. New York: Dover, 1890.

Jamison, Kay Redfield. *Robert Lowell: Setting the River on Fire: A Study of Genius, Mania, and Character*. New York: Knopf, 2017.

Jaynes, Julian. *The Origin of Consciousness in the Breakdown of the Bicameral Mind*. 1976. Boston, MA: Mariner, 2000.

Jensen, Rolf. *The Dream Society: How the Coming Shift from Information to Imagination Will Transform Your Business*. New York: McGraw-Hill, 2001.

Jerving, Sara, Katie Jennings, Masako Melissa Hirsch, and Susanne Rust. "What Exxon Knew about Warming in the Arctic." *Los Angeles Times*, October 11, 2015.

Judt, Tony. *Ill Fares the Land: A Treatise on Our Present Discontents*. London: Penguin, 2010.

Kelly, Raymond C. *The Nuer Conquest: The Structure and Development of an Expansionist System*. Ann Arbor: University of Michigan Press, 1985.

Kidd, David Comer, and Emanuele Castano. "Reading Literary Fiction Improves Theory of Mind." *Science* 342, no. 6156 (October 18, 2013): 377–80. doi:10.1126/science.1239918.

Kimball, Bruce. *Orators and Philosophers*. New York: Teachers College Press, 1986.

King, Rev. Martin Luther, Jr. "Beyond Vietnam." In *Voices of a People's History of the United States*, 2nd ed. Edited by Howard Zinn and Anthony Arnove. New York: Seven Stories Press, 2004).

Kinney, Arthur F. *Shakespeare and Cognition: Aristotle's Legacy and Shakespearean Drama*. New York: Routledge, 2006.

Klein, Naomi. *The Shock Doctrine*. New York: Penguin, 2008.

Klein, Naomi. *This Changes Everything: Capitalism vs. the Climate*. New York: Simon & Schuster, 2014.

Klein, Sheldon. "The Invention of Computationally Plausible Knowledge Systems in the Upper Paleolithic." In *The Origins of Human Behaviour*, edited by R. A. Foley. London: Unwin Hyman, 1991.

Kleinman, Arthur. *The Illness Narratives: Suffering, Healing, and the Human Condition*. New York: Basic Books, 1988.

Kolozi, Peter. *Conservatives against Capitalism: From the Industrial Revolution to Globalization*. New York: Columbia University Press, 2017.

Kringelbach, Morten L. and Kent C. Berridge. "New Pleasure Circuit Found in the Brain." *Scientific American* 307, August, 2012. https://www.scientificamerican.com/article/new-pleasure-circuit-found-brain.

Kuhn, Thomas. *The Structure of Scientific Revolutions*. Chicago, IL: University of Chicago Press, 1962.

Kuper, Adam. "If Memes Are the Answer, What Is the Question?" In *Darwinizing Culture*, edited by Aunger, 175–88. Oxford: Oxford University Press, 2001.

Lagemann, Ellen Condliffe. *Liberating Minds: The Case for College in Prison*. New York: Free Press, 2016.

Laland, Kevin N. *Darwin's Unfinished Symphony: How Culture Made the Human Mind*. Princeton, NJ: Princeton University Press, 2017.

Laland, Kevin N., and John Odling-Smee. "The Evolution of the Meme." In *Darwinizing Culture*, edited by Aunger, 121–42. Oxford: Oxford University Press, 2001.

Landau, Mark, Jeff Greenberg, Sheldon Solomon, Tom Pyszcynski, and Andy Martens. "Windows into Nothingness." *Journal of Personality and Social Psychology* 90, no. 6 (June 2006): 879–92.

Lanier, Jaron. *You Are Not a Gadget*. New York: Knopf, 2011.

Laor, Yuval, and Eva Jablonka. "The Evolution and Development of Culture." Review of *Cultural Evolution: How Darwinian Theory Can Explain Human Culture and Synthesize the Social Sciences*, by Alex Mesoudi. *History and Theory* 52, no. 2 (May 2013): 290–99.

Lear, Jonathan. *Radical Hope: Ethics in the Face of Cultural Devastation*. Cambridge, MA: Harvard University Press, 2006.

Lehrer, Jonah. "Groupthink: The Brainstorming Myth." *The New Yorker*, January 30, 2012.

Lem, Stanislaw. *Imaginary Magnitude*. Translated by Mark E. Heine. New York: Harcourt Brace, 1984.

Leonard, Andrew. "Conservatives Declare War on College." *Salon*, February 22, 2013. www.salon.com/2013/02/22/conservatives_declare_war_on_college/.

Lepani, Katherine. *Islands of Love, Islands of Risk: Culture and HIV in the Trobriands*. Nashville, TN: Vanderbilt University Press, 2012.

Levitin, Daniel J. *The Organized Mind*. New York: Penguin, 2014.

Lieberman, Philip. *The Unpredictable Species: What Makes Humans Unique*. Princeton, NJ: Princeton University Press, 2013.

Liu, Alan. "Drafts for *Against the Culturally Singularity* (book in progress)." *Alan Liu*, May 2, 2016. http://liu.english.ucsb.edu/drafts-for-against-the-cultural-singularity.

Lorenz, Chris. "If You're So Smart, Why Are You under Surveillance? Universities, Neoliberalism, and New Public Management." *Critical Inquiry* 38, no. 3 (Spring 2012): 599–629.

Lorraine, Ali. "Inside the Minds of U.S. Jihadis." *Los Angeles Times*, March 25, 2017.

Loukola, Olli J., Clint J. Perry, Louie Coscos, and Lars Chittka. "Bumblebees Show Cognitive Flexibility by Improving on an Observed Complex Behavior." *Science* 355, no. 6327 (February 24, 2017): 833–36. doi:10.1126/science. aag2360.

Louv, Richard. *Last Child in the Woods*. New York: Algonquin, 2005.

Lucky, Robert. *Silicon Dreams: Information, Man, and Machine*. New York: St. Martins, 1989.

Marcus, Greil. *The Old, Weird America*. New York: Picador, 2011.

Marcuse, Herbert. *One-Dimensional Man*. 1964; rpt. New York: Routledge Classics, 2002.

Martel, Yann. *The Life of Pi*. New York: Houghton Mifflin, 2002.

Martin, Andrew. "The Scientific A-Team Saving the World from Killer Viruses, Rogue AI and the Paperclip Apocalypse." *The Guardian*, August 30, 2014. www.theguardian.com/technology/2014/aug/30/saviours-universe-four-unlikely-men-save-world.

Marx, Karl. "The German Ideology." In *Knowledge and Postmodernism in Historical Perspective*, edited by Joyce Oldham Appleby, Elizabeth Covington, David Hoyt, Michael Latham, and Allison Sneider, 180–88. Hove: Psychology Press, 1996.

Mayer, Jane. *Dark Money: The Hidden History of the Billionaires behind the Rise of the Radical Right*. New York: Doubleday, 2016.

McAuliffe, Kathleen. *This Is Your Brain on Parasites: How Tiny Creatures Manipulate Our Behavior and Shape Society*. Boston, MA: Houghton Mifflin, 2016.

McCaslin, Nellie. *Creative Drama in the Classroom and Beyond*. Boston, MA: Pearson, 2006.

McGinn, Colin. "The Problem of Philosophy." *Philosophical Studies* 76 (1994): 133–156.

McGreal, Chris. "'The S-word': How Young Americans Fell in Love with Socialism." *The Guardian*, September 2, 2017, www.theguardian.com/us-news/2017/sep/02/socialism-young-americans-bernie-sanders.

McKibben, Bill. *The Age of Missing Information*. New York: Random House, 2006.

McKibben, Bill. Eaarth. New York: Random House, 2006.

McKibben, Bill. *The End of Nature.* 1989. Reprinted with new introduction by the author. New York: Random House, 2006.

McKinnon, Susan. *Neo-Liberal Genetics: The Myths and Moral Tales of Evolutionary Psychology.* Chicago, IL: Prickly Paradigm Press, 2005.

McLuhan, Marshall. *From Cliché to Archetype.* New York: Penguin, 1970.

Menand, Louis. *The Marketplace of Ideas: Reform and Resistance in the American University.* New York: Norton, 2010.

Menand, Louis. *The Metaphysical Club: A Story of Ideas in America.* New York: Farrar, Straus and Giroux, 2002.

Meskin, Aaron, Mark Phelan, Margaret Moore, and Matthew Kieran. "Mere Exposure to Bad Art." *British Journal of Aesthetics* 53, no. 2 (April 2013): 139–64.

Mesoudi, Alex. *Cultural Evolution: How Darwinian Theory Can Explain Human Culture and Synthesize the Social Sciences.* Chicago, IL: University of Chicago Press, 2011.

Metzl, Jonathan. *The Protest Psychosis: How Schizophrenia Became a Black Disease.* Boston, MA: Beacon Press, 2010.

Milder, Robert. "The Radical Emerson?" In *Cambridge Companion to Ralph Waldo Emerson,* edited by Joel Porte and Saundra Morris, 49–75. Cambridge: Cambridge University Press, 1999.

Mill, John Stuart. *Autobiography.* London, 1873. Reprinted. Oxford: Oxford University Press, 1924.

Mithen, Steven. *The Singing Neanderthals: The Origins of Music, Language, Mind, and Body.* Cambridge, MA: Harvard University Press, 2011.

Modell, Arnold H. *Imagination and the Meaningful Brain.* Boston, MA: MIT Press, 2006.

Mohr, Nicholasa. *Growing Up Inside the Sanctuary of My Imagination.* New York: Simon & Schuster, 1994.

Montaigne, Michel de. *Essays.* Translated by John Florio. London, 1603.

Morrison, Patt. "We Couldn't Save Cecil the Lion, But Can We Save the Planet?" *Los Angeles Times,* August 12, 2015. www.latimes.com/opinion/op-ed/la-oe-morrison-kareiva-20150812-column.html.

Morton, Timothy. *Dark Ecology: For a Logic of Future Coexistence.* New York: Columbia University Press, 2016.

Mounk, Yascha. *The People Versus Democracy: Why Our Freedom Is in Danger and How to Save It.* Cambridge, MA: Harvard University Press, 2018.

Muir, John. "The Hetch Hetchy Valley." *Sierra Club Bulletin* 6, no. 4 (1908).

Muller, Jerry Z. "The Tyranny of Metrics." *Chronicle of Higher Education,* January 21, 2018.

Murray, Penelope, and Peter Wilson. *Music and the Muses: The Culture of 'mousikē' in the Classical Athenian City.* New York: Oxford University Press, 2004.

Nagoshi, Julie L. *et alia.* "Deconstructing the Complex Perceptions of Gender Roles, Gender Identity, and Sexual Orientation among Transgender Individuals." *Feminism & Psychology.* October 10, 2012. Accessed June 6, 2018.

Nelson, Libby. "Yale's Big Fight over Sensitivity and Free Speech, Explained." *Vox,* November 7, 2015, www.vox.com/2015/11/7/9689330/yale-halloween-email.

Neuroscience News. "How LSD Affects Language." August 22, 2016. http://neurosciencenews.com/language-lsd-neuroscience-4883/.

Newfield, Christopher. *The Great Mistake: How We Wrecked Public Universities and How We Can Fix Them*. Baltimore, MD: Johns Hopkins University Press, 2016.

Newfield, Christopher. *Unmaking the Public University*. Cambridge, MA: Harvard University Press, 2008.

Nicholson, Helen. *Applied Drama: The Gift of Theatre*. New York: Palgrave Macmillan, 2005.

Nietzsche, Friedrich. *Beyond Good and Evil: Prelude to a Philosophy of the Future*. Translated by Walter Kaufmann. New York: Vintage, 1989.

Nisbett, Richard E., and Dov Cohen. *Culture of Honor: The Psychology of Violence in the South*. Boulder, CO: Westview Press, 1996.

Nussbaum, Martha C. *Not for Profit: Why Democracy Needs the Humanities*. Princeton, NJ: Princeton University Press, 2010.

Oakley, Francis. *Community of Learning: The American College and the Liberal Arts Tradition*. New York: Oxford University Press, 1992.

Oatley, Keith, Raymond A. Mar, and Maja Djikic. "The Psychology of Fiction: Present and Future." In *Cognitive Literary Studies*, edited by Isabel Jaén and Julien Jacques Simon. Austin, TX: University of Texas Press, 2012. 235–49.

Obama, Barack. "Remarks of the President to the United States Hispanic Chamber of Commerce." March 10, 2009, http://obamawhitehouse.archives.gov/the-press-office/remarks-president-united-states-hispanic-chamber-commerce.

O'Neil, Cathy. *Weapons of Math Destruction: How Big Data Increases Inequality and Threatens Democracy*. New York: Crown, 2016.

Orwell, George. *Nineteen Eighty-Four*. London: Secker & Warburg, 1949.

Orwell, George. "Notes on Nationalism." *Polemic*, May, 1945.

Packer, George. *The Unwinding*. London: Faber & Faber, 2014.

Parfit, Derek. *Reasons and Persons*. Oxford: Oxford University Press, 1986.

Parmentier, Richard. "Untitled." *Chicago Journals* 43, no. 2 (2003): 162–64.

Pattani, Aneri. "They Were Shorter and at Risk for Arthritis, but They Survived an Ice Age." *New York Times*, July 6, 2017.

Paul, Annie Murphy. "Your Brain on Fiction." *New York Times*, March 18, 2012.

Perreault, Charles. "The Pace of Cultural Evolution." *PLoS ONE* 7, no. 9 (September 2012): e45150. doi:10.1371/journal.pone.0045150.

Petersen, Alexander M., Joel Tenenbaum, Shlomo Havlin, and H. Eugene Stanley. "Statistical Laws Governing Fluctuations in Word Use from Word Birth to Word Death." *Scientific Reports* 2, no. 313 (2012). doi:10.1038/srep00313.

Philipps, Dave. "At Veterans Hospital in Oregon, a Push for Better Ratings Puts Patients at Risk, Doctors Say." *New York Times*, January 1, 2018, www.nytimes.com/2018/01/01/us/at-veterans-hospital-in-oregon-a-push-for-better-ratings-puts-patients-at-risk-doctors-say.html.

Picketty, Thomas. *Capital in the Twenty-First Century*. Cambridge, MA: Belknap, 2013.

Pinker, Steven. *The Better Angels of Our Nature: Why Violence Has Declined*. New York: Penguin, 2011.

Pinker, Steven. *How the Mind Works*. New York: Norton, 1997.

Plato, "The Apology of Socrates." In *The Apology, Phaedo, and Crito of Plato*. Vol. 2. Translated and edited by Benjamin Jowett, Hastings Crossley, and George Long, 3–29. New York: Collier, 1909.

Plato, *Laws*. Translated by R. G. Bury. Loeb Classical Library. Cambridge, MA: Harvard University Press, 1926.

Plimpton, George. *The Bogey Man: A Month on the PGA Tour*. New York: HarperCollins, 1968.

Plotkin, Henry. *Evolutionary Worlds without End*. Oxford: Oxford University Press, 2010.

Polanyi, Karl. "The Essence of Fascism." In *Christianity and the Social Revolution*. Edited by John Lewis, Karl Polanyi, and Donald K. Kitchin, 359–94. London: Victor Gollancz Ltd, 1935.

Pollan, Michael. *How to Change Your Mind: What the New Science of Psychedelics Teaches Us about Consciousness, Dying, Addiction, Depression, and Transcendence*. New York: Penguin, 2018.

Pollan, Michael. "Some of My Best Friends Are Bacteria." *New York Times Sunday Magazine*, May 12, 2013.

Pollan, Michael. *The Omnivore's Dilemma: A Natural History of Four Meals*. New York: Penguin, 2006.

Popper, Karl. "Natural Selection and the Emergence of Mind." Lecture Delivered at Darwin College, Cambridge. November 8, 1977. www.informationphilosopher.com/solutions/philosophers/popper/natural_selection_and_the_emergence_of_mind.html.

Popper, Karl. *The Open Society and Its Enemies*. 2nd ed. Rev. Princeton, NJ: Princeton University Press, 1950.

Postman, Neil. *Amusing Ourselves to Death: Public Discourse in the Age of Show Business*. New York: Penguin, 1986.

Postman, Neil, and Charles Weingartner. *Teaching as a Subversive Activity*. New York: Delacorte, 1969.

Pringle, Heather. "The Origins of Creativity." *Scientific American*, March, 2013.

Professor Watchlist. "About Us." Accessed November 25, 2016. www.professorwatchlist.org/about-us/.

Puchner, Martin. *The Written Word*. New York: Random House, 2017.

Quammen, David. *Spillover: Animal Infections and the Next Human Pandemic*. New York: Norton, 2012.

Raichle, Marcus E. "Two Views of Brain Function." *Trends in Cognitive Sciences* 14, no. 4 (April 2010): 180–90. doi:10.1016/j.tics.2010.01.008.

Rauch, Jonathan. "Seeing Around Corners." *The Atlantic*, April, 2002.

Rawls, John. *A Theory of Justice*. Cambridge, MA: Harvard University Press, 1999.

Redman, Charles. *Human Impact on Ancient Environments*. Tucson: University of Arizona Press, 1999.

Rhodes, Richard. *The Making of the Atomic Bomb*. New York: Simon and Schuster, 2012.

Rich, Frank. "Karl Rove Beats the Democrats Again." *New York Times*, June 18, 2006.

Richerson, Peter J., and Morten H. Christiansen, eds. *Cultural Evolution: Society, Technology, Language, and Religion*. Cambridge, MA: MIT Press, 2013.

Richerson, Peter J., and Robert Boyd. *Not by Genes Alone: How Culture Transformed Human Evolution.* Chicago, IL: University of Chicago Press, 2005.

Rider, Sharon. "The Future of the European University: Liberal Democracy or Authoritarian Capitalism?" *Culture Unbound* 1 (2009): 83–104, www.cultureunbound.ep.liu.se/v1/a07/cu09v1a07.pdf.

Roth, Michael. *Beyond the University: Why Liberal Education Matters.* New Haven, CT: Yale University Press, 2014.

Rothstein, Richard. *The Color of Law: A Forgotten History of How Our Government Segregated America.* New York: Liveright, 2017.

Ruder, Debra Bradley. "The 'Water Cooler' Effect." *Harvard Magazine*, May–June, 2011.

Rynard, Pat. "Senator Mark Chelgren Aims to Purge Democrats from Iowa Universities." *Iowa Starting Line*, February 20, 2017, http://iowastartingline.com/2017/02/20/senator-chelgren-aims-purge-democrats-iowa-universities/.

Said, Edward W. *Humanism and Democratic Criticism.* New York: Columbia University Press, 2004.

Said, Edward W. *Representations of the Intellectual.* New York: Vintage, 1996.

Salmond, John A. *The Conscience of a Lawyer: Clifford J. Durr and American Civil Liberties, 1899–1975.* Tuscaloosa: University of Alabama Press, 1990.

Samet, Elizabeth D. "Mouse-Boys, Literate Spiders, and the Security of Imagination." In *What Is Education*, edited by Lee Oser and Rosanna Warren, 14–17. Boston, MA: ALSCW, 2012.

Sapir, Edward. "The Status of Washo." *American Anthropologist* 19, no. 3 (July–September 1917): 449–50.

Sapolsky, Robert M. "Rich Brain, Poor Brain." *Los Angeles Times*, October 18, 2013. www.latimes.com/opinion/op-ed/la-oe-sapolsky-cognitive-load-poverty-20131018-story.html#axzz2t544uGt5.

Scarry, Elaine. "Poetry, Injury, and the Ethics of Reading." In *The Humanities and Public Life.* Edited by Peter Brooks, with Hilary Jewett, 41–48. New York: Fordham University Press, 2014.

Schelling, Thomas. "Dynamic Models of Segregation." *Journal of Mathematical Sociology* 1, no. 2 (1971), 143–86.

Scheppele, Kim Lane. "Responses and Discussion." In *The Humanities and Public Life.* Edited by Peter Brooks, with Hilary Jewett, 123–25. New York: Fordham University Press, 2014.

Schjeldahl, Peter. "The Anti-Modernists." *The New Yorker*, March 24, 2014.

Schwartz, Barry. *Why We Work.* New York: Simon and Schuster, 2015.

Scott, Charlotte. *The Child in Shakespeare.* Oxford: Oxford University Press, 2018.

Scott, James C. *Domination and the Arts of Resistance.* New Haven, CT: Yale University Press, 1990.

Scott, James C. *Weapons of the Weak: Everyday Forms of Peasant Resistance.* New Haven, CT: Yale University Press, 1985.

Seeley, Thomas D. *The Wisdom of the Hive: The Social Physiology of Honey Bee Colonies.* Cambridge, MA: Harvard University Press, 1995.

Sender, Ron, Shai Fuchs, and Ron Milo. "Are We Really Vastly Outnumbered? Revisiting the Ration of Bacterial to Host Cells in Humans." *Cell* 164, no. 3 (January 2016): 337–40. doi:10.1016/j.cell.2016.01.013.

Shakespeare, William. *The Riverside Shakespeare.* 2nd ed. Edited by G. Blakemore Evans. Boston, MA: Houghton Mifflin, 1997.

Shea, Christopher. "The New Science of the Birth and Death of Words." *Wall Street Journal*, March 17, 2012.

Shennan, Stephen. *Genes, Memes and Human History: Darwinian Archaeology and Cultural Evolution.* London: Thames and Hudson, 2002.

Shepard, Roger N. "The Perceptual Organization of Colors: An Adaptation to Regularities of the Terrestrial World?" In *The Adapted Mind*, edited by Jerome H. Barkow, Leda Cosmides, and John Tooby, 495–532. New York: Oxford University Press, 1992.

Shirky, Clay. *Cognitive Surplus: Creativity and Generosity in a Connected Age.* New York: Penguin, 2010.

Shklovsky, Viktor. *Theory of Prose.* 1925; rpt. Elmwood Park, IL: Dalkey Archive Press, 1991.

Shore, Bradd. *Culture in Mind: Cognition, Culture, and the Problem of Meaning.* New York: Oxford University Press, 1996.

Sidney, Sir Philip. *Defence of Poesy.* London, 1595

Silk, Joan B., Susan C. Alberts, and Jeanne Altmann. "Social Bonds of Female Baboons Enhance Infant Survival." *Science* 302, no. 5648 (2003): 1231–34.

Simonton, Dean Keith. *Greatness: Who Makes History and Why.* New York: The Guilford Press, 1994.

Simpkin, Arabella L., and Richard M. Schwartzstein. "Tolerating Uncertainty —— The Next Medical Revolution?" *New England Journal of Medicine* 375 (November 3, 2016): 1713–15.

Singal, Jesse. "This Is What a Modern-Day Witch Hunt Looks Like." *New York Magazine*, May 2, 2017, http://nymag.com/daily/intelligencer/2017/05/transracialism-article-controversy.html.

Smail, Daniel Lord. *On Deep History and the Brain.* Berkeley: University of California Press, 2008.

Small, Gary, Teena D. Moody, Prabha Siddarth, and Susan Y. Bookheimer. "Your Brain on Google: Patterns of Cerebral Activation during Internet Searching." *The American Journal of Geriatric Psychiatry* 17, no. 2 (February 2009): 116–26.

Small, Helen. *The Value of the Humanities.* Oxford: Oxford University Press, 2013.

Smith, Adam. *An Inquiry into the Nature and Causes of the Wealth of Nations.* Edited by J. R. McCulloch. Edinburgh: Adam and Charles Black, 1863.

Smith, Daniel et al. "Cooperation and the Evolution of Hunter-Gatherer Storytelling." *Nature Communications* 8, no. 1853 (2017), doi:10.1038/s41467-017-02036-8.

Snyder, Timothy. *Bloodlands: Europe Between Hitler and Stalin.* New York: Basic Books, 2012.

Sorokin, Pitirim. *Society, Culture, and Personality: Their Structure and Dynamics.* New York: Cooper Square, 1969.

Sperber, Dan. *Explaining Culture: A Naturalistic Approach.* Oxford: Blackwell, 1996.

Stannard, David. *American Holocaust: The Conquest of the New World.* Oxford University Press, 1993.

Stanovich, Keith E. *The Robot's Rebellion: Finding Meaning in the Age of Darwin*. Chicago, IL: University of Chicago Press, 2004.

Sterelny, Kim. *The Evolved Apprentice: How Evolution Made Humans Unique*. Cambridge, MA: MIT Press, 2012.

Sterelny, Kim. *Thought in a Hostile World: The Evolution of Human Cognition*. London: Blackwell, 2003.

Stevens, Wallace. "The Man with the Blue Guitar" and "The Idea of Order at Key West." *The Collected Poems of Wallace Stevens*. New York: Knopf, 1954.

Steward, Julian H. *Theory of Culture Change: The Methodology of Multilinear Evolution*. Urbana: University of Illinois Press, 1955.

Stille, Alexander. "Holy Orders." *The New Yorker*, September 14, 2015.

Stock, Jay T. "Are Humans Still Evolving?" *EMBO Reports* 9 (2008): S51–S54. doi:10.1038/embor.2008.63.

Stout, Lynn. *The Shareholder Value Myth: How Putting Shareholders First Harms Investors, Corporations, and the Public*. San Francisco, CA: Berrett-Koehler, 2012.

Sugiyama, Michelle Scalise. "Narrative Theory and Function: Why Evolution Matters." *Philosophy and Literature* 25, no. 2 (2001): 233–50.

Sullivan, William. *Work and Integrity: The Crisis and Promise of Professionalism in America*. Stanford, CA: Jossey-Bass, 2004.

Sunstein, Cass R. "Social Norms and Social Roles." *Program in Law and Economics Working Paper*, no. 36 (1996). doi:10.2307/1123430.

Suskind, Ron. "Faith, Certainty, and the Presidency of George W. Bush." *The New York Times Magazine*, October 17, 2004.

Swed, Mark. "Is Streaming a Threat to Music?" *Los Angeles Times*, August 9, 2015.

Talbot, Margaret. "The Addicts Next Door." *The New Yorker*, June 5 and 12, 2017.

Tang, Guomei et al. "Loss of mTOR-Dependent Macroautophagy Causes Autistic-like Synaptic Pruning Deficits." *Neuron* 83, no. 5 (September 3, 2014): 1131–43. doi:10.1016/j.neuron.2014.07.040.

Tattersall, Ian. *The Monkey in the Mirror: Essays on the Science of What Makes Us Human*. New York: Mariner Books, 2003.

Taub, Amanda. "How 'Islands of Honesty' Can Crush a System of Corruption." *New York Times*, December 9, 2016.

Tawney, Richard Henry. *Religion and the Rise of Capitalism*. New York: Harcourt Brace, 1926.

Taylor, Charles. *Sources of the Self*. Cambridge, MA: Harvard University Press, 1992.

Taylor, Gary. *Cultural Selection: Why Some Achievements Survive the Test of Time and Others Don't*. New York: Basic Books, 1996.

Thompson, George. *Aeschylus and Athens*. 1941. Reprinted. London: Beekman, 1980.

Tocqueville, Alexis de. Alexis de Tocqueville to Ernest de Chabrol, New York, June 9, 1831. In *The Tocqueville Reader: A Life in Letters and Politics*, edited by Olivier Zunz and Alan S. Kahan, 40–41. Oxford: Blackwell, 2002.

Tocqueville, Alexis de. *Democracy in America*. Translated by George Lawrence. New York: Harpers, 2000.

Tolkien, J. R. R. *The History of Middle-earth.* Edited by Christopher Tolkien. Vol. 10, *Morgoth's Ring.* Boston: Houghton, 1993.

Tooby, John, and Leda Cosmides. "Does Beauty Build Adapted Minds?" In *Evolution, Literature, and Film: A Reader,* edited by Brian Boyd, Joseph Carroll, and Jonathan Gottschall, 174–83. New York: Columbia University Press, 2010.

Tooby, John, and Leda Cosmides. "The Psychological Foundations of Culture." In *The Adapted Mind,* edited by Jerome Barkow, Leda Cosmides, and John Tooby, 19–136. New York: Oxford University Press, 1992.

Toplak, Maggie E., and Keith E. Stanovich. "Associations between Myside Bias on an Informal Reasoning Task and Amount of Post-Secondary Education." *Applied Cognitive Psychology* 17, no. 7 (2003): 851–60. doi:10.1002/acp.91.

Turkle, Sherry. "Stop Googling. Let's Talk." *The New York Times,* September 26, 2015.

Van Tilburg,Wijnand Adriaan Pieter, and Eric Raymond Igou. "From Van Gogh to Lady Gaga: Artist Eccentricity Increases Perceived Artistic Skill and Art Appreciation." *European Journal of Social Psychology* (2014). doi:10.1002/ejsp.1999.

Vergese, Abraham. "Machine Medicine." *New York Times Magazine,* May 20, 2018.

Waal, Frans de. *Primates and Philosophers.* Princeton, NJ: Princeton University Press, 2016.

Walker, Scott. "UW Flexible Degree." Office of the Governor, State of Wisconsin, June 2012. www.uwgb.edu/sofas/structures/governance/senate/agendas/Flexible%20Degree%20Proposal%20Packet1.pdf.

Warner, Jeremy L, Robert M. Najarian, and Lawrence M. Tierney, Jr. "Uses and Misuses of Thresholds in Diagnostic Decision Making." *Academic Medicine* 85 (2010): 556–68.

Watkins, Calvert. *How to Kill a Dragon: Aspects of Indo-European Poetics.* New York: Oxford University Press, 1995.

Watkins, Vernon. *Poems for Dylan.* Wales: Gomer Press, 2003.

Watson Barbara B. "On Power and the Literary Text." *Signs* (Autumn, 1975), 111–18.

Watson, Dana Cairns. *Gertrude Stein and the Essence of What Happens.* Nashville, TN: Vanderbilt University Press, 2005.

Watson, Robert N. *Back to Nature: The Green and the Real in the Late Renaissance.* Philadelphia: University of Pennsylvania Press, 2006.

Watson, Robert N. "Coining Words on the Elizabethan and Jacobean Stage." *Philological Quarterly* 88 (2009): 49–75.

Watson, Robert N. "Coriolanus and the 'Common Part.'" *Shakespeare Survey* 69 (2016): 181–97.

Watson, Robert N. "The Humanities Really Do Produce a Profit." *Chronicle of Higher Education,* March 21, 2010.

Watson, Robert N. "Lord Capulet's Lost Compromise: Editing and the Binary Dynamics of *Romeo and Juliet.*" *Renaissance Drama* 43, no. 1 2015: 53–83.

Watson, Robert N. "*Midsummer Night's Dream* and the Ecology of Human Being." In *Ecocritical Shakespeare,* edited by Lynne Bruckner and Dan Brayton, 33–56. London: Routledge, 2011.

Watson, Robert N. "Protestant Animals: Puritan Sects and English Animal-Protection Sentiment, 1550–1650." *ELH* 81, no. 4 (2014): 1111–48.

Watson, Robert N. "Shakespeare's New Words." *Shakespeare Survey* 65 (2012): 358–77.

Weber, Max. *The Protestant Ethic and the Spirit of Capitalism*. London: Unwin Hyman, 1905.

Wharton, David. "Poll Vaulting." *Los Angeles Times*, September 7, 2016.

Whitman, Walt. *Democratic Vistas*. In *Complete Prose Works*. Boston: Small, Maynard & Company, 1902.

Wilde, Oscar. "The Soul of Man under Socialism." In *Collected Works of Oscar Wilde*. Ware, Hertfordshire: Wordsworth Editions, 2007.

Wilford, Hugh. *The Mighty Wurlitzer: How the CIA Played America*. Cambridge, MA: Harvard University Press, 2009.

Wilson, David Sloan. *Darwin's Cathedral: Evolution, Religion, and the Nature of Society*. Chicago, IL: University of Chicago Press, 2002.

Wilson, David Sloan. *Evolution for Everyone: How Darwin's Theory Can Change the Way We Think about Our Lives*. New York: Delta, 2007.

Wilson, David Sloan. "Evolutionary Social Constructivism." In *The Literary Animal: Evolution and the Nature of Narrative*, edited by Jonathan Gottschall, David Sloan Wilson, E. O. Wilson, and Frederick C. Crews, 20–37. Evanston, IL: Northwestern University Press, 2005.

Wilson, E. O. "How to Unify Knowledge." *Annals of the New York Academy of Sciences* 935 (2001): 12–17.

Withrock, Isabelle C. et al. "Genetic Diseases Conferring Resistance to Infectious Diseases." *Genes & Diseases* 2, no. 3 (September 2015): 247–54. doi:10.1016/j.gendis.2015.02.008.

Wong, Lisa, and Robert Viagas. *Scales to Scalpels: Doctors Who Practice the Healing Arts of Music and Medicine*. New York: Pegasus, 2012.

Wood, Graeme. "Anthropology Inc." *The Atlantic*, March, 2013.

Zapf, Hubert. *Literature as Cultural Ecology*. London: Bloomsbury, 2016.

Zimmer, Carl. "Our Microbiome May Be Looking Out for Itself." *New York Times*, August 14, 2014. www.nytimes.com/2014/08/14/science/our-microbiome-may-be-looking-out-for-itself.html.

Zimmer, Carl. "The Purpose of Sleep? To Forget, Scientists Say." *New York Times*, February 2, 2017. www.nytimes.com/2017/02/02/science/sleep-memory-brain-forgetting.html.

Zimmerman, Frederick J., Dimitri A. Christakis, and Andrew N. Meltzoff. "Associations between Media Viewing and Language Development in Children under Age 2 Years." *Journal of Pediatrics* 151, no. 4 (August 7, 2007): 364–68. doi:10.1016/j.jpeds.2007.04.071.

Zucchino, David. "An Afghan Uprising of One." *Los Angeles Times*, June 2, 2013.

Index

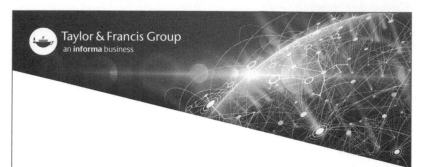